PREVENTION'S
FOOD AND
NUTRITION

By the Editors of
PREVENTION
Magazine Health Books

PREVENTION'S
FOOD AND
NUTRITION

The Most Complete Book Ever Written on Using Food and Vitamins to Feel Healthy and Cure Disease

BERKLEY BOOKS, NEW YORK

The table on page 74 is reprinted with permission from *Recommended Dietary Allowances, 10th edition,* copyright © 1989 by the National Academy of Sciences. Published by National Academy Press, Washington, D.C.

The table on page 652 was adapted from *The Power of Your Plate* by Neal D. Barnard, M.D. Copyright © 1990 by Dr. Neal Barnard. Reprinted by permission.

The tables on pages 723 and 726 were adapted from *The Living Heart Brand Name Shopper's Guide* by Michael E. Debakey, M.D., Antonio M. Gotto, Jf., M.D., D.P.H., Lynne W. Scott, M.A., R.D./L.D., and John P. Foreyt, Ph.D. Copyright © 1992 by MasterMedia Limited. Reprinted by permission.

PREVENTION'S FOOD & NUTRITION

A Berkley Book / published by arrangement with
Rodale Press, Inc.

PRINTING HISTORY
Rodale Press edition published 1993
Berkley edition / October 1996

All rights reserved.
Copyright © 1993 by Rodale Press, Inc.
Prevention is a registered trademark of Rodale Press, Inc.
This book may not be reproduced in whole or in part,
by mimeograph or any other means, without permission.
For information address: The Berkley Publishing Group,
200 Madison Avenue, New York, New York 10016.

The Putnam Berkley World Wide Web site address is
http://www.berkley.com/berkley

ISBN: 0-425-15520-X

BERKLEY ®
Berkley Books are published by The Berkley Publishing Group,
200 Madison Avenue, New York, New York 10016.
BERKLEY and the "B" design
are trademarks belonging to Berkley Publishing Corporation.

PRINTED IN THE UNITED STATES OF AMERICA

10 9 8 7 6 5 4 3 2 1

NOTICE

This book is intended as a reference volume only, not as a medical guide or manual for self-treatment. If you suspect that you have a medical problem, we urge you to seek competent medical help. Keep in mind that nutritional needs vary from person to person, depending on age, sex, health status and total diet. Information here is intended to help you make informed decisions about your diet, not to substitute for any treatment that may have been prescribed by your physician.

Contents

PART 5: HEALING DIETS

PART 6: IMPROVING YOUR EATING STYLE

PART 1

NUTRITION BASICS

CHAPTER 1

The Nutrition Revolution

An Introduction

No doubt about it, it's an exciting time in nutrition. Okay, "exciting" and "nutrition" may not be two words you've ever linked together before—unless you count diving into Aunt Anne's Delectable Double Fudge Cake at the annual family reunion. But if there was ever a time to call nutrition exciting, it's now.

We all have at least a vague idea that good nutrition is important for good health. And we definitely know what happens when we eat *too* much: that uncomfortable stuffed feeling, which, if repeated too often, leads to the search through the recesses of our closets for roomier clothing.

So we've always recognized—to a certain extent—that there is a correlation between what we put in our mouths and how we look and feel (although we don't always let that *influence* what we put in our mouths). But never before has there been so much compelling evidence that what we eat has a direct relation to the occurrence of serious diseases ranging from cataracts to cardiovascular disease to cancer.

3

Food to prevent disease? Once most people would have hooted at the concept. "Just another crazy gimmick," they would have sniffed. But with the publication of numerous carefully controlled studies by respected researchers, the idea that nutrients can not only treat but prevent disease has moved steadfastly forward into the realm of acceptable science. And it's not just that good nutrition can let us live longer. It can also let us live *better*.

"As we go forward, we see more and more things that are nutritionally related that have to do with the quality of life, not just longevity," says Daniel B. Menzel, Ph.D., chairman of the Department of Community and Environmental Medicine at the University of California at Irvine.

NUTRIENTS TO THE RESCUE

They sound like something you should have studied in chemistry class, but they may turn out to be some of the best friends you'll ever make. "Antioxidants are probably one of the hottest areas in the coming decade," says Harinder S. Garewal, M.D., Ph.D., assistant director for cancer prevention and control at the University of Arizona Cancer Center in Tucson. "Excitement is high."

The antioxidants that have scientists and nutritionists so excited include beta-carotene—the stuff that makes carrots orange and that converts to vitamin A in the body—and vitamins C and E. In brief, antioxidants can scavenge and render harmless the free radicals in your body that are a result of normal bodily processes as well as exposure to x-rays, sunlight, ozone, smoke and other environmental pollutants. These free radicals may be part of what causes much of the deterioration we associate with aging—and our increased exposure to environmental pollutants such as nitrogen dioxide or ozone may *increase* our need for the antioxidants that can neutralize these free radicals, says Dr. Menzel.

A NEW ROLE FOR A NEW VITAMIN D

Antioxidants, move over. Vitamin D is attracting new attention.

With the development of a new form of vitamin D that appears to circumvent a potentially serious side effect from large doses, the door may have opened to greatly expand this vitamin's use as a treatment.

"There are new roles for vitamin D that go way beyond its original activities in partnership with calcium," says Hector DeLuca, Ph.D., chairman of the Department of Biochemistry at the University of Wisconsin in Madison and a pioneer in vitamin D research. "Vitamin D isn't just for bones any more."

The classical role for vitamin D has been to help the body utilize calcium and build and maintain strong bones and teeth. Since 1985, scientists have suspected that vitamin D could also help fight cancer—but its use as a treatment was strictly limited because of side effects.

The problem is that high doses of vitamin D can raise blood calcium to excessive levels, which in severe cases can cause calcification of soft tissue, kidney failure and coma. "The window of safety between treatment and harm was very narrow," says Dr. DeLuca.

But this new form of D—technically referred to as an analog of dihydroxyvitamin D_3—*doesn't* mobilize calcium. This alleviates the risk of high blood calcium, dramatically increasing the feasibility of using vitamin D as a treatment.

The possibility of treating cancer is, of course, of primary interest, and research by Dr. DeLuca and others shows that D does help suppress the growth of cancer cells. But vitamin D has also been used to successfully treat psoriasis, a skin disorder, and it has a role in helping prevent osteoporosis. Other uses for this vitamin may be right around the corner.

Harvard Medical School researchers turned up astounding proof of the power of beta-carotene in a ten-year study of 22,000 male physicians: They found that men with a history of heart problems who received beta-carotene supplements every other day had *half as many* heart attacks, strokes and deaths as those who didn't take beta-carotene. (And *no* heart attacks occurred in a group who took both beta-carotene and aspirin.)

The antioxidants are also valiant anti-cancer crusaders. Some of Dr. Garewal's work showed that daily beta-carotene drastically reduced abnormal changes in the mouth that could lead to cancer. Another study of 189 women with cervical cancer and 227 cancer-free women showed that the risk of cervical cancer was only about half as great for those with high intakes of vitamin E, vitamin C and beta-carotene.

"The antioxidants really do work to reduce the incidence of cancer," says Dr. Menzel. "And people from all over the world in all different kinds of environmental circumstances showed these substances have very positive anti-cancer activities."

A LONG LIST OF PROTECTORS

Other nutrients have remarkable protective and healing powers as well. Folate, a B vitamin, can help fight cancer and has dramatically cut the rate of devastating birth defects.

Osteoporosis can be a crippling problem for the elderly, particularly women. But studies show that getting adequate amounts of dietary calcium can help women retain bone mass and possibly fend off this bone-weakening disease.

Vision-impairing cataracts are another plague associated with growing older, but just eating more fruits and vegetables may help prevent this problem. A U.S. Department of Agriculture (USDA) study found that people eating less than 1½ servings of fruit or less than 2 servings of vegetables daily were $3\frac{1}{2}$ times more likely to develop cataracts than those who ate more.

"As you grow older, your risk for developing cataracts grows larger and larger," says Paul F. Jacques, D.Sc., an epidemiologist with the USDA's Human Nutrition Research Center on Aging at Tufts University in Boston. "Eating a healthy diet may delay the usual aging of the lens of the eye, and so delay cataracts." Dr. Jacques thinks the secret may be the nutrient combination found in fruits and vegetables.

The list goes on. Zinc improves the immune system. There are some indications magnesium might help chronic fatigue syndrome. Vitamins E and C have slowed the progression of Parkinson's disease for some patients. Some physicians recommend eating more potassium-rich foods to control blood pressure and avoid stroke. Increased fiber in the diet may help lower cholesterol levels and cut risks of colon cancer and other gastrointestinal disorders.

"TAKE TWO ORANGES AND CALL ME IN THE MORNING"

Does all this mean that one day our doctors will be prescribing fruits, vegetables, whole-grain breads or nutrient supplements instead of drugs?

It's not a farfetched concept. In fact, the first line of attack for many problems is already diet-centered. Treatment for high blood pressure, high cholesterol and diabetes often depends heavily on dietary changes. And the American Cancer Society advocates a low-fat, high-fiber diet to help avoid cancer.

Some physicians actually prescribe specific nutrients for certain health problems. "Doctors use niacin to treat high triglycerides and high cholesterol," says Adrianne Bendich, Ph.D., senior clinical research coordinator in the Human Nutrition Research Division of Hoffmann-La Roche in Nutley, New Jersey. "They routinely use vitamin E to reduce the adverse effects of many cancer chemotherapies. Both calcium and vitamin D have a role to play against osteoporosis. There are strong indications that children hospitalized with measles should be given vitamin A to prevent complications. And I think the use of nutrients as preventive medicine is growing."

ALL THIS, AND CUT CANCER RISKS, TOO?

It was the ultimate controlled experiment—no late-night sneaking out to a 7-Eleven for a candy bar or Big Gulp. While at sea for six months, crew members of the U.S. Navy's USS *Scott* were fed a diet that met the American Cancer Society's guidelines: low in fat, high in fiber, with lots of variety and plenty of fruits and vegetables. (No one expected to assess cancer risks during the six-month trial; the goal of the study was merely to test how well the guidelines could be adapted to everyday diets.)

The results:

- The crew averaged a weight loss of 12 pounds, while crew members of a sister ship served regular Navy fare *gained* 7 pounds.
- Average waist size decreased 2 inches, compared to an *increase* of 1½ inches on crew members of the sister ship.
- Seventy-four percent of those weighing 200 pounds or more lost weight, compared to 26 percent of the large-size group on the sister ship.
- Eighty-nine percent of crew members with above-acceptable body fat percentages showed a fat percentage decline.

You might not expect results this marked from a stay at an expensive health spa! And as a side benefit, more than half the crew members liked their new diet, and many of them planned to continue similar eating habits on dry land.

WHAT IT MEANS TO YOU

Despite all the breakthroughs in nutritional research, deciding what and how to eat can still be enormously confusing. We're bombarded with information and misinformation about food and nutrition. One specialist says you can get all the nutrients you need in your daily diet; another one says you can't. Health food stores display a range of products that promise to replenish sexual vigor, vanquish migraines and a whole lot more. Meanwhile, supermarkets sell new food products for those concerned about heart disease and cancer. Cute tykes on television commercials lisp about the dangers of cholesterol, and "fat-free" has become the sell line of the decade. Many of us, confused by the barrage of information, abandon plans to renovate our diets.

And today is a hectic time. Just like 50 years ago, most of our meals are prepared by Mom—but today Mom is probably also juggling a 9-to-5 job, evening classes and workouts at the gym. Finding time to go to the supermarket can be a major task, let alone planning and preparing nutritious meals. More and more, we reach for prepared foods, or we dine out.

And the best of intentions, we all know, can fly out the window when you're faced with that all-you-can-eat breakfast buffet, the sumptuous potluck church supper or the fancy dinner at the boss's house.

But many of us are genuinely concerned about our health and the health of our families, and we want to eat better. If only we had more time . . . if only it were easier to keep track of nutrients . . . if only good nutrition didn't seem so complicated.

EATING BETTER CAN BE EASY

We're not saying that nutrition is a simple issue, but eating healthy doesn't have to be complicated. Unless you're on a medically restricted diet, you don't have to carry a

HOW WE'RE EATING NOW

Think about what you've eaten during the past week or two. Do you think you got your quota of vitamins and minerals, fruits and vegetables, protein and whole grains—and have you kept your fat intake down? Or do you *know* your diet is, well, less than perfect, but you just don't have the time or energy to do any better?

About a fourth of us are already very careful about what we eat, according to the Survey of American Dietary Habits, conducted by the American Dietetic Association. Another 38 percent of us know we should eat better, but either we don't want to give up our chips and ice cream or we think that a healthy diet takes too much time.

Another huge chunk of the population—presumably no one reading this book—just doesn't care what they eat. Thirty-six percent of American adults don't try to manage their diets. They eat out frequently and skip meals often.

The survey also showed that many of us are concerned about cholesterol, fat and vitamins and minerals—and while 52 percent knew that the recommended blood cholesterol is under 200, only 7 percent knew that the ceiling on fat intake recommended by the American Dietetic Association is 30 percent of calories.

So as a nation how are we doing, consumption-wise? A Nationwide Food Consumption Survey showed that most of us are consuming at least the Recommended Dietary Allowance of vitamins A, C, B_{12}, thiamine and riboflavin. We are a bit low on vitamin B_6 and vitamin E, but we're in no great danger of deficiency.

Our mineral status is more iffy, however. Females aged 12 to 50 take in only about two-thirds of the recommended iron levels; men and women both fall short on zinc and copper. Adult women consume less than the recommended amounts of calcium, and both men and women consume less magnesium than recommended.

When it comes to protein, we eat more than we need. Fat? It's no surprise that we overdo it in this category, considering our love affair with such fatty fare as ice cream and french fries. We average 35 to 37 percent of our daily calories from fat. Carbohydrate consumption is about one-fifth lower than recommended, and we don't get enough fiber.

In other words, while many of us are definitely *concerned* about nutrition, many of us also still need to improve our diets.

notepad and keep track of the nutrient content of everything you eat.

What's important, however, is understanding the basics of good nutrition so you can make good choices throughout the day. That means altering your shopping, cooking and dining-out habits—but a little bit at a time.

In this book we explain today's hot issues: How nutrition really affects your heart, your brain, your blood pressure, your stamina and more. We examine all of the essential nutrients in foods, what they do and who needs more of what.

Ever enter the grocery store armed with a list of healthy foods and exit with things you really didn't intend to buy? We offer a guide for supermarket shopping and another for health food stores, plus tips on growing your own good foods. Wish you had an array of quick-and-easy healthy recipes? They're here. A week-by-week blueprint for improving your diet in all the critical areas? You've got it. A comparison of special diet programs offered by top clinics and spas? It's here.

It's all here, and more. You're holding in your hand a book that can guide you to enjoyable healthy eating—and a lifetime of good nutrition.

CHAPTER 2

The Basic Three

Protein, Carbohydrate
and Fat

Oat bran won't do it, oranges won't do it, eggs won't do it. And neither will milk, cheese, steak, chicken, pretzels, potato chips, lima beans, peas, carrots or spaghetti. Even a sweet, soothing bowl of sherbet or a tempting tray of truffles won't do it. It's a basic fact of life: No single food can meet all of your nutritional needs.

"There is no one miracle food that has it all," says Elaine Kvitka, R.D., a nutrition consultant in Scottsdale, Arizona. "You need more than 40 different nutrients in your diet every day. In order to get those, you need to eat a wide variety of foods."

Even a breastfed baby isn't getting all the necessary nutrients from Mom's milk. "Babies are born with built-up reserves of nutrients in their bodies that supplement breastfeeding," says Andrea Gardiner, R.D., a dietitian at the Hospital of the Good Samaritan in Los Angeles. "But after about four months, those reserves are depleted and the baby needs to begin eating food in order to survive."

There's no doubt that food is vital to our survival. That's because food does two important things. First, it provides us with essential nutrients, substances that the body can't produce for itself. Without those nutrients, we'd literally have no way of repairing cells or growing new ones. Without them, our bones would be brittle, our nerves and muscles wouldn't work well and thousands of other crucial jobs in our bodies, ranging from wound repair to heartbeat regulation, wouldn't get done.

Second, food serves as the fuel our bodies need to create heat and energy, says George Seperich, Ph.D., a food scientist and associate professor of agribusiness at Arizona State University in Tempe.

Without an adequate food supply, the body starts to burn anything, including muscle, to keep itself alive. If a person is undernourished for long enough, the body will even start breaking down muscle in the heart to feed itself.

"Your body actually starts to digest itself from the inside out," Dr. Seperich says. "Once it starts converting muscle cells to fuel, it gradually loses its ability to discriminate between heart muscle and less vital muscle. And of course, the minute you start weakening the heart muscle, you're in big trouble."

While famine and malnutrition are still facts of life in some parts of the world, most cultures long ago developed diets that have successfully fed millions. While these cuisines are diverse and often seem to have little in common, scientists now know that each contains the same basic components that every person needs to grow and stay healthy. If any one of these vital components is missing from a diet in sufficient quantities, it can lead to malnourishment and disease.

In some cases, scientists have determined that a lack of just one essential nutrient can cause disorders such as anemia or scurvy. In other instances, an excessive amount of one nutrient can actually cause malabsorption and deficiency of another nutrient. So eating well is a balancing act that requires not only that we consume all the necessary nutrients but also that all those nutrients work together as a team in our bodies so that we can live active and fulfilling lives.

In this chapter, we'll be looking at three of the most basic diet components: protein, carbohydrate and fat.

THE PROS AND CONS OF PROTEIN

In a sense, protein is the body's repairman and jack-of-all-trades. Found in every cell, protein builds and repairs everything from muscles and bones to blood vessels, hormones, hair and fingernails, says George L. Blackburn, M.D., Ph.D., associate professor of surgery at Harvard Medical School and chief of the Nutrition/Metabolism Laboratory at the Cancer Research Institute of New England Deaconess Hospital in Boston. Protein helps create enzymes that enable us to digest food and antibodies that fight off infections. In a pinch, it also can be used as a fuel by the body.

Chemically, protein is composed of varying combinations of 22 amino acids. Amino acids are compounds that contain carbon, hydrogen, oxygen and nitrogen, which happen to be the four elements necessary for life. To get a feeling for what a protein looks like, Dr. Seperich suggests that you imagine that you're making a bracelet and each amino acid is like a pop-it bead.

"Each bead has a little bulb that snaps into a hole in the bead next to it," he says. "When you snap all the beads together, you have a complete protein."

Most of these amino acids can be manufactured by the body, but nine essential ones can only be obtained from the foods that we eat. Lysine, one of these essential amino acids, is needed for the absorption of calcium, a mineral that strengthens bones and teeth. Others, such as phenylalanine, are needed for the production of important nerve hormones in the brain involved in learning and memory.

Animal proteins—meats, eggs and fish—were once considered superior protein sources because they have large amounts of proteins, and most contain all the amino acids. But scientists now believe that a mixture of animal and vegetable proteins is most useful to the body.

Eggs, for example, were once considered to be the perfect protein source. But scientists have found that if you replace a third of the egg protein with potato protein, the body actually uses the combination more efficiently than egg protein alone to build tissue or burn as fuel.

Although vegetable foods such as grains and beans also have some protein, they are considered lower-quality sources because they contain less of the nutrient than animal foods. In addition, most plant proteins contain just a few of the essential amino acids. The amino acids in plant proteins are still important, however. Rice and corn, for example, contain threonine, an amino acid needed for the formation of collagen, the substance that holds skin together. Beans and peanuts have significant amounts of methionine, an amino acid that promotes healthy skin and nails.

While any single plant food isn't likely to have all the essential amino acids, you can still get all the protein and essential amino acids you need from vegetables, fruits, beans and grains if you mix them right. Try to imagine making that bracelet of amino acids beads in the example given by Dr. Seperich. Only this time, you don't have enough beads to do the job.

"Each individual vegetable doesn't quite contain all of the beads you need to make a complete bracelet or protein. But if you use the amino acids from several plant foods, you can," he says.

If, for example, you take kidney beans, which are high in some amino acids and low in others, and combine them with

A USER'S GUIDE TO PROTEIN

Here's a sampling of protein amounts in common foods. A food is considered a good source of protein if it has at least 25 grams of the nutrient.

Food	Portion	Protein (g.)	Calories	Percent of Calories from Protein
Pork chop	3 oz.	30	231	52
Top round beef	3 oz.	30	178	67
Veal shoulder	3 oz.	29	169	69
Chuck roast	3 oz.	28	179	63
Chicken breast, roasted	3 oz.	27	142	76
Bluefin tuna	3 oz.	25	156	64
Tuna, canned in water	3 oz.	25	111	90
Turkey breast, roasted	3 oz.	25	133	76
Ground beef, lean	3 oz.	24	238	40
Ham	3 oz.	24	183	52

rice, which is high in the amino acids that are lacking in kidney beans, then you'll end up eating a high-quality protein, says Elizabeth Somer, R.D., coauthor of *The Nutrition Desk Reference*. Rice and beans, in fact, is a dish served in the West Indies with the main meal.

But you don't necessarily have to eat those vegetable foods together, Dr. Seperich says. Thanks to the time it takes for your body to digest nutrients, the protein in the oatmeal you eat at breakfast can be combined with the corn you eat at lunch and the spaghetti you eat at dinner to create a high-quality protein containing all the essential amino acids.

Food	Portion	Protein (g.)	Calories	Percent of Calories from Protein
Porterhouse steak	3 oz.	24	185	52
Coho salmon	3 oz.	23	157	59
Shrimp	3 oz.	18	84	86
Low-fat (1 %) cottage cheese	½ cup	14	82	68
Tofu, firm	3 oz.	13	117	43
Parmesan cheese	1 oz.	12	128	38
Skim milk	1 cup	10	100	40
Lentils, boiled	½ cup	9	115	31
Peanut butter	2 tbsp.	8	188	17
Spanish peanuts	1 oz.	8	162	20
Swiss cheese	1 oz.	8	105	30
Egg	1 large	6	75	32
Egg substitute, liquid	¼ cup	6	60	40
Yogurt, nonfat, plain	½ cup	6	63	38
Ice milk, vanilla	1 cup	5	184	11

How to Get the Right Amount

More than 700 million people are believed to suffer from protein deficiency worldwide, mostly in developing countries. Kwashiorkor and marasmus, two common diseases caused by inadequate amounts of protein, can inhibit growth and impair mental capabilities. Symptoms include weight loss, irritability, swelling of the stomach and skin sores.

Both diseases are rare in the United States, Gardiner says. If anything, we're probably eating too much protein.

"I think that the myth that we have to have some protein

at every meal is still around," says Melanie Polk, R.D., consulting nutritionist and author from North Potomac, Maryland. "Americans are probably eating twice as much protein as they really need."

The Recommended Dietary Allowance (RDA) of protein varies based on your age and weight. A 45-year-old woman weighing 139 pounds, for example, needs about 50 grams of protein daily. For a man of the same age weighing 174 pounds, the recommendation is for about 63 grams.

However, according to the National Research Council, adult women are consuming up to 70 grams of protein a day and some men are eating more than 90 grams. That's probably because it's easy to overload on protein on the typical American diet, Kvitka says. Just by eating an egg and a slice of sausage for breakfast, a quarter-pound hamburger for lunch and a three-ounce porterhouse steak for dinner, you've consumed 59 grams of protein that day.

Even if you eat more prudently, it's not hard to meet or exceed your RDA for protein. If you just eat ½ cup wheat cereal with 1 cup skim milk and two pieces of toast for breakfast, then have an apple, two ounces of cottage cheese, a three-ounce serving of salmon and ½ cup peas for lunch, you'll consume 60 grams of protein. That's nearly 120 percent of the RDA for a 25- to 50-year-old woman and easily meets the RDA for a similarly aged man. And you haven't touched your dinner yet.

So what are the consequences of eating too much protein? High-protein foods, particularly meats, often are rich in calories and loaded with fat. If you meet your daily protein requirements, most of that protein will be used to build and repair muscle and some may be used as fuel by the body. But if you eat excessive amounts, any leftover protein that isn't burned for fuel will be stored as fat.

A diet high in animal protein may interfere with absorption of certain minerals such as calcium and may cause the excretion of more minerals in the urine.

Excessive protein also can overwork your kidneys. "If you give your kidneys more protein than they can handle—particularly animal protein, which is more difficult to process—it wears them down," Dr. Blackburn says. "Americans' obsession with getting enough protein may explain the fact that kidney disease is so common here." Here are a couple of tips to help you get the right amount of protein, but not too much.

Remember the 15 percent rule. Try to limit your protein consumption to less than 15 percent of your total calories, Dr. Blackburn suggests. To do that, women should eat no more than two three- to four-ounce servings of meat, poultry or fish a day. (A three-ounce serving roughly translates into one loin lamb chop, one-half chicken breast or four steamed jumbo shrimp.) Men need a bit more protein, but still should eat no more than two four- to six-ounce servings of meat, poultry or fish daily.

Take the spotlight off meat. Stop making meat the centerpiece of your meals, Somer says. In addition to all its protein, meat contains saturated fat and cholesterol, two things that contribute to heart disease. So instead of giving steak, pork chops and that teen idol—hamburger—a starring role in every meal, let meats play a bit part while dishes like spaghetti and beans make your taste buds swoon. "If we stopped planning our meals around meat and started planning them around grains and vegetables, we'd be much better off," Somer says.

FUEL UP ON CARBOHYDRATES

If you drove a high-performance racing car, would you fuel it with a sub-standard grade of gasoline? Of course not. Well, in a way your body is like that racing car, and the best fuel for it is carbohydrates.

"Your body works best when it's running on carbohydrates," Gardiner says. "Carbohydrates are like premium gasoline. They're the most efficient fuel your body can get."

Carbohydrates are sugars and starches that your body can easily break down into fuel. They also help break down fat and team up with proteins to form compounds that are essential for combating infections, lubricating joints and maintaining health of skin, bones and nails. Carbohydrates are found almost exclusively in plant foods such as beans, fruits and vegetables.

Unlike protein, which isn't broken down until it reaches the stomach, a carbohydrate begins to be digested almost immediately after it enters the mouth. Saliva begins the process of breaking down the carbohydrate into glucose, the major form of sugar in the blood and your body's primary fuel. "Your nervous system and red blood cells will only use glucose. They won't use any other fuel. They need to have it," Gardiner says.

SIMPLE VERSUS COMPLEX

Basically, carbohydrates can be divided into two broad categories. Simple carbohydrates are tiny single or twin molecules of sugar found in such foods as table sugar, honey and molasses. The most common of these simple carbohydrates is glucose. Other types of simple carbohydrates include fructose, which is found in fruit, and lactose, which is found in milk. Simple sugars are a good energy source because they're already broken down into their component parts and are absorbed quite quickly into the bloodstream, Dr. Seperich says.

Natural sugars such as those found in fruit are the best form of simple carbohydrates because they have vitamins and minerals, which are not found in sugars used in soft drinks, candies and other sweets, Somer says. Unfortunately, most of the sugar that we consume in this country is refined.

"The refined sugars are generally found in nutrient-poor foods. They typically are in foods that are high in fat and have a minimal amount of vitamins and minerals," Somer says. "The American diet is already marginal in terms of vitamins and minerals. So high-sugar foods just worsen that trend."

Complex carbohydrates, also known as starches, also supply your body with glucose. Commonly found in vegetables, fruits, beans and grains, complex carbohydrates are composed of groups of simple sugars stuck together in long molecular chains. To give you an idea of the size difference, think of a simple sugar as a tugboat. In comparison, a complex carbohydrate is like an aircraft carrier.

It takes your body longer to digest a complex carbohydrate because your digestive system must break it down into simple sugars. Because of that, complex carbohydrates also slow the absorption of glucose into the bloodstream. That's important for people with diabetes, who need to avoid extreme fluctuations in blood sugar levels.

In addition, complex carbohydrates are particularly important because they provide us with fiber, an indigestible substance in plant food that has a powerful punch. Researchers believe that fiber does a number of important things in the body, including help decrease constipation, lower cholesterol, and prevent colon and breast cancer.

Because it is indigestible, fiber goes through your digestive system like a big cotton ball absorbing water and sweeping stool, bile acids (which are made from cholesterol) and other fluids out of the body, Dr. Seperich says. Better yet, fiber may help you control your weight because it provides added bulk that fills your stomach and curbs your appetite.

MORE CARBS ARE NEEDED

Unfortunately, dietary experts say we eat fewer carbohydrates than we should.

THE WORLD'S BEST FOOD PROCESSOR

It slices. It dices. It even mashes, chops and churns. But your digestive system does something even the most expensive food processor can't do. It breaks food down into vital nutrients and absorbs them into your bloodstream.

This complex process is a bit like running an assembly line in reverse. "As we go along this disassembly line, there are different places where nutrients are broken down and absorbed," says Ronald L. Hoffman, M.D., medical director of the Hoffman Center for Holistic Medicine in New York and author of *Seven Weeks to a Settled Stomach.* Some carbohydrates, for example, can be easily disassembled by enzymes in the mouth, while most proteins need to be broken down by potent acids in the stomach. Fat, another major dietary component, isn't digested until after it is drenched with bile acid in the small intestine.

The first stop on this journey is the mouth, where your teeth chop the food into small bits and saliva mixes and softens the food into a digestible mush. After less than a minute, it enters the esophagus, a ten-inch-long muscular tube that connects the mouth to the stomach. In the esophagus, the food is mixed with more secretions that aid digestion. The trip through the esophagus can be quick—liquids often zip down it in less than ten seconds. Once in the stomach, the food is bathed in powerful secretions of hydrochloric acid, a substance so strong that it can burn holes in thick carpet. (Fortunately, your stomach

At the beginning of the century, carbohydrate consumption in the United States and Europe hovered around 70 percent of our caloric intake. But since 1920, carbohydrate consumption in the United States has dropped by about 20

has a self-protective mechanism that stops this acid from harming you). After six to eight hours of bombardment from these secretions, the food is transformed into a creamy, souplike substance called chyme. However, despite what you might think, the stomach doesn't absorb that many nutrients.

"Some absorption does occur in the mouth, and alcohol and some small chemical substances are absorbed to some extent in the stomach. But most of the absorption occurs in the small intestine," Dr. Hoffman says.

The small intestine is actually the major organ in the digestive tract. About 20 feet long, it is only called the small intestine because its diameter is less than that of the large intestine. After chyme leaves the stomach, it enters the small intestine, where most of the nutrients are extracted and absorbed into the bloodstream. That process can take more than nine hours.

Finally, the residue tumbles into the large intestine. About five feet long, the large intestine doesn't digest food, but it does absorb water and other fluids. It also is home to a variety of useful bacteria, yeasts and fungi that manufacture nutrients, such as vitamin K, that your body needs. As the waste travels through your large intestine, water is extracted and it becomes more and more solid until it is excreted from your body one to three days later.

The whole digestive process, depending on the meal and your metabolism, can take less than 18 hours or up to five days, Dr. Hoffman says.

percent. Today, the average American diet consists of 46 percent calories from carbohydrates. And of those carbohydrates, half are the less desirable simple sugars. Not surprisingly, there also has been a sharp decrease in the proportion of energy provided by starches and a significant increase in the amount of fats and meats in our diet.

"One hundred years ago, we ate more carbohydrates than we do now. In particular, we ate fewer sweets and more starches. But social changes such as affluence have made it easier to get sweet things into our diet," says Maria Linder, Ph.D., a professor of biochemistry at California State University, Fullerton.

Some people have avoided carbohydrates because they have an undeserved bad reputation, Polk says.

"Many people still have a negative image of carbohydrates because they think if they eat lots of pasta, breads or potatoes, they're going to get fat," Polk says. "In reality, it's not those foods, but it's what you put on them that gets you in trouble."

"Carbohydrates are only fattening if you do things like load up your baked potato with butter and sour cream or if you smear cream cheese on your bagel," Kvitka says.

The consensus of the U.S. Department of Agriculture and the National Research Council is that at least 55 percent of your calories should come from carbohydrates. Here's how you can meet that goal.

It's simple—eat complex. The first thing you should eat at a meal should be a complex carbohydrate, Dr. Blackburn says. A small serving of pasta or soups that contain noodles or potatoes are good examples. Doing that might lessen your cravings for fatty foods, particularly if you eat slowly so that your meal lasts at least 20 minutes. That gives the carbohydrates time to activate enzymes in your intestinal tract, liver and brain, so you won't feel as much of a craving for fat.

Develop a passion for fruits, grains and vegetables. You should try to eat five or more ½-cup servings of vegetables and fruits daily and at least six servings of breads, cereals and beans.

"Six servings of grains sounds like a lot," Somer says. "But if you have a bowl of oatmeal and a couple pieces of toast for breakfast, you've already had three servings of grains. Then if you have a sandwich for lunch, that's two more servings. Finally if you have a baked potato or a ½-cup serving of rice with dinner, you have your six servings of grains for that day. It's really not as much as it sounds like."

A MUSCLE-BUILDING MEAL PLAN

If you believe the gym is the only place to start building muscle, think again. Replacing high-fat foods with lots of breads, grains, fruits and vegetables might help you create a solid, muscular body.

We know that a high-carbohydrate, low-fat diet can help us lose fat without the rigors of crash dieting. But research suggests a more unexpected benefit: It may boost lean body mass—muscle.

When researchers put 18 women on a high-fat diet for 4 weeks, and then on a low-fat, high-carbohydrate diet for 20 weeks, they found an 11 percent decrease in fat weight. But surprisingly, the women also had a 2 percent increase in lean body mass. Somehow the women had created new lean tissue without exercise.

"This is a very intriguing finding," says T. Elaine Prewitt, R.D., Ph.D., of the Department of Nutrition and Medical Dietetics at the University of Illinois at Chicago, who headed the study.

No, we're not suggesting that you drop your hand weights and pick up a fork instead. If anything, exercise adds even more to these benefits and helps maintain them over time.

FAT: FRIEND OR FOE?

There's no doubt that fat can be your enemy. But it may surprise you to know that fat, if eaten in moderate amounts, can be an important ally in your effort to stay healthy.

"It's absolutely essential that we have some fat in our bodies," Dr. Seperich says. "We spend a lot of time trying to get rid of it, but, in reality, your body needs a certain percentage of it to function properly."

Fats, also known as lipids, are hard to avoid because they're found in some form in virtually every food. In general, foods such as cheese or butter that are high in saturated fats are solid at room temperature, while unsaturated fats like vegetable oils are usually liquids.

Saturated fats—which have been linked to heart disease and high cholesterol—are primarily found in animal foods such as meat, poultry and dairy products.

The two types of unsaturated fat, polyunsaturated and monounsaturated, are usually found in plants and fish. Research suggests that these unsaturated fats, particularly omega-3 fatty acids found in fish, may help lower blood cholesterol levels and prevent heart attacks.

While there is no established RDA for fats, there are essential fatty acids that your body can't produce and that you must get from your diet. Of these, linoleic acid is the most important. Found in vegetable oils, nuts and seeds, this polyunsaturated fat is important for growth and development as well as the production of hormonelike substances that regulate blood pressure. However, because we do eat so much fat, essential fatty acid deficiencies are extremely rare.

Of course, most of us have heard about the downside of fat. Eating excessive amounts of it has been linked to high cholesterol, heart disease, obesity and some types of cancer.

Yet fat still accounts for 43 percent of the total calories the average American is eating. That's about 80 to 100 grams of

HOW FATS MEASURE UP

This table lists the percentage of saturated and unsaturated fat in commonly used cooking oils and fats. (The percentages may not add up to 100 percent since many of these fats have small amounts of other fatty substances.)

Oil Fat	Saturated Fat (%)	Mono-unsaturated Fat (%)	Poly-unsaturated Fat (%)
11 TERRIFIC COOKING OILS AND FATS . . .			
Canola oil	7	60	30
Safflower oil	9	13	76
Walnut oil	9	23	65
Sunflower oil	11	20	67
Corn oil	13	25	59
Olive oil	14	76	9
Soybean oil	15	24	59
Peanut oil	17	47	32
Rice oil	19	42	38
Wheat germ oil	19	15	63
Margarine	20	48	32
. . . PLUS 7 TO AVOID			
Coconut oil	89	6	2
Butter	64	29	4
Palm oil	50	36	9
Lard	39	45	11
Chicken fat	30	45	20
Cottonseed oil	26	18	53
Vegetable shortening	25	45	20

fat—equivalent to almost a whole stick of butter—every day.

"The number one thing that people can do to improve their waistlines, heart and overall health is cut the amount of fat in their diets," Somer says. "If that was the only thing they did, they would solve a wealth of problems."

But while dietitians stress that it's important to *cut* fat consumption to no more than 30 percent of your total calories, you shouldn't eliminate it from your diet entirely. That's because fat does some terrific things for you.

WHAT'S GOOD ABOUT FAT

Fat is a compact way for the body to store lots of energy until we need it, Dr. Seperich says. In fact, fats are capable of storing more than twice as much energy per gram as the same amount of carbohydrates.

"If we didn't have fat and stored all our energy as carbohydrates, we'd all have to be 12 feet tall and weigh 700 pounds to do it," Dr. Seperich says.

We also need fat for healthy skin and hair. And without it, we'd have a hard time regulating our body temperature. Fat deposited just below the skin acts like a thermal blanket to keep our body temperature constant, Dr. Seperich says.

Fat surrounds vital organs, such as the kidneys and the heart, protecting them from blows and trauma. Fat is also important to the nervous system because it acts like an insulator, coating nerves in a protective covering.

To squeeze the most benefits out of the fat you do eat, yet avoid the damage too much fat can cause, try these strategies.

Read between the grams. Probably the easiest way to ensure that you really are cutting the total fat in your diet to less than 30 percent of calories is to read labels on food packages, Kvitka says. In particular, be aware of the grams of fat in a food. "Percentage of fat is such a difficult concept for some people," she says. "But as you begin to read labels and become aware of fat grams, you'll learn that you can get to your goal by keeping your portions of meat down to two three-ounce servings a day, choosing low-fat or nonfat dairy products and getting five or six servings of fruits or vegetables a day."

A MENU WITH THE RIGHT MIX

Here's a sample menu that illustrates how to fit the right proportions of carbohydrate, protein and fat into your day. For a total of 1,960 calories, this menu supplies 61 percent of calories from carbohydrate, 24 percent from fat and 15 percent from protein. This is in line with experts' recommendations that at least 55 percent of daily calories come from carbohydrates. You also should try to limit your protein consumption to 15 percent and reduce your fat intake to less than 30 percent of calories.

Food	Portion	Calories
BREAKFAST		
Cranberry juice	½ cup	65
Oatmeal	1 cup	145
Blueberries	½ cup	41
Yogurt, low-fat	1 cup	200
LUNCH		
Sandwich made with:		
Wheat bread, light	2 slices	123
Tuna salad w/light mayonnaise	4 oz.	136
Alfalfa sprouts	¼ cup	3
Romaine lettuce	¼ cup	2
Tomato	½	13
Black bean soup	1 cup	218
Apple	1	81
SNACK		
Air-popped popcorn, light	3 cups	75
DINNER		
Tossed salad	1 cup	32
Italian dressing	1 Tbsp.	32
Vegetable lasagna	11 oz.	400
Italian bread	2 slices	170
Margarine, diet	2 tsp.	33
Pear	1	98
SNACK		
Raspberry frozen yogurt, nonfat	½ cup	93

Keep an immediate goal in sight. Take a long-term goal like reducing your fat consumption to 30 percent of calories and break it down into smaller goals, Somer says.

"Some people might want to start by eliminating butter from their toast in the morning. Others might prefer eating smaller portions of meat with every meal," Somer says. "There are a million ways to do it."

Cut back on all obvious fats in your diet. Bake, steam, broil or microwave your food, Kvitka says, and choose fried foods only occasionally. "High-fat foods like pizza and ice cream should only be eaten in moderate amounts," she says. "For example, have just one small scoop of ice cream, not an entire banana split. Better yet, try low-fat or nonfat frozen dairy desserts."

CHAPTER 3

Vitamins and Minerals

The Essential Facts

So you pop your once-a-day every morning and never give the matter of vitamins and minerals another thought. Or maybe you just assume you get all the nutrients you need in the food you eat, and you don't think about vitamins and minerals at all.

But there's a lot more to vitamins and minerals than a little column of numbers running down the side panel of your cereal box.

The basic facts are easy: There are 13 essential vitamins. Recommended Dietary Allowances, or RDAs, have been established by the National Research Council for 11 of them: vitamin A, six of the B vitamins—B_6, B_{12}, folate, niacin, riboflavin (B_2) and thiamine (B_1)—vitamin C, vitamin D, vitamin E and vitamin K. There's less information for the two remaining vitamins, biotin and pantothenate, so instead of RDAs, there are "estimated safe and adequate" daily dietary intakes for these. In this chapter, values given for RDAs are those for women and men aged 25 to 50.

There's an established RDA for seven minerals—calcium, phosphorus, magnesium, iron, zinc, iodine and selenium—and suggested intakes for potassium, copper, manganese, fluoride, chromium and molybdenum. (Sodium is also essential, but as we generally consume too much of it, rather than not enough, deficiencies are rare.)

What's *not* so evident about vitamins and minerals is exactly what each nutrient does, who may need more, what happens if you don't get enough (or if you get too much) and what the best food sources are. In some cases it's also important to know a nutrient's protective intake range—usually a ballpark number that research suggests should put you in the right range for protective purposes. So here's your A-to-Z guide—from vitamin A to zinc.

Vitamins

VITAMIN A AND BETA-CAROTENE

Chances are you've read a lot about beta-carotene in the news. Studies have shown that this substance can prevent oral cancer, delay cataracts and reduce the risk of heart attack and lung cancer. It's an antioxidant, a compound that may protect against disease by neutralizing unstable oxygen molecules, called free radicals, within the body.

Beta-carotene is a carotenoid (one of the group of compounds that makes up the red, orange and yellow pigments in plants) that's converted into vitamin A in the body. Unlike the preformed vitamin A from animal food sources, you essentially can't overdose on beta-carotene. It's converted to vitamin A on an as-needed basis, which is one reason it's the best way to get your vitamin A.

UNITS OF MEASUREMENT EXPLAINED

Vitamin and mineral amounts are usually expressed in *milligrams* (one-thousandth of a gram) or even smaller units called *micrograms* (one-thousandth of a milligram). These are commonly abbreviated *mg.* and *mcg.*, respectively. Another common measure is *international units* (I.U.). Vitamin D amounts, for example, are expressed in either mcg. or I.U. One microgram of vitamin D equals 40 I.U. Vitamin E is expressed in either I.U. or *alpha-tocopherol equivalents* (α-TE). One alpha-tocopherol equivalent equals 1 milligram of d-alpha-tocopherol (natural vitamin E). You may see vitamin A values expressed in a number of different ways. This nutrient was originally measured in I.U., but in 1974 the United States began using a measurement called *retinol equivalents* (REs). One RE equals either 3.3 I.U. of retinol (preformed vitamin A) or 6 micrograms of beta-carotene.

VITAMIN A SOURCES

Superior food sources of vitamin A include:

Food	Portion	Vitamin A (RE)
Sweet potato, baked	1	2,488
Carrot, raw	1	2,025
Spinach, boiled	½ cup	737
Butternut squash, baked	½ cup	714
Fresh tuna, cooked, dry heat	3 oz.	643
Cantaloupe	1 cup cubes	515
Beet greens, boiled	½ cup	367

What does vitamin A do? It's involved in vision, growth, cell differentiation and reproduction. Night blindness and problems in bone growth can be caused by a vitamin A deficiency. It also shows dramatic effects in reducing the death rate from measles, and derivatives of vitamin A such as the drugs Accutane and tretinoin can help clear up acne and psoriasis.

And even one daily serving of fruit or vegetables rich in beta-carotene may cut your risk for heart attack or stroke. "We've found a 22 percent reduction in the risk of heart attack and a 40 percent reduction in stroke for those women with high intakes of fruit and vegetables rich in beta-carotene compared with those with low intakes," says JoAnn E. Manson, M.D., project director for Brigham and Women's Hospital and Harvard Medical School.

Sources: For beta-carotene, fruit and vegetables (the deeper the color, the more vitamin A they provide); for pre-formed vitamin A, fish-liver oil, meat and milk.

RDA: 800 RE (4,000 I.U.) for women; 1,000 RE (5,000 I.U.) for men.

Protective range: As beta-carotene, 15 to 30 milligrams.

People with special needs: Those who are poorly nourished, have diabetes or are exposed to high levels of toxic chemicals and pollutants. Nursing mothers need an additional 400 to 500 RE daily.

Signs of deficiency: Night blindness, dry or rough skin, weak tooth enamel, diarrhea, loss of appetite.

Cautions: Very high doses of vitamin A (more than 50,000 I.U. in adults and 20,000 I.U. in children) can cause side effects such as headache, vomiting, blurred vision, hair loss, liver damage and aching bones. Vitamin A derivatives may cause birth defects if taken while pregnant.

VITAMIN B$_6$

Of all the B vitamins, B$_6$, or pyridoxine, may be the most important for maintaining a strong immune system. A study of eight healthy elderly adults by the U.S. Department of Agriculture's (USDA) Human Nutrition Research Center on

Aging at Tufts University in Boston found that deficiencies of B_6 adversely affected the immune system, but normal function returned when B_6 intake was increased.

VITAMIN B_6 SOURCES

Superior food sources of vitamin B_6 include:

Food	Portion	Vitamin B_6 (mg.)
Banana	1	0.7
Potato, baked	1	0.7
Chick-peas, canned	½ cup	0.6
Chicken breast, roasted	½	0.5
Fresh tuna, cooked, dry heat	3 oz.	0.4

B_6 is needed to help many enzymes function and for protein and nucleic acid synthesis. Severe deficiencies can cause anemia, nervous disorders and skin problems.

One study found that premenstrual symptoms were relieved in 21 of 25 women receiving 500 milligrams of B_6 daily—*and* that B_6 appeared to boost chances of conception. (Such a large dosage should only be taken under medical supervision.) Some women also find that B_6 alleviates morning sickness.

Some people have reported relief from carpal tunnel syndrome—a painful condition affecting the nerve that runs through the wrist—with B_6, but there's little medical evidence to confirm that.

Sources: Fortified cereals, whole grains, fish, chicken, soybeans, oats, peanuts, fruits and vegetables.

RDA: 1.6 milligrams for women; 2.0 milligrams for men.

Protective range: 2 to 10 milligrams.

People with special needs: Those taking oral contraceptives or those with carpal tunnel syndrome or diabetes. Women need an additional 0.6 milligrams if pregnant, 0.5 milligrams if nursing.

Signs of deficiency: Anemia, confusion, weakness, irritability, nervousness, poor coordination, insomnia, skin lesions, muscle twitching.

Cautions: Large amounts (2,000 milligrams a day) have resulted in nerve damage—consult a doctor before exceeding 50 milligrams daily. Reduces the therapeutic effect of levodopa, a drug for Parkinson's disease.

VITAMIN B$_{12}$

In the early 1900s, if you suffered from pernicious anemia, a blood disease that causes nerve tissue to degenerate, you were out of luck: The disease is fatal, and there was no cure. In 1926, however, researchers discovered an amazing cure—raw liver.

The curative powers of liver came from vitamin B$_{12}$, also called cobalamin. We need B$_{12}$ to synthesize DNA (which carries the code of genetic information) and help make blood. Studies have also linked it to helping prevent heart disease, cancer and neurological problems.

If you're low in either B$_{12}$ or folate (another B vitamin), your blood levels of an amino acid called homocysteine increase, notes Joel B. Mason, M.D., assistant professor in the divisions of clinical nutrition and gastroenterology at Tufts University School of Medicine—and high homocysteine is associated with an increased risk of cardiovascular disease. "Very modest increases in homocysteine can increase the risk of disease," says Dr. Mason.

What about cancer? A study of 73 men who smoked at least the equivalent of a pack of cigarettes per day for 20 years found that supplementing with vitamin B$_{12}$ and folate decreased the number of precancerous bronchial cells.

VITAMIN B$_{12}$ SOURCES

Superior food sources of vitamin B$_{12}$ include:

Food	Portion	Vitamin B$_{12}$ (mcg.)
Clams, steamed	20 small	89.0
Mackerel, cooked, dry heat	3 oz.	16.2
Oysters, steamed	6 med.	16.1
Atlantic herring, cooked, dry heat	3 oz.	11.2
Fresh tuna, cooked, dry heat	3 oz.	9.3

Allergic to sulfites? One study showed that B$_{12}$ can also help alleviate reactions to this common food additive.

Vitamin B$_{12}$ deficiencies can cause some psychological problems and changes in mental function—and may be one of the reasons some older people seem confused, less alert and not well coordinated. Some people can't absorb vitamin B$_{12}$ at a normal rate; doctors estimate that one in five people over age 60 just doesn't manufacture enough stomach acid to absorb B$_{12}$.

Vitamin B$_{12}$ is found almost exclusively in animal food products. If you don't eat meat, fish, dairy products or eggs, you may need a B$_{12}$ supplement. (There's some B$_{12}$ in tempeh, a fermented soybean product, but amounts can vary and are small.) Vegetarian children are particularly at risk because they have no stores of B$_{12}$.

Sources: Fish, dairy products, eggs, beef and pork. While liver and other organ meats are rich in B$_{12}$, they are not recommended for frequent consumption because of their high cholesterol content.

RDA: 2 micrograms.

Protective range: 2 to 10 micrograms.

People with special needs: Strict vegetarians and alcohol or drug abusers. Women need an extra 0.2 micrograms daily if pregnant and 0.4 micrograms daily if nursing.

Signs of deficiency: Anemia, neurological problems, sore tongue, weakness.

TWO KINDS OF VITAMINS

Nutrition scientists divide vitamins into two categories: fat-soluble and water-soluble. What's the difference?

Fat-soluble vitamins dissolve in fat, of course, and water-soluble ones dissolve in water. The significance of this is that the fat-soluble vitamins—vitamins A, D, E and K—are stored in your body, and because they accumulate, you can overdose on these vitamins if you take excessive amounts of supplements.

It's tougher to overdose on the water-soluble vitamins—vitamins C, B_6 and B_{12}, biotin, folate, niacin, pantothenate, riboflavin and thiamine—because excess intakes of these vitamins are excreted in your urine. This doesn't mean, however, that you *can't* overdose on a water-soluble vitamin: Nutritionists warn that doses more than ten times the RDA may cause problems.

BIOTIN

Biotin, a B vitamin, is produced in our intestines, so normally we have plenty of it. It's involved in the synthesis of fatty acids and glucose and the metabolism of several amino acids.

Deficiencies in biotin can cause skin problems and loss of hair, but there's no scientific evidence that biotin can help control normal hair loss.

Sources: Milk, vegetables, nuts, whole grains, organ meats, brewer's yeast and tuna.

Estimated safe and adequate daily intake: 30 to 100 micrograms.

People with special needs: Those who smoke, eat a lot of raw egg white, are on a poorly balanced diet or are taking oral antibiotics.

Signs of deficiency: Fatigue, depression, nausea, sleepiness, loss of appetite, muscle pain, hair loss, dermatitis.

VITAMIN C

C is for colds and cancer—fighting them, that is. Or so research scientist and Nobel laureate Linus Pauling has claimed for decades, and the latest evidence indicates that there's some truth to these claims.

Vitamin C's historical role, however, was alleviating scurvy, a serious disease marked by bleeding gums and swollen limbs that crippled navies and explorers. Also known as ascorbic acid, vitamin C helps form the dentin layer (just under the enamel) of our teeth and collagen in our connective tissue. It's also involved in amino acid metabolism and helps us use iron, calcium and folate.

There's strong evidence that vitamin C, an antioxidant that helps protect cells from damage by destructive oxygen molecules, helps prevent some forms of cancers. Vitamin C may act in conjunction with carotenoids and other substances in fruit and vegetables, according to Gladys Block, Ph.D., a professor of public health nutrition at the University of California in Berkeley. And colds: Studies at the University of Torino in Italy found that vitamin C protected against colds, hay fever and exposure to air pollution.

Meeting the RDA of 60 milligrams daily should be no problem. "If you meet the National Academy of Sciences guidelines and eat at least five servings of fruit and vegetables each day, you can't help but take in 120 milligrams of vitamin C," says Paul F. Jacques, D.Sc., an epidemiologist at Tufts University.

Vitamin C also may help prevent heart disease. Studies by Dr. Jacques found that women with higher levels of vitamin C in their blood were more likely to have higher levels of HDL (high-density lipoprotein) cholesterol, the "good" cholesterol—possibly because of C's work as an antioxidant.

Vitamin C helps protect against cataracts, a vision robber that affects nearly half of Americans aged 75 to 85. Eating 3½ servings of fruit and vegetables a day is enough to help lower the risk.

VITAMIN C SOURCES

Superior food sources of vitamin C include:

Food	Portion	Vitamin C (mg.)
Orange juice, fresh	1 cup	124
Broccoli, fresh, boiled	1 cup	116
Brussels sprouts, fresh, cooked	1 cup	97
Red bell peppers, raw	½ cup	95
Cranberry juice cocktail	1 cup	90
Cantaloupe	1 cup cubes	68

Sources: Citrus fruits, broccoli, spinach, strawberries and melons.

RDA: 60 milligrams.

Protective range: 100 to 500 milligrams.

People with special needs: Smokers and alcohol abusers. Women need an additional 10 milligrams daily if pregnant, 30 to 35 milligrams if nursing.

Signs of deficiency: Scurvy (weak muscles, swollen or bleeding gums, loss of teeth, fatigue, depression), shortness of breath, easy bruising, nosebleeds, anemia, frequent infections.

Cautions: Huge doses can cause side effects in some people; consult a doctor.

VITAMIN D

The great thing about vitamin D is that you can make it yourself: Your body forms vitamin D when your skin is exposed to the ultraviolet rays of the sun. You can also get D from foods such as fatty fish, liver, egg yolks and fortified milk.

The primary role of this vitamin is to help build and maintain strong bones and teeth (D is essential to help us absorb calcium, the bone-building mineral). The classic sign of deficiency is rickets, a disease that causes stunted, bowed limbs and unhealthy teeth in growing children. Deficiency has also been linked to osteomalacia, a bone formation defect.

Some studies have found that vitamin D helps in the treatment of psoriasis and may boost resistance to tuberculosis.

Vitamin D may have many other functions, however, which researchers are just starting to uncover. Some studies indicate that D may protect against colorectal and breast cancer and may help in treating other cancers.

"We can look for many new treatments and new functions of vitamin D in the future," says Hector DeLuca, Ph.D., chairman of the Department of Biochemistry at the University of Wisconsin in Madison. Research by Dr. DeLuca indicates that the hormonal form of vitamin D can suppress growth of cancer cells.

Who's likely to be deficient in D? The elderly tend to be at risk because they may have limited exposure to sunlight, eat few vitamin D-rich foods or take medications that interfere with vitamin D uptake or metabolism. Other high-risk categories are alcoholics, people who live in areas without much sun and people who don't eat dairy products. Studies have found cases of rickets in vegetarian children who did not eat eggs or drink milk.

You can get your vitamin D from food. Or you can give yourself a "dose" of sunshine three times a week: Spend five or ten minutes outdoors with your face, arms and hands exposed to the morning or late-afternoon sun, says Michael Holick, M.D., Ph.D., director of the Vitamin D and Bone Research Laboratory at the Boston University School of Medicine. Another option is a multivitamin supplement that supplies 200 to 400 I.U.

VITAMIN D SOURCES

Superior food sources of vitamin D include:

Food	Portion	Vitamin D (I.U.)
Herring, pickled	3 oz.	578
Atlantic sardines, canned in oil	3 oz.	231
Salmon, chum, canned	3 oz.	190
Fortified milk	8 oz.	100
Edam cheese	3 oz.	72

It is possible to get too much vitamin D, so read labels carefully if you use supplements. Too much D can cause hypercalcemia—high levels of calcium in the blood. If you have elevated blood calcium already, *don't* take supplemental D.

Sources: Fatty fish (mackerel, sardines, salmon), liver, egg yolks, fortified milk and sunlight.

RDA: 5 micrograms (200 I.U.).

People with special needs: Vegetarians, the elderly, alcoholics and those who avoid the sun or have kidney failure. Women need an additional 200 I.U. if pregnant or nursing.

Signs of deficiency: Rickets in children (bowed legs, malformed joints or bones, retarded growth, weak muscles, late development of teeth), osteomalacia in adults (pain in ribs, spine, pelvis, legs; muscle weakness; brittle bones).

Cautions: Overdoses may cause high blood levels of calcium (hypercalcemia). If you have elevated blood calcium, take supplemental D only under a doctor's direction.

VITAMIN E

Vitamin E, or tocopherol, is another of those magical antioxidants that protects your cells from damage by destructive oxygen molecules. Evidence is growing that it plays a role in preventing heart disease, cataracts and cervical cancer and improving the immune system. There's some suggestion that treatment with E can help people with Parkinson's disease and tardive dyskinesia, a movement disorder.

Most of us don't have to worry about actual deficits of vitamin E: The only people prone to deficiency are some premature babies and people who don't absorb fat normally.

But a Nurses Health Study involving more than 87,000 women found that about 100 I.U. of supplemental vitamin E daily was associated with a 36 percent drop in the risk of heart attacks. Low levels of E may also double the risk of angina, according to another study.

Another study showed that vitamin E can protect strenuously used muscles from damage. Vitamin E seemed to invigorate the substances that help repair the muscles. This protective process also occurs when your body fights an infection, says William J. Evans, Ph.D., chief of the Human Physiology Laboratory at Tufts University and coauthor of *Biomarkers: The 10 Determinants of Aging You Can Control.*

VITAMIN E SOURCES

Superior food sources of vitamin E include:

Food	Portion	Vitamin E (mg. α-TE)
Sunflower seeds, dried	¼ cup	18
Sweet potatoes, boiled	1 cup	15
Kale, fresh, boiled	1 cup	10
Yams, boiled or baked	1 cup	6
Spinach, boiled	1 cup	4

Sources: Vegetable oil, mayonnaise, corn-oil margarine, peanuts, whole grains, wheat germ and spinach.

RDA: 12 I.U. (8 milligrams α-TE) for women; 15 I.U. (10 milligrams α-TE) for men.

Protective range: 100 to 400 I.U. (67 to 268 milligrams α-TE).

People with special needs: Those over 55 and those who abuse alcohol or drugs or have hyperthyroidism. Women need an additional 2 milligrams α-TE daily if pregnant, 3 to 4 milligrams α-TE if nursing.

Signs of deficiency: Anemia, lethargy, apathy, inability to concentrate, muscle weakness, decreased sexual performance.

Cautions: High doses deplete vitamin A stores. Very high doses may impair sex functions, alter hormone metabolism and produce a bleeding tendency. Don't take vitamin E supplements if you are on anticoagulant drugs or have a vitamin K deficiency (which impairs blood clotting).

FOLATE

This B vitamin, also called folic acid, is involved in metabolism and all biological reactions in your body. A defi-

FOLATE SOURCES

Superior food sources of folate include:

Food	Portion	Folate (mcg.)
Lentils, boiled	½ cup	179
Pinto beans, boiled	½ cup	146
Spinach, boiled	½ cup	131
Wheat germ, toasted	¼ cup	100
Orange juice, fresh	1 cup	75

ciency causes anemia similar to vitamin B_{12} anemia, with symptoms of weakness, fatigue and cramps, and possibly depression and schizophrenia.

In some patients with atherosclerosis, folate prevented the recurrence of heart attacks. And in several studies, folate supplementation improved the eyesight of elderly patients.

Low folate concentrations in the blood have also been linked with cervical cancer, points out C. E. Butterworth, Jr., M.D., with the Department of Nutrition Sciences at the University of Alabama in Birmingham. Research there also showed that oral doses of ten milligrams of folate plus 500 micrograms of B_{12} decreased the number of precancerous bronchial cells.

Sources: Fresh leafy green vegetables, wheat germ, mushrooms, oranges, beans, rice, brewer's yeast and liver.

RDA: 180 micrograms for women; 200 micrograms for men.

Protective range: 400 to 800 micrograms.

People with special needs: The elderly, those with sickle cell anemia or any condition involving high production of red blood cells, alcoholics, women taking oral contraceptives, people with intestinal malabsorption problems.

Women need an additional 220 micrograms daily if pregnant, 80 to 100 micrograms if nursing.

Signs of deficiency: Anemia, irritability, weakness.

Cautions: People with B_{12} deficiency anemia should not take folate until the B_{12} deficiency is treated.

VITAMIN K

K is for *koagulation*—the Danish word for coagulation. As you might suspect, vitamin K—which was discovered by a Danish scientist in 1934—plays a crucial role in blood clotting.

This vitamin can also help control bleeding in the brain of premature babies, whose immature blood vessels evidently can't handle the pressure surges that occur during birth. In one study of 92 pregnant women who were expected to deliver prematurely, half received vitamin K injections every five days until delivery. Of the babies born to mothers receiving vitamin K, only 16 percent suffered brain bleeding and none had severe bleeding. Thirty-six percent of the babies of mothers who didn't receive vitamin K had bleeding, however, and 11 percent had severe bleeding.

Vitamin K also plays a role in maintaining healthy bones and helping fractures to heal. "We think K may have a positive effect on bone transformation," says Cees Vermeer, Ph.D., of the Department of Biochemistry at the University of Limburg in the Netherlands. Many elderly people have an inadequate intake of vitamin K, he says. One Japanese study found that supplemental K reduced the loss of calcium—essential for healthy bones—by 18 to 50 percent in three postmenopausal women with osteoporosis. However, high doses of vitamin K can cause allergic skin reactions or liver problems, and supplementation above 100 micrograms daily is not encouraged.

Sources: Green leafy vegetables, fruits, root vegetables, seeds, eggs, dairy products, meat and alfalfa. Also synthesized by intestinal bacteria.

RDA: 65 micrograms for women; 80 micrograms for men.

People with special needs: Those with malabsorption problems, on very low calorie diets or being fed intravenously.

Signs of deficiency: Defective blood coagulation (can lead to nosebleeds, blood in urine and spontaneous black-and-blue marks).

Cautions: Doses over 500 micrograms may cause rashes, itching, flushing or possibly liver problems.

NIACIN

When scores of residents of small southern towns in the early 1900s fell prey to a disease marked by an uncomfortable combination of symptoms—dermatitis, diarrhea and dementia—at first no one suspected that the culprit was something missing from their diets.

The disease was pellagra, and the missing nutrient was niacin. This B vitamin is involved in the synthesis of protein and fat and the formation of DNA. It helps maintain your skin, nerves and digestive system. Niacin has other important uses: One study found that it reduces cholesterol and the recurrence of heart attacks by nearly 30 percent.

There are two forms of niacin: nicotinic acid and nicotinamide. Nicotinic acid, however, can cause "niacin flush"—a burning, itching feeling in the face, neck, arms or chest—when taken in large doses.

Sources: Brewer's yeast, meats, poultry, halibut, salmon, swordfish, tuna, peanut butter, sunflower seeds and legumes.

RDA: 15 milligrams for women; 19 milligrams for men.

People with special needs: Those over 55, alcoholics, those who participate in vigorous physical activity or have diabetes or hyperthyroidism. Women need an additional 2 milligrams daily if pregnant, 5 milligrams if nursing.

Signs of deficiency: Muscle weakness; fatigue; loss of appetite; red, swollen tongue; headaches; skin lesions; nausea and vomiting; diarrhea; irritability.

Cautions: Doses of nicotinic acid over 100 milligrams can cause burning; itching and tingling in face, neck, arms and upper chest; nausea; headache; cramps; diarrhea and altered heart rate. Extremely large doses may cause liver problems. People with diabetes, gout or gallbladder or liver disease should consult a doctor before taking niacin.

NIACIN SOURCES

Superior food sources of niacin include:

Food	Portion	Niacin (mg.)
Chicken breast, roasted	½	11.8
Light tuna, canned in water	3 oz.	10.5
Fresh tuna, cooked, dry heat	3 oz.	9.0
Halibut, cooked, dry heat	3 oz.	6.1
Turkey white meat, roasted	3 oz.	5.8

PANTOTHENATE

This B vitamin, also called pantothenic acid, is easy to find—all food groups contain some. It's involved in metabolizing carbohydrate, fat and protein. Deficiency may lower resistance to infection, and higher intakes may help you fight stress.

Sources: Organ meats, most fish, whole grains, blue cheese, brewer's yeast, corn, eggs, lentils, wheat germ, sunflower seeds, peanuts and peas.

Estimated safe and adequate daily intake: 4 to 7 milligrams.

People with special needs: Drug or alcohol abusers, athletes, pregnant or nursing women, those over 55, those on inadequate or low-calorie diets or smokers.

Signs of deficiency: May include fatigue, sleeping problems, loss of appetite, nausea, lowered resistance to infection.

Cautions: More than 10 grams daily could cause diarrhea and bloating. Don't take pantothenate if you are taking medication for Parkinson's disease.

RIBOFLAVIN

This B vitamin, also known as vitamin B_2, is essential for growth and tissue repair. Deficiencies have been linked to esophageal cancer.

Deficiency may be fairly common, particularly in youngsters who drink less than one cup of milk a day. Two cups of milk daily supply sufficient riboflavin, but you can also get it from fruit, vegetables and cereals.

If you do take a riboflavin supplement, take it with meals to dramatically increase the amount you'll absorb.

Sources: Milk, yogurt, cheese, wheat germ, whole grains, chicken, leafy green vegetables, almonds and fruit.

RIBOFLAVIN SOURCES

Superior food sources of riboflavin include:

Food	Portion	Riboflavin (mg.)
Beef liver, braised	3 oz.	3.5
King mackerel, cooked	3 oz.	0.5
Nonfat yogurt	1 cup	0.5
Skim milk	1 cup	0.5
Swiss cheese	1 oz.	0.1

RDA: 1.3 milligrams for women; 1.7 milligrams for men.

People with special needs: Those who exercise regularly, eat only processed foods or are on low-calorie diets, have hypothyroidism or are alcoholics. Women need an additional 0.3 milligrams daily if pregnant, 0.4 to 0.5 milligrams if nursing.

Signs of deficiency: Cracks in corners of mouth, inflamed tongue and lips, sensitive eyes, itching and scaling of skin, trembling, dizziness, insomnia.

THIAMINE

This B vitamin, also called vitamin B_1, is involved in converting blood sugar into energy. It also helps form red blood cells and maintain skeletal muscle.

What it's most known for is preventing beriberi, a serious deficiency disease that causes confusion, weakened muscles, loss of appetite and quickened heartbeat. If not halted, the disease progresses either to "wet" beriberi, which causes swelling, accumulation of fluid in the heart muscle and eventual death, or "dry" beriberi, which causes serious nervous system problems and wasting away.

This was a common health problem in the mid-nineteenth century, particularly in countries where polished white rice was a staple of the diet. In the Philippines, where most of the thiamine present in rice is lost in milling, washing and cooking, beriberi is still the fourth leading cause of death.

Most of us in the United States get ample thiamine in our diets, but one group at risk for deficiency is alcoholics, because alcohol interferes with the absorption of thiamine *and* impairs the ability to store it. Many of the classic outward symptoms of alcoholism—confusion, vision problems and eye muscle paralysis—may be caused by thiamine deficiency.

But even marginal deficiencies can cause an array of unpleasant symptoms in older people. A study of 80 Irish women with moderate deficiency found that thiamine supplements improved their sleep patterns, decreased fatigue and restored appetite and sense of general well-being. The researchers suggest having your doctor check your thiamine levels with a blood test if you are over 65 and have these symptoms.

Sources: Pork, whole grains, wheat germ, brewer's yeast, legumes and seafood.

RDA: 1.1 milligrams for women; 1.5 milligrams for men.

People with special needs: Those on low-calorie diets, heavy coffee or tea drinkers, the elderly or alcoholics. Women need an additional 0.4 milligrams daily if pregnant, 0.5 milligrams if nursing.

Signs of deficiency: Loss of appetite, fatigue, nausea, vomiting, confusion, depression, gastrointestinal problems, fluid accumulation in arms and legs.

THIAMINE SOURCES

Superior food sources of thiamine include:

Food	Portion	Thiamine (mg.)
Pork center loin, roasted	3 oz.	0.8
Sunflower seeds, dried	1 oz.	0.7
Florida pompano, cooked, dry heat	3 oz.	0.6
Wheat germ, toasted	¼ cup	0.5
Spinach noodles, enriched, cooked	1 cup	0.4

Minerals

CALCIUM

So you know all about calcium, you say. Try this quiz.

Calcium can help: (a) build and maintain strong bones and teeth, (b) lower blood pressure, (c) cut colon cancer risks, (d) ease menstrual discomfort, (e) reduce the number of premature births or (f) all of the above.

The correct answer is (f) all of the above.

People who miss out on enough calcium in their younger, bone-forming years may pay the piper years later. Around age 40, we begin to lose this mineral from our bones faster than it can be replaced. Women face especially large losses during menopause because of the lack of estrogen, which is necessary for their bones to absorb calcium. The result can be osteoporosis, with bones so weakened that they can break while just walking. Some studies have indicated that calcium can help even after the bone-forming years, however. According to several studies, calcium can help people with mild high blood pressure lower their levels to normal.

What role does calcium play in cancer prevention? For colon cancer, calcium may bind with possible cancer-causing bile acids that are produced in the colon.

A study of pregnant teenagers found that mothers who received supplemental calcium had markedly fewer premature births. And a 5½-month study by the USDA found that women who received higher calcium than a control group had fewer menstrual and premenstrual symptoms such as mood changes, cramps and backaches.

Sources: Dairy products, canned salmon and sardines (with bones), soybeans, tofu, kale, turnip greens and kelp.

RDA: 800 milligrams.

Protective range: 1,200 to 1,500 milligrams.

People with special needs: Those who avoid milk and other dairy products, are over 55 (especially women), are on low-calorie diets or are alcoholics. Women need an additional 400 milligrams daily if pregnant or nursing.

Signs of deficiency: Frequent fractures, hump in spine, seizures, muscle cramps, low backache.

Cautions: Avoid supplemental calcium if you have kidney stones or high blood calcium.

CALCIUM SOURCES

Superior food sources of calcium include:

Food	Portion	Calcium (mg.)
Skim milk	1 cup	302
Sardines, canned	6	275
Mozzarella cheese	1 oz.	181
Salmon, canned (with bones)	3 oz.	181
Figs, dried	5	135

CHROMIUM

Yep, this is the stuff used to make the trim on your car glitter—but it's also an essential mineral linked to glucose tolerance, the ability to process blood sugar.

Glucose *intolerance* is a precursor of diabetes, and controlling it may prevent the development of that disease. In one study, glucose tolerance improved in 10 of 12 elderly people who were given chromium. Another study showed that supplementing with 200 micrograms daily improved glucose tolerance in people who were mildly glucose-intolerant.

What this means is that adequate chromium could keep many people who have mild glucose intolerance from becoming diabetic, says Richard A. Anderson, Ph.D., a biochemist with the USDA's Human Nutrition Research Center in Beltsville, Maryland. It's tough to get enough chromium in your foods, says Dr. Anderson. And he recommends a supplement. Another way to increase your chromium intake is to eat fewer foods that *deplete* chromium—such as cookies and pastries, with their simple carbohydrates. Complex carbohydrates such as pasta and potatoes, on the other hand, help *preserve* chromium.

You don't have to worry about overdosing on the chromium you get in foods. Toxicity can result, however, from overexposure to industrial processes involving chromium, such as electroplating, steel making and glassmaking.

Sources: Vegetables, whole grains, fruit, meat, cheese, oysters, fish, dairy products, beef, chicken and brewer's yeast.

Estimated safe and adequate daily intake: 50 to 200 micrograms.

Protective range: 100 to 200 micrograms.

People with special needs: Those who use alcohol or are on low-calorie diets, the elderly, pregnant women, athletes.

Signs of deficiency: Diabetes-like symptoms (overweight, fatigue, excessive thirst, frequent urination, urinary tract infections, yeast infections).

COPPER

Copper is necessary for the formation of red blood cells; it's also a catalyst for the storage and release of iron. It's involved in the production of collagen, the protein that makes bone, cartilage, skin and tendons all work. Copper also helps produce melanin, the pigment that gives color to our hair and skin. In animals, supplementary copper has been shown to protect against some cancers.

Some research indicates that copper deficiency is linked to heart disease. Leslie M. Klevay, M.D., research leader of the Clinical Nutrition Laboratory with the USDA Human Nutrition Research Center at the University of North Dakota in Grand Forks, notes that copper deficiency can raise cholesterol levels, lead to glucose intolerance, produce heart rhythm problems and increase blood pressure.

Many of us may not be getting enough copper: Two-thirds of Americans get less than the suggested minimum.

Sources: Nuts, fruit and legumes, oysters and other shellfish.

Estimated safe and adequate daily intake: 1.5 to 3.0 milligrams.

People with special needs: Premature babies and those taking high levels of zinc or vitamin C.

Signs of deficiency: Anemia, bone demineralization, low white blood cell count.

COPPER SOURCES

Superior food sources of copper include:

Food	Portion	Copper (mg.)
Oysters, cooked	12 med.	7.5
Alaskan king crab, steamed	3 oz.	1.0
Potatoes, baked, with skin	7 oz.	0.6
White beans, boiled	1 cup	0.5
Apricots, dried	½ cup	0.3

FLUORIDE

Scientists know that fluoride is incorporated into bones and tooth enamel, but they're not yet positive that it's nutritionally essential.

What they do know is that fluoride reduces dental cavities, particularly in children eight and younger, so many communities have fluoride added to the public water supply for that purpose. There's also some suggestion that fluoride may help protect bones in adults, apparently stimulating new bone growth and helping to make bone stronger.

Fluoridated water has one milligram of fluoride or less per liter; you can also get fluoride from foods, although the content varies.

Sources: Tea, canned salmon (with bones), mackerel and fluoridated water.

Estimated safe and adequate daily intake: 1.5 to 4.0 milligrams.

Cautions: High levels have caused mottling of children's teeth; huge doses may be toxic.

IODINE

You may have noticed that the salt you buy is fortified with iodine, but have you ever wondered why you need this mineral? Most of the iodine in your body is in your thyroid gland, and you need ample iodine to keep your thyroid hormones on track.

Deficiency can cause many disorders, including thyroid enlargement (known as goiter) and mental retardation. Iodine is present in both soil and water, but in some areas of the world levels are so low that iodine deficiency is common. The introduction of iodine into the salt supply in the United States in 1924 greatly decreased the occurrence of goiter, but it continues to be a major problem in Africa, Asia and South America.

Some studies suggest that iodine may help relieve fibrocystic breasts, painful or sore breasts common in premenopausal women.

Most North Americans get plenty of iodine in their diets,

even without iodized salt. An exception may be people who eat lots of cruciferous vegetables such as rutabagas, cabbage, brussels sprouts and cauliflower. These foods are iodine antagonists—they block uptake of the mineral.

Sources: Seaweed, fish, shrimp, oysters and iodized salt.

RDA: 150 micrograms.

People with special needs: Those on low-calorie diets, who live in areas where soil is deficient in iodine and eat mostly locally grown produce, or those who eat lots of cruciferous vegetables. Women need an additional 25 micrograms daily if pregnant, 50 micrograms if nursing.

Signs of deficiency: Chronic fatigue, weight gain, intolerance to cold, goiter (enlarged thyroid gland).

Cautions: Too much iodine during pregnancy can result in thyroid enlargement, dwarfism or mental deficiency in the baby. Don't take supplements if you have elevated serum potassium or myotonia congenita (a hereditary disease that makes the muscles stiff). More than 50 milligrams daily can cause inflammation of the salivary glands.

IRON

Having trouble sleeping at night? You may not be consuming enough iron.

An insomnia study by the USDA found that people consuming one-third the recommended amount of iron woke more frequently during the night than people taking in adequate iron.

But contributing to a sound night's sleep is a minor role for iron. Iron produces the red blood cells that transport oxygen in our bodies. That's why a shortage of iron causes anemia. Low iron intake has been linked to learning problems in young children, and one study suggested that low iron levels adversely affected short-term memory and attention span in young women.

IRON SOURCES

Superior food sources of iron include:

Food	Portion	Iron (mg.)
Clams, steamed	20 small	26.2
Cream of Wheat, cooked	¾ cup	7.7
Tofu	4 oz.	6.2
Soybeans, boiled	½ cup	4.4
Pumpkin seeds, hulled, dried	1 oz.	4.3

And iron deficiency is more common than you may think: Experts estimate that one-third to one-half of young American women are iron deficient. Even mild iron-deficiency anemia may cause you to feel depressed or lethargic. "If you're tired, listless and apathetic in a way you're not used to, you'd better check your iron levels," says Ernesto Pollitt, Ph.D., professor of human development at the University of California at Davis.

You should check with your doctor before taking iron supplements: One in 300 people may suffer from a genetic defect that causes iron overload, says James D. Cook, M.D., professor of medicine and director of the Division of Hematology at the University of Kansas Medical Center in Kansas City.

Sources: Red meat, clams, garbanzos, tomato juice and raisins.

RDA: 15 milligrams for women; 10 milligrams for men.

Protective range: 15 milligrams.

People with special needs: Menstruating women, those on restricted diets. Pregnant women need an additional 15 milligrams daily.

Signs of deficiency: Listlessness, heart palpitations on exertion, irritability, fatigue, pale skin, cracked lips and tongue.

Cautions: Don't take iron supplements if you have acute hepatitis, excess iron in your body, hemolytic anemia, or have had many blood transfusions. Iron supplements formulated for adults can be lethal for small children.

MAGNESIUM

Without magnesium, we wouldn't be here: This mineral is involved in every major biologic function in our bodies. It also may help prevent heart disease, kidney stones and gallstones, chronic fatigue syndrome and menstrual problems. Magnesium also acts as an antacid in small doses and as a laxative in large doses, and helps strengthen tooth enamel. Low magnesium can cause problems such as depression, irritability and confusion, says Daniel Kanofsky, M.D., assistant professor of psychiatry at the Albert Einstein College of Medicine of Yeshiva University in New York City.

Some researchers believe magnesium deficiency is a cause of cardiovascular disease. Death rates from heart disease are higher in areas with soft water—which, unlike hard water, doesn't contain appreciable amounts of magnesium. And magnesium given intravenously does help save the lives of heart attack victims.

Promising news for people who suffer from chronic fatigue syndrome (CFS) comes from a study in the United Kingdom. Of 15 CFS patients receiving a weekly intramuscular shot of magnesium sulfate for six weeks, 12 showed marked improvement—while only 3 of 17 patients who didn't receive magnesium said they felt better. "It may be worthwhile to check for magnesium deficiency in the blood—and if it's there, take the proper steps to fix it," says M. J. Campbell, Ph.D., senior lecturer at the University of Southampton General Hospital in the United Kingdom.

Sources: Wheat germ, sunflower seeds, leafy green vegetables, seafood, nuts, dairy products and meats.

RDA: 280 milligrams for women; 350 milligrams for men.

Protective range: 400 milligrams.

People with special needs: The elderly; those with diabetes, on low-calorie diets, taking diuretics or digitalis; alcohol drinkers; those who engage in regular strenuous exercise. Women need an additional 20 milligrams daily if pregnant, 60 to 75 milligrams if nursing.

Signs of deficiency: Nausea, muscle weakness, irritability, mental derangement.

Cautions: People with kidney problems, certain heart problems or ileostomy (a surgical opening in the small intestine) should not take magnesium supplements.

MAGNESIUM SOURCES

Superior food sources of magnesium include:

Food	Portion	Magnesium (mg.)
Pumpkin seeds, hulled, dried	1 oz.	152
Tofu	4 oz.	120
Sunflower seeds, dried	1 oz.	101
Wheat germ, toasted	¼ cup	91
Almonds	1 oz.	84

MANGANESE

There's still a lot of mystery about what manganese does for us, but scientists *do* know that it's essential. In animals, manganese is required for normal bone structure and glucose metabolism, and animals that are deficient in manganese sometimes have trouble reproducing.

Manganese helps enzymes break down carbohydrates and

fats into fuel, and animal experiments suggest that it also works as an antioxidant, protecting cells from damage from destructive oxygen molecules. "Because manganese functions as an antioxidant, your intake may be important in terms of preventing a number of degenerative diseases like heart disease," says Sheri Zidenberg-Cherr, Ph.D., research nutritionist and lecturer at the University of California at Davis.

Most of us get adequate manganese in our diets, but if you're taking large doses of calcium or iron supplements, you could be significantly interfering with your manganese levels. There's some evidence that magnesium and phosphorus can partially block manganese absorption as well.

Overdosing on manganese in foods is unlikely, but people exposed to manganese dust—such as mine workers—can actually experience "manganese intoxication." Symptoms include delusions and hallucinations, followed by deep depression and an inability to stay awake.

Sources: Whole grains, nuts, shellfish, milk and organ meats.

Estimated safe and adequate daily intake: 2 to 5 milligrams.

People with special needs: Those on low-calorie diets or being fed intravenously or by tube. High intake of magnesium, calcium, iron or phosphate may decrease absorption of manganese.

Signs of deficiency: Slow growth and development in children.

Cautions: Consult a doctor before taking supplemental manganese if you have liver disease.

MOLYBDENUM

This mineral with the funny name is a part of the body's enzyme system. It also becomes a part of bones, liver and kidneys.

Molybdenum may play a vital role in protecting against esophageal cancer. A small region in China with soil very deficient in molybdenum has the highest rate of esophageal cancer in the world. Molybdenum is necessary for nitrates in the soil to change to the amines that are needed to nourish plants; without molybdenum, the nitrates change to cancer-causing forms instead. People in the region were also deficient in vitamin C, which helps detoxify those cancer-causing forms.

The happy ending to this story is that since molybdenum has been added to the soil and diets have been supplemented with vitamin C, the rate of esophageal cancer appears to be declining in China.

Molybdenum deficiency is quite rare, however. Studies show that most American diets supply between 75 and 250 micrograms, so chances are you're getting plenty.

Sources: Whole grains; legumes; dark green, leafy vegetables; milk; beans and organ meats.

Estimated safe and adequate daily intake: 75 to 250 micrograms.

People with special needs: Those on low-calorie diets or being fed intravenously or by tube.

Cautions: Don't take over 500 micrograms a day without a doctor's prescription. Consult a doctor before taking supplements containing molybdenum if you have high levels of uric acid or gout. Intake of 10 to 15 milligrams daily is associated with goutlike symptoms.

PHOSPHORUS

This mineral regulates the release of energy, helps transport nutrients involved in calcification of bones and teeth and helps regulate the acidity of body fluids.

It's an essential mineral, but because it's so plentiful in foods—daily intake in the American diet ranges from 800 to

1,500 milligrams—deficiency is rare. Phosphorus deficiency has resulted from taking antacids containing aluminum hydroxide, which binds with phosphorus and makes it unavailable for absorption.

Sources: Almost all foods.

RDA: 800 milligrams.

People with special needs: Alcoholics, those with gastrointestinal and kidney problems or diabetic ketoacidosis. Women need an additional 400 milligrams daily if pregnant or nursing.

Signs of deficiency: Bone loss, weakness, anorexia, pain.

POTASSIUM

We need potassium for many things—including maintaining a regular heartbeat and normal muscle contraction—but the exciting news is that, in some cases, this mineral can evidently lower blood pressure and help prevent heart disease and stroke.

"Strong evidence from a number of studies suggests that a diet low in potassium may lead to high blood pressure," says George Webb, Ph.D., associate professor of physiology and biophysics at the University of Vermont College of Medicine in Burlington.

In one study of 37 men and women with high blood pressure, one group took 2,340 milligrams of potassium daily, another group took the potassium plus magnesium, while a third group received a blank pill. After eight weeks, the blood pressure of both groups taking potassium dropped dramatically.

"A low potassium intake may substantially increase your risk of getting hypertension or, we now suspect, may make existing high blood pressure worse," says G. Gopal Krishna, M.D., associate professor of medicine at the University of Pennsylvania in Philadelphia.

Another study suggests that just one extra serving of fresh vegetables or fruit daily could reduce your risk of fatal stroke by 40 percent. That study, involving 859 southern Californian men and women ranging in age from 50 to 79, found that the 24 people who suffered stroke-related deaths had a markedly lower potassium intake than the others.

And if you're low in potassium, you actually retain more sodium—one of the enemies in the blood pressure battle—and *lose* more calcium, necessary to maintain strong bones.

Sources: Fresh vegetables and fruit, meat and milk.

Estimated minimum daily intake: 1,600 to 2,000 milligrams.

People with special needs: Those taking diuretics.

Signs of deficiency: Weakness, paralysis, low blood pressure, irregular or rapid heartbeat.

Cautions: People with impaired kidney function should avoid foods and supplements rich in potassium.

POTASSIUM SOURCES

Superior food sources of potassium include:

Food	Portion	Potassium (mg.)
Potato, baked	1	844
Apricots, dried	10 halves	482
Lima beans	1/2 cup	478
Banana	1	451
Skim milk	1 cup	447
Chicken breast, roasted	3 oz.	220

SELENIUM

We need this mineral only in very tiny quantities, but those minute amounts appear to help prevent some serious diseases—cancer and stroke.

Take a look at Rapid City, South Dakota, with the lowest rate of deaths from cancer in the United States. Rapid City *also* has the highest amount of selenium in its soil (and its crops). Now look at Ohio, with almost double the cancer rate as South Dakota and—you guessed it—the lowest soil selenium levels. Experiments show reduced rates of liver, skin, mammary and colon cancers in animals given selenium—and one study showed the cancer-fighting effect was more dramatic when rats received *both* selenium and garlic.

"From a practical standpoint, this means that people should eat foods that give them an adequate level of selenium," says Cornell University toxicologist Donald Lisk, Ph.D.

Areas of Georgia and North and South Carolina also have very low soil selenium—plus the highest rates of stroke and heart disease.

Like beta-carotene and vitamins C and E, selenium is an antioxidant. It latches onto harmful oxygen molecules, which may help explain its disease-fighting potential. Selenium may also increase immune responses, and it plays a role in sperm production and movement. Studies in China showed that supplementing with selenium can stop Keshan disease, which involves the degeneration of heart muscles.

Even moderately low levels of selenium can cause anxiety and tiredness. Researchers at the University College in Swansea, Wales, found that a supplement of 100 micrograms daily improved moods and anxiety levels.

Sources: Brewer's yeast, grains, fish, broccoli, cabbage, celery, cucumbers, onions, garlic, radishes and mushrooms.

RDA: 55 micrograms for women; 70 micrograms for men.

Protective range: 70 to 200 micrograms.

People with special needs: Women need an additional 10 micrograms daily if pregnant, 20 micrograms if nursing.

Signs of deficiency: Heart muscle disorders.

Cautions: Inorganic selenium (sodium selenite) may decrease absorption of vitamin C, so don't take them together.

Toxicity has resulted from taking 1,000 micrograms of sodium selenite daily.

SELENIUM SOURCES

Superior food sources of selenium include:

Food	Portion	Selenium (mcg.)
Tortilla chips	1 oz.	284
Corn chips	1 oz.	182
Tuna, canned	3 oz.	99
Cracked wheat bread	3 slices	67
Salmon, canned	3 oz.	64

ZINC

You can think of zinc as the bodyguard of your immune system, stalwartly fighting off invaders that threaten your heath. But zinc moonlights at various other jobs, ranging from protecting your vision to reducing the duration of your colds.

Zinc is essential for normal growth and development; deficiencies can limit growth and delay sexual maturity. Zinc appears to slow down the advance of macular degeneration, a major cause of vision loss in the elderly. Low levels of the mineral have been linked with pregnancy complications and with low birth weight. Zinc may improve wound healing, particularly in people with a prior deficiency.

While serious zinc deficiency is rare, marginal deficiency may not be. Pregnant women are particularly at risk, and surveys show that zinc intakes of children are below minimal requirements. Many ingredients in our food—including fiber and other substances in plant foods, plus iron, calcium and copper—can reduce the availability of zinc. (On the other hand, protein and red wine can enhance zinc absorption.)

Because it can be difficult to consume enough zinc, Sheldon Saul Hendler, M.D., Ph.D., assistant clinical professor of medicine at the University of California at San Diego and author of *The Doctors' Vitamin and Mineral Encyclopedia*, recommends a daily supplement of 15 to 30 milligrams for adults and 10 milligrams for children. Because zinc can interfere with the absorption of copper and selenium, he suggests that along with zinc you take 1.5 to 3.0 milligrams of copper and 50 to 200 micrograms of selenium.

Sources: Wheat germ, wheat bran, whole grains, brewer's yeast, seafood, poultry and meat.

RDA: 12 milligrams for women; 15 milligrams for men.

People with special needs: Vegetarians, the elderly, athletes, dieters. Women need an additional 3 milligrams daily if pregnant, 4 to 7 milligrams if nursing.

Signs of deficiency: Moderate deficiencies can cause loss of smell and taste, slowed growth in children, rashes, loss of hair, vision impairment, irregular muscle movement, skin lesions, sterility, low sperm count, delayed wound healing. Serious deficiency can result in delayed bone maturity, enlarged liver or spleen, shrunken testicles, dwarfism.

Cautions: High doses (18 to 25 milligrams daily) of zinc may cause a copper deficiency; huge doses (300 milligrams daily) have adversely affected the immune system. Don't take supplemental zinc if you have stomach ulcers.

ZINC SOURCES

Superior food sources of zinc include:

Food	Portion	Zinc (mg.)
Oysters, steamed	6 med.	76.4
Beef blade roast, braised	3 oz.	8.7
Alaskan king crab, steamed	3 oz.	6.5
Ribeye steak, broiled	3 oz.	5.9
Wheat germ, toasted	¼ cup	4.7

CHAPTER 4

Meeting Your Nutrient Needs

The RDAs and Beyond

It would be great if we all arrived on Earth with "care and feeding" tags like the ones that come with houseplants, listing exactly how much iron and vitamin A and selenium and so forth we need each day.

Unfortunately, we don't. Yes, much of our packaged food comes with little charts explaining nutrient content, and we can find larger charts telling us just how much of each nutrient we should be getting—but for most of us that still leaves plenty of unanswered questions.

What exactly do these figures mean? Are these *minimum* amounts or *maximum* amounts? And what about the exciting headlines on the newsstands about vitamins and minerals that might help prevent cancer, cataracts, high cholesterol, heart attacks and more?

Once we might have dismissed these headlines as farfetched and, well, *nuts*—but no one's laughing anymore.

"There was a lot of quackery in this field," says Harinder S. Garewal, M.D., Ph.D., assistant director for cancer prevention and control at the University of Arizona Cancer Center in Tucson. "But the work being done now is very sophisticated. It's now swinging back into acceptable science."

WHO DECIDES HOW MUCH?

The Recommended Dietary Allowances (RDAs) were established in 1941 to provide standards to serve as a goal for good nutrition.

These figures have been periodically revised by the Food and Nutrition Board of the National Research Council. A lot of different information is used to come up with these amounts, including studies that show how much of a nutrient is required to correct a deficiency and how much of a nutrient is normally consumed by people in good health. The figures also take into account that not all of each vitamin or mineral you ingest is actually usable by your body.

Because researchers are constantly getting new information from new studies, the RDAs evolve over time. The actual amounts may be raised or lowered, age groupings may be changed or nutrients may be added to the list. The 1989 RDAs, for example, included vitamin K and selenium for the first time, lowered folate and B_{12} requirements and increased calcium amounts for certain age groups. New tables are released every five to ten years.

WHEN MORE MIGHT BE BETTER

But what about going *beyond* the RDAs? These figures are judged to be adequate to meet the nutrient needs of most healthy people, but they often don't come close to the amounts that some scientists and nutritionists suggest could prevent or even help cure specific ailments. And it's possible that certain groups, such as the elderly—who often process nutrients less efficiently—have special needs.

"There is a growing number of studies that suggest that the RDAs are not really appropriate or sensitive to the changing nutritional needs of aging adults. Nor are they focused on the most important public health objective today—preventing chronic diseases like cancer and heart disease," says Jeffrey Blumberg, Ph.D., associate director of the U.S. Department of Agriculture's (USDA) Human Nutrition Research Center on Aging at Tufts University in Boston.

Some nutritionists believe that instead we should be given safe *ranges* of nutrients that we can consume in levels *beyond* the RDAs. "The American public should be advised about the reasonable doses of each of the vitamins—doses that have been associated with no adverse effects. I think the public is bright enough to use vitamin supplements safely," says Adrianne Bendich, Ph.D., senior clinical research coordinator in the Human Nutrition Research Division of Hoffman-La Roche in Nutley, New Jersey.

"My own feeling is that there is a good likelihood that if all these studies continue to point in the same direction, then recommendations could be made for disease prevention in general," says Dr. Garewal.

THOSE AMAZING ANTIOXIDANTS

The unquestioned stars in the nutrient-as-treatment arena are the antioxidants—beta-carotene (which converts in the body to vitamin A), vitamin C and vitamin E. We all have within us something called free radicals, unstable molecules that can wreak havoc on cells and tissues. These harmful free radicals may be formed by natural processes in the body or by environmental influences such as cigarette smoke, sunlight or pollution. Antioxidants, however, neutralize these free radicals—and apparently help prevent (and in some cases treat) cancers, heart disease and respiratory problems.

Beta-carotene versus cancer. Some of Dr. Garewal's work has showed convincing results in the use of beta-carotene in fighting oral leukoplakia, premalignant lesions that may become cancerous. Seventeen of 24 people who took 30 milligrams of beta-carotene per day for six months showed major improvement. This is far more beta-carotene than the 4.8 milligrams (for women) and 6 milligrams (for men) needed to provide the RDA for vitamin A.

And there's an array of other convincing studies. Beta-carotene intake of over 6.2 milligrams per day in a Latin American study was associated with a 32 percent lower risk of cervical cancer than an intake of less than 2.3 milligrams per day. And in a Harvard Medical School study beta-carotene also dramatically cut risks of heart attack, stroke and death among men with prior heart problems.

"In my own mind, I like to get the very last trial nailed in before making definitive recommendations," says Dr. Garewal. "But there's a lot of convincing data about beta-carotene and other antioxidants that continues to accumulate. Hopefully, in the next few years evidence on which to base definitive recommendations will become available."

Vitamin C against colds and cancer. Vitamin C is another potential cancer blocker, according to Gladys Block, Ph.D., a professor of public health nutrition at the University of California at Berkeley. Thirty-three of 46 studies she reviewed found that C offered significant protection against cancers of the esophagus, larynx, pancreas, stomach, rectum, breast and cervix. "I do think the evidence is strong enough for me to say that for prevention of some cancers, vitamin C probably makes a difference," says Dr. Block.

And evidence suggests that vitamin C also helps protect against infections of the upper respiratory tract as well as bronchial problems caused by exposure to air pollutants. Researchers found that two grams (2,000 milligrams) of vitamin C daily helped protect people from the common cold, hay fever and effects of exposure to traffic fumes. (The RDA for men and women over age 25 is 60 milligrams.)

Research conducted in Torino, Italy, found that short-term exposure to air pollution decreases lung function and that treatment with C may counteract its effects. The research also indicates that vitamin C can help alleviate airway irritability, protect against the effects of air pollution and improve the prognosis for patients with chronic lung disease.

Vitamin E has many roles. Vitamin E has been nominated for a number of starring roles, including fighting cancer, helping heart attack victims and improving immune response. There are suggestions that it may slow Parkinson's disease, help control epilepsy and reduce symptoms of premenstrual syndrome.

One study found that a group of nurses who took about 100 I.U. of vitamin E a day had 36 percent less risk of heart attack. And there's a possibility that E protects heart attack victims from further injury after the blood clots that triggered their attacks are dissolved. How? A major cause of heart attack and stroke is blood platelet blockage of arteries. But supplements of 400 I.U. a day of vitamin E greatly reduced the chance that platelets would stick to artery walls.

Vitamin E also apparently is involved in maintaining a healthy immune system. In one study of 32 healthy older adults, those who received 800 I.U. of E daily for 30 days—more than 50 times the RDA—showed markedly improved immune response. And other research showed that cervical cancer risk was about one-half lower for women who consumed high levels of vitamin E.

THOSE BUSY B VITAMINS

Not all the excitement in nutritional treatment is on the antioxidant front, however. The B-complex group of nutrients is also gaining a lot of attention.

Folate fights birth defects. One exciting role for this B vitamin is the prevention of neural tube defects. These can lead to spina bifida, a serious birth defect in which the covering of the spinal cord does not close completely, and anencephaly, where much of the brain is missing. When 81 Cuban women who had previously had children with neural tube defects (and hence were statistically more likely to have another child with the problem) were given five milligrams of folate daily from a month before conception to ten weeks after, *none* of them had babies with neural tube defects.

Large doses of folate may also help brighten the day for people with clinically diagnosed depression. Forty-one of 123 patients at an English hospital who were diagnosed with either major depression or schizophrenia were found to have some degree of folate deficiency. Twenty-two of the 41 were given a daily dose of 15 milligrams of a form of folate (the RDA for men is 200 *micrograms*, or 0.2 milligrams) and the other 19 were given blank pills. Over six months, the group supplemented with folate showed much greater improvement than the group without folate. (The patients were all receiving standard drug treatment as well.)

Some parts of the body may need more folate than others, according to Douglas C. Heimburger, M.D., of the Departments of Nutrition Sciences and Medicine at the University of Alabama at Birmingham. The result can be a localized deficiency in that part of the body even though the folate level in the blood is normal. Such deficiencies can occur in smokers and may be a contributing factor in certain types of cancer, says Dr. Heimburger.

Move over, gelatin. Biotin is a B vitamin you may not have given a second thought to—unless you're troubled by splitting nails. Swiss research has showed that daily doses of biotin strengthen thin, fragile nails. In the study of 32 men and women, nail thickness increased by 25 percent in the

RECOMMENDED DIETARY ALLOWANCES

Do you want to know specifically how much of each major nutrient you should be getting? Here are the amounts recommended by the Food and Nutrition Board of the National Research Council for various age groups, based on median heights and weights. These are average daily intakes—meaning that some days you could eat

Category	Age (yr.) or Condition	Weight (lb.)	Height (in.)	Protein (g.)	Vitamin A (mcg. RE)*
Infants	0.0–0.5	13	24	13	375
	0.5–1.0	20	28	14	375
Children	1–3	29	35	16	400
	4–6	44	44	24	500
	7–10	62	52	28	700
Males	11–14	99	62	45	1,000
	15–18	145	69	59	1,000
	19–24	160	70	58	1,000
	25–50	174	70	63	1,000
	51+	170	68	63	1,000
Females	11–14	101	62	46	800
	15–18	120	64	44	800
	19–24	128	65	46	800
	25–50	138	64	50	800
	51+	143	63	50	800
Pregnant				60	800
Lactating	1st 6 months			65	1,300
	2nd 6 months			62	1,200

*RE = Retinol Equivalent
†-TE = Alpha-Tocopherol Equivalent
‡NE = Niacin Equivalent

more and some days less—that are considered adequate to maintain good nutrition for healthy people under normal environmental stresses. The board recommends that you get these nutrients from a variety of foods to help supply other important nutrients for which RDAs have not been established.

VITAMINS

VITAMIN D (mcg.)	VITAMIN E (mg. -TE)†	VITAMIN K (mcg.)	VITAMIN C (mg.)	THIAMINE (mg.)	RIBOFLAVIN (mg.)	NIACIN (mg. NE)‡
7.5	3	5	30	0.3	0.4	5
10	4	10	35	0.4	0.5	6
10	6	15	40	0.7	0.8	9
10	7	20	45	0.9	1.1	12
10	7	30	45	1.0	1.2	13
10	10	45	50	1.3	1.5	17
10	10	65	60	1.5	1.8	20
10	10	70	60	1.5	1.7	19
5	10	80	60	1.5	1.7	19
5	10	80	60	1.2	1.4	15
10	8	45	50	1.1	1.3	15
10	8	55	60	1.1	1.3	15
10	8	60	60	1.1	1.3	15
5	8	65	60	1.1	1.3	15
5	8	65	60	1.0	1.2	13
10	10	65	70	1.5	1.6	17
10	12	65	95	1.6	1.8	20
10	11	65	90	1.6	1.7	20

		VITAMINS		
CATEGORY	AGE (yr.) OR CONDITION	Vitamin B$_6$ (mg.)	FOLATE (mcg.)	Vitamin B$_{12}$ (mcg.)
Infants	0.0–0.5	0.3	25	0.3
	0.5–1.0	0.6	35	0.5
Children	1–3	1.0	50	0.7
	4–6	1.1	75	1.0
	7–10	1.4	100	1.4
Males	11–14	1.7	150	2.0
	15–18	2.0	200	2.0
	19–24	2.0	200	2.0
	25–50	2.0	200	2.0
	51+	2.0	200	2.0
Females	11–14	1.4	150	2.0
	15–18	1.5	180	2.0
	19–24	1.6	180	2.0
	25–50	1.6	180	2.0
	51+	1.6	180	2.0
Pregnant		2.2	400	2.2
Lactating	1st 6 months	2.1	280	2.6
	2nd 6 months	2.1	260	2.6

group that received, 2,500 micrograms of biotin daily for six to nine months. (Although no RDA has been set for biotin, it's estimated that a daily intake of 30 to 100 micrograms is normally adequate.)

"Biotin is absorbed into the bed of the nail, where it may encourage a better, thicker nail to grow," says Richard K. Scher, M.D., head of the Nail Section at Columbia Presbyterian Medical Center in New York City. But he recom-

MINERALS

CALCIUM (mg.)	IODINE (mcg.)	IRON (mg.)	MAGNESIUM (mg.)	PHOSPHORUS (mg.)	SELENIUM (mcg.)	ZINC (mg.)
400	40	6	40	300	10	5
600	50	10	60	500	15	5
800	70	10	80	800	20	10
800	90	10	120	800	20	10
800	120	10	170	800	30	10
1,200	150	12	270	1,200	40	15
1,200	150	12	400	1,200	50	15
1,200	150	10	350	1,200	70	15
800	150	10	350	800	70	15
800	150	10	350	800	70	15
1,200	150	15	280	1,200	45	12
1,200	150	15	300	1,200	50	12
1,200	150	15	280	1,200	55	12
800	150	15	280	800	55	12
800	150	10	280	800	55	12
1,200	175	30	300	1,200	65	15
1,200	200	15	355	1,200	75	19
1,200	200	15	340	1,200	75	16

mends checking with your doctor before trying biotin supplements to cure your brittle nails.

The cholesterol fighter. Niacin has been used since the 1950s to lower cholesterol and triglycerides in the blood. Very huge doses were used at first, but results have been good with amounts ranging from 1,200 to 2,000 milligrams, still far higher than the RDA of 19 milligrams for men aged 25 to 50 (15 milligrams for women). Annoying side effects tended to limit its use, but researchers have found that enclosing the niacin in a wax honeycomb minimizes side effects. "Rapid absorption of the necessary high dose was what caused side effects," says Joseph M. Keenan, M.D., assistant professor and director of geriatric programs of the University of Minnesota in Minneapolis. "But waxed niacin greatly reduces those problems. Now it's the most effective slow-release form of the vitamin known."

A boost for your immune system. Supplements of B_6 can improve immunity in the elderly. In a study of eight healthy elderly adults at the U.S. Department of Agriculture's (USDA) Human Nutrition Research Center on Aging at Tufts University in Boston, the amounts of B_6 to correct immune impairments in most people were more than the RDA.

The RDA may be low for older Americans, particularly women, say USDA researchers. In another study they measured B_6 levels of 12 people aged 61 to 71 and found that women had to take in 1.9 milligrams a day to have enough B_6 in their bodies (the RDA is only 1.6 milligrams). For men, the RDA of 2.0 milligrams a day proved adequate—but might not be enough for people who are ill or who have increased needs.

TWO MORE VERSATILE VITAMINS

Researchers are also finding new uses for old standbys—in this case vitamins A and K.

A way to save lives. The death rate among hospitalized children suffering from measles drops substantially when they are supplemented with vitamin A. One study found that only about 2 percent of children with severe measles who received vitamin A died, compared with 10 percent of children receiving a blank pill. "Vitamin A status is one of the primary determinants affecting the virulence of measles," says Greg Hussey, senior specialist in the Department of Pediatrics and Child Health at the University of Cape Town in South Africa. "Our recommendation is that vitamin A be given as part of standard therapy to all children with measles in a hospital setting."

And a vitamin A–derived drug called tretinoin appears to help age cancer cells and hasten their demise. Nine of ten people with leukemia experienced complete remission when treated with tretinoin. When tretinoin was combined with chemotherapy, no patients relapsed. "This unique mechanism has broad implications for other types of cancer," says Raymond Warrell, Jr., M.D., at the Memorial Sloan-Kettering Cancer Center in New York City.

Extra help for bones. Vitamin K, which is involved in the formation and maintenance of bone, may also have a role in preventing and treating osteoporosis. Postmenopausal women who received vitamin K supplements showed much less loss of calcium in the urine, suggesting their bone mass was being depleted at a reduced rate. "This has implications for the RDA," says Cees Vermeer, Ph.D., of the Department of Biochemistry at the University of Limburg in the Netherlands. "We have to carefully re-examine this figure. We will probably find that the real need is much higher."

MORE BENEFITS FROM MINERALS

Minerals, too, are proving helpful in exciting new ways, often in amounts that challenge traditional thinking about RDAs.

Calcium to ease PMS. We've long known of calcium's role in building and maintaining strong bones and preventing osteoporosis, but this mineral appears to have significant other jobs as well. Strong evidence supporting calcium's role in curtailing symptoms of menstrual discomfort came

THE ALPHABET SOUP OF NUTRIENT REQUIREMENTS

So the label says the cereal you're eating is providing 100 percent of your RDA for seven important nutrients. Better make that U.S. RDA. Or maybe RDI. Are we confusing you?

The basic measure of daily nutrient intake is the RDA, or Recommended Dietary Allowance. If you take a closer look at that panel on the side of your cereal box, however, you'll see that nutrient amounts are listed as *percentage of U.S. Recommended Daily Allowances (U.S. RDAs)*. Actual RDAs vary according to how old you are, whether you're male or female and if you're pregnant or nursing. So how could one percentage be correct for everyone eating this cereal?

The answer is that it isn't. The U.S. RDAs were developed in 1968 by the Food and Drug Administration to give consumers some information about the nutritional content of the food they buy. But because it would be too awkward to list all the breakdowns by age and sex for each nutrient, the U.S. RDAs were pegged to the *highest* recommendation for any age and sex group (usually a male aged 15 to 18). So the percentage on your cereal box is most likely a percentage of the RDA for a teenaged male: Your own needs could very well be lower.

Following this so far? The RDAs are updated periodically to reflect new findings: Since 1974 they were changed twice, in 1980 and 1989. Logically, you'd think

from a 5½-month, live-in study by the USDA involving ten women who alternately received daily doses of either 1,300 or 600 milligrams of calcium. (The RDA for women aged 25 to 50 is 800 milligrams.) When women received the higher dosage, they reported fewer mood swings, cramps and back

that the U.S. RDAs would have changed as well, to reflect the new values.

Wrong. The U.S. RDAs were never changed, presumably because of the amount of relabeling of products that would be required. So at least up until 1992, if your cereal box said that a serving supplied 10 percent of the U.S. RDA of protein, what it actually meant was that it supplied 10 percent of the amount of protein scientists thought a teenaged boy needed in 1968.

But in 1990, the Food and Drug Administration proposed replacing the U.S. RDAs with something called the Reference Daily Intake (RDI). Instead of being based on the highest possible need for any group, the RDIs would be based on an *average* of the needs of adults and children over the age of three. In most cases, the RDI would be lower than the previous U.S. RDAs. Many nutritionists didn't like the idea of the change, however, and wanted to stick with the old U.S. RDAs.

By the time you read this book, this issue may have been resolved one way or another: You'll either still be facing the U.S. RDA on the side panel of your cereal box, or you'll be looking at new RDI figures.

All this doesn't mean that the figures on your food labels are useless—only that they should be used as a guideline, never an absolute. They provide a valuable tool for comparing one processed food to another. If you want to know *specifically* how much of each nutrient is recommended for your age group and sex, check the RDA table on page 74.

aches; when these same women received less calcium, they had more problems with work efficiency and concentration.

Hiking HDLs with chromium. Beta-blocking drugs are used to treat angina, hypertension and cardiac arrhythmias, but the beta-blockers can cause an undesirable drop in levels

HIGH DOSES MAY BE HAZARDOUS

While in most cases it's difficult to overdose on vitamins and minerals in foods, you *can* overdose on supplements—with serious or even fatal consequences. Here are some areas of potential concern.

Vitamin A. Amounts even a few times greater than the RDA can be toxic, according to Jack Zeev Yetiv, M.D., Ph.D., author of *Popular Nutritional Practices: A Scientific Appraisal.* (And this is one nutrient you can overdose on from food, by eating large amounts of liver.) Effects can range from headache, vomiting, weakness and dry, rough skin to more serious problems such as liver damage, increased pressure in the brain, and bone and joint pain and damage. Toxicity is usually seen only with over 50,000 I.U. in adults and 20,000 I.U. in children, but how you react to high doses of vitamin A can depend on your health in general and particularly the health of your liver.

If you're taking A supplements, stop *immediately* if you have any symptoms such as nagging headaches, blurry vision, hair loss, nausea or aching bones, according to Sheldon Saul Hendler, M.D., Ph.D., assistant clinical professor of medicine at the University of California at San Diego

of high-density lipoprotein, or HDL, (good) cholesterol. Chromium, however, can *increase* HDL levels in people receiving beta-blockers, according to a North Carolina study of 63 men. One group received 600 micrograms of chromium daily—the estimated adequate daily intake is 50 to 200 micrograms—while the other group received look-alike pills with no chromium. The chromium-supplemented group showed significant increases in HDL levels.

Saving eyesight with zinc. A study of 151 patients with

and author of *The Doctors' Vitamin and Mineral Encyclopedia*. It's safer to consume beta-carotene instead, preferably in food, because studies have shown that it's not toxic, even in large amounts.

Vitamin D. This nutrient can be toxic in large doses, particularly for young children. It can cause high levels of calcium in the blood and excess calcium in the urine, deposits of calcium in soft tissues and kidney and cardiovascular damage. A dose as low as 45 micrograms (1,800 I.U.) per day has caused problems in children.

Niacin. Overdosing on niacin may cause flushing, headache and itching—or more serious problems such as heartbeat abnormalities, low blood pressure, liver damage and aggravation of peptic ulcers. Niacin also tends to increase blood sugar levels, which may cause problems for people with diabetes.

Vitamin B$_6$. Megadoses of 2,000 to 6,000 milligrams per day have caused nerve damage. You should stop taking supplemental B$_6$ if you have symptoms such as numb hands or feet or unsteadiness while walking.

Iron. This mineral can poison children who take adult supplements formulated for adults.

macular degeneration, a common eye problem that causes blindness, found that patients receiving 100 milligrams of zinc twice a day with their meals lost less of their vision than patients who received pills with no zinc. (The RDA is 12 milligrams for men and 15 milligrams for women.)

A WORD TO THE WISE

Enthused by all these studies, you may feel the urge to rush out and begin stocking up on vitamin and mineral supplements. Hold it right there. You should realize that all these studies were carefully controlled, and the people taking supplements were meticulously monitored. While some nutrients can generally be safely consumed in doses higher than the RDAs, there are others that are dangerous when taken in excess. On the other hand, certain conditions or drugs can affect your vitamin and mineral status and mean that you need *more* of certain nutrients. For these reasons, you should always consult your doctor before considering supplementation at levels above the RDA.

And certainly don't think that practicing superb nutrition or taking preventive supplements will protect you against all ills or make up for other unhealthy lifestyle habits. "A nutrient is not a magic bullet," says Dr. Garewal. If you smoke cigarettes, for example, taking beta-carotene isn't the primary line of defense against disease, he says—stopping smoking is the more important change.

CHAPTER 5

Nutrient Robbers

You Can Guard Against Them

As you go unsuspectingly about your daily life, a stealthy band of thieving hoods is stalking you. And when they strike—deliberately or inadvertently—they'll inevitably deprive you of something valuable. We're talking about the nutrient robbers.

Sometimes they masquerade as a friend, such as aspirin, yet cat burgle with deliberate precision, snatching a single vital vitamin. Other times, such as when you're in the kitchen cooking, they loot and pillage indiscriminately, stealing varieties of nutrients. Often, as is the case with pollutants, they take from you the very key you need to lock your doors, latch your windows and protect yourself from their onslaught.

You're not defenseless against the nutrient robbers. You just have to know when they strike and what they're after.

SMOG ALERT

Coal, oil, shale, gasoline, diesel fuel—we depend on them for energy, transportation and light. "By far, cars are the dirtiest of the lot," says Daniel B. Menzel, Ph.D., chairman of the Department of Community and Environmental Medicine at the University of California at Irvine. As we tool down the road, nitrogen oxide and a little bit of unburned fuel dumps out of the tailpipe. Radiated by light, especially that from the ultraviolet spectrum, the mixture turns into nitrogen dioxide and ozone.

These potent poisons, Dr. Menzel says, are free radicals, meaning they have an extra electron attached to their molecular structure. Once free radicals get inside the body, they wreak havoc, initiating a chain reaction of damaged cells.

Nitrogen dioxide, the most common pollutant and the one found in the highest concentration, rapidly oxidizes vitamin C, Dr. Menzel says. Ozone seems to aim its destruction at fatty acids in cell membranes, where vitamin E is located. Both nutrients give themselves up to neutralize the free radicals so that body tissues either are saved or not injured as much.

So what should you do if you're regularly exposed to high levels of air pollution?

Replace what's been stolen. "Take some vitamin C, and take some vitamin E," says Dr. Menzel.

No one knows how much of the vitamins should be taken for best protection against pollution, he says. Studies he has conducted on animals suggest that adults should be taking between 150 and 200 international units (I.U.) of vitamin E every day. Compare that to the Recommended Dietary Allowance (RDA) of 15 I.U. for men and 12 I.U. for women.

As for vitamin C, while the government recommends ingesting 60 milligrams a day, Dr. Menzel personally feels that several hundred milligrams would be closer to reality, for better protection against pollution. You should check with your doctor, however, before taking any nutritional supplement at levels in excess of the RDA.

How Heat Can Deplete

If you really want to cook your goose nutritionally, turn the heat way up and let it bake for a long, long time.

That's the recipe for nutrient immolation. The higher the temperature and the longer the cooking time, the more you deprive yourself of the vitamins and minerals packed away in food. "Many are inactivated by heat," says Gertrude Armbruster, Ph.D., an associate professor in the Division of Nutritional Sciences at Cornell University in Ithaca, New York. "Heat changes the nature of nutrients so that they're not absorbed as well by the body." And nutrients may also leach out in cooking liquid.

Those emerald green broccoli florets, then, may not be quite the storehouses of vitamin C you believe them to be, depending on how you've cooked them. Anytime food is cooked—no matter what the method—nutrients are lost. Once in the kitchen, though, some cooking methods are more destructive than others. In general, "the less time food is cooked, the more nutritious it is," Dr. Armbruster says.

Of the dry-heat cooking methods, baking and grilling probably have the most negative impact on nutrients, Dr. Armbruster says. "They're long-time processes that expose food to high temperatures." All heat-sensitive nutrients—vitamin C, for example, some of the B vitamins, and possibly minerals—are vulnerable under those conditions. Broiling also subjects food to high heat, she says, "but it's a shorter cooking time, so it may not be as destructive."

Don't bake foods to a crisp. People often bake, broil and grill to brown food or make it crispy. While perhaps more appealing to the eyes and the palate, crispy brown food is less nutritious, according to Dr. Armbruster. "The browning process transforms protein in meat," she says. "It's effectively 'burned' and not absorbed as well as unburned protein."

Use wet heat wisely. Wet-heat cooking methods can be

just as destructive to vitamins and minerals as baking and grilling. "In addition to the high heat, now you're adding water, which is another source of loss for all the water-soluble nutrients," Dr. Armbruster says.

Generally, pressure cooking preserves more nutrients in vegetables that otherwise would require a longer cooking time. Steaming, a wonderful no-fat alternative to frying, spares more vitamins and minerals than pressure cooking or boiling, but losses do occur.

When steamed, spinach, for example, loses almost 50 percent of its vitamin C, the most vulnerable of all vitamins. But boiling or pressure cooking destroys 60 percent. Broccoli loses about 55 percent of its vitamin C when boiled but only about 25 percent when steamed.

The B vitamin family is more thermally insulated. In most vegetables, niacin barely is affected by any cooking method. Thiamine, riboflavin, vitamin B_6 and folate are lost in smaller amounts when foods are steamed than when they are boiled.

Minerals in vegetables are especially susceptible. Even steaming can decrease availability of the potassium and calcium in spinach by half or more. Half of the iron and magnesium may be made unavailable, while the loss of zinc is about 30 percent. Boiling and draining remove even higher percentages of those minerals.

Perhaps the ultimate way to preserve nutrients is to eat vegetables raw in salads, Dr. Armbruster says. When that's not practical or desirable, steam them just until soft or boil them in as little water as possible. And make sure the water is boiling before you add the food.

Save that cooking liquid. When you steam carrots, do you pour the remaining orangish water down the sink? If you do, you're dumping cancer-combating carotenoids into the sewer system. After boiling potatoes, do you discard the broth? You're permitting valuable vitamin C to drip down the drain.

No matter how unappetizing it may initially look, use the

nutrient-rich cooking water in other preparations. "There wouldn't really be significant losses if you keep that water," Dr. Armbruster says. "Although we recommend that, I'm told hardly anyone does it." The liquid can be used in soups, beverages, gravies and sauces.

WAVE BYE-BYE TO COOKING LOSSES

Conventional stoves can drive off vitamins in droves. What's a health-conscious cook to do? Ride the microwave to the nutritional future.

"In some cases, you can get close to 100 percent nutrient retention with a microwave," according to Gertrude Armbruster, Ph.D., of Cornell University in Ithaca, New York. "It really minimizes nutrient losses."

Microwaves target water molecules in food, forcing them to vibrate and give off heat, which then cooks the food. "The energy gets to where it's supposed to go," Dr. Armbruster says. But when you cook on the stove, you're heating a lot more than you need to, and it takes a long time.

"Only 40 to 60 percent of the vitamins remain in vegetables cooked conventionally on the stove. Microwave cooking preserves significantly more, up to 50 to 100 percent. It makes a big difference."

STRESS: A NUTRITIONAL MESS

If you haven't stewed and steamed off your vitamins and minerals on the stovetop, you may once they enter your body. The frantic, frustrating exasperation of stress can rob you of nutrients at the same time it's increasing the need for them. "I wish we knew specifically how stress increases free-radical generation in the body, but there's evidence it does," says John Milner, Ph.D., head of the Department of Nutrition at Pennsylvania State University in University Park. The mental strain forces the body to secrete more hormones that speed up metabolism and the turnover of cells, he says. Fats also are altered and begin to turn rancid. Here's how to fight back.

Stick to a regular meal plan. Stress may send you to the refrigerator to soothe savaged nerves, so overeating could be a concern, Dr. Milner says. But under mental duress you also may skip meals or grab quick bites on the run. So in addition to worrying about whatever it is you're worrying about, you also must worry about maintaining your regular eating routine.

Fortify yourself with E, C and beta-carotene. To counteract any free radicals formed by stress, meals should provide adequate amounts of the antioxidant vitamins A, E and C, Dr. Milner says. "During stressful situations, the antioxidants serve as scavengers for free radicals generated in the body," he says.

Bounce back after trauma. Physiologic stress is an even greater danger to nutritional well-being. "The body's response to serious injury, complicated surgery or chronic inflammation such as rheumatoid arthritis creates a significant drain on energy and protein stores," says Joel B. Mason, M.D., an assistant professor in the divisions of clinical nutrition and gastroenterology at Tufts University School of Medicine in Boston. "It is not uncommon for a serious bodily injury to result in a loss of ten pounds of muscle and other critical organ tissues within a week; such a drain is not only harmful by itself but makes it considerably more difficult for the body to recover from the complications associated with the injury or disease.

"A common misconception, even among doctors, is that overweight patients have plenty of 'excess stores' to draw from and are therefore immune to the adverse nutritional effects associated with physiologic stress," says Dr. Mason. It is very important for anyone who has sustained a serious physiologic stress, regardless of whether or not they are overweight, to receive the additional calories and protein demanded by their condition.

Similarly, a person who has lost more than 10 percent of usual body weight due to disease and who is anticipating surgery will benefit from an aggressive attempt to correct some of the malnourishment before surgery. Adequate nutrient stores will improve the chances of a successful outcome. A well-trained dietitian can provide guidelines.

SOME HEALERS ARE STEALERS

What's worse—high blood pressure or impotence? Arthritis pain or anemia?

Many commonly used over-the-counter and prescription drugs can profoundly affect your nutrient needs. Some accelerate excretion of vitamins and minerals; others impede absorption. But if you understand how certain drugs interact with nutrients, you need not face damned-if-you-do-damned-if-you-don't alternatives.

ASPIRIN

Aspirin can ease pain and may even play a role in decreasing the chances of heart disease, Dr. Milner says. But if you're taking aspirin regularly, you may want to call your citrus supplier. That's because prolonged or excessive use forces the kidneys to excrete more vitamin C and potassium. In addition to depleting the body of those nutrients, you run the risk of developing iron-deficiency anemia, because aspirin can irritate the stomach lining and cause minor bleeding.

Aspirin also displaces folate in the body, and that could create a deficiency in those with poor diets, according to John Pinto, Ph.D., director of the Nutrition Research Laboratory at Memorial Sloan-Kettering Cancer Center in New York City. "Arthritic individuals who take a lot of aspirin should be especially cautious," he says.

HIGH FIBER: AN EXTRA CHALLENGE

We know how fiber helps us. The natural laxative eases food through the body and reduces the possibility of colon and intestinal diseases. It also helps lower blood sugar levels in people with diabetes. But by rushing food through the system, fiber also cuts into the time the body needs to absorb nutrients.

"Especially at the extremes of life, for the very young and the old, fiber may create problems by interfering with absorption," says Benjamin Caballero, M.D., director of the Center for Human Nutrition at Johns Hopkins University in Baltimore.

The most significant interference is with calcium, needed in greater amounts by growing children and women to prevent later development of osteoporosis. "If you're just barely fulfilling the recommended calcium intake, a high-fiber diet will certainly affect calcium status," he says. "And it's not easy anyway to get all the calcium you need from foods. Women need at least 800 milligrams of calcium a day to prevent osteoporosis and probably should be taking supplements if they eat a lot of high-fiber foods."

Fiber also promotes excretion of vitamin B_6 and, at extremely high doses, causes out-and-out deficiencies of zinc, even if the diet contains adequate amounts of the mineral. But most healthy adults who eat well-balanced diets have little cause for concern, Dr. Caballero says. "The typical American diet has generous amounts of most nutrients and the fact that fiber decreases the efficiency of absorption probably has little relevance for healthy adults consuming a variety of foods."

To counter depletion: Eat foods high in vitamin C, iron and folate.

LAXATIVES

Mineral oil, that old constipation cure, is a nutritional damnation in disguise. A lot of older people remain regular users of this regularity regulator, which also still is found in many commercial preparations, according to Arthur I. Jacknowitz, Pharm.D., chairman of the Department of Clinical Pharmacy in the School of Pharmacy at West Virginia University in Morgantown. Three other ingredients commonly found in laxatives—bisacodyl, phenolphthalein and senna—also can cause severe deficiencies in frequent users.

After ingesting laxatives containing any of these substances, among the things passing through your intestines more quickly will be all the fat-soluble vitamins—A, E, D and K—as well as phosphorus and calcium. Mineral oil traps fat-soluble vitamins and prevents their absorption, Dr. Jacknowitz says; the other drugs force the intestines to contract involuntarily, speeding food through too rapidly for proper absorption.

To counter depletion: Don't use mineral-oil laxatives frequently. Don't take a laxative containing any of the other three medications within two hours of any meal.

DIURETICS

What some laxatives do to fat-soluble vitamins, diuretics and other high blood pressure drugs do to their water-soluble counterparts—flush them from your system. "If you are well nourished, you shouldn't see appreciable vitamin deficiencies with diuretics," Dr. Pinto says, "but you could have a definite problem if you aren't or if your diet is at all marginal."

Potassium and magnesium are lost quickly through use of diuretics. Some medications, such as furosemide (sold under the brand name Lasix) and hydrochlorothiazide (sold as Esidrix) also speed the excretion of zinc, calcium and thiamine, Dr. Pinto says. Thiamine depletion alone caused by use of these drugs could cause cardiovascular problems. Regular use of diuretics also can elevate blood sugar levels by disrupting enzymes necessary for carbohydrate metabolism. Hydralazine, another high blood pressure medication, disrupts vitamin B_6 absorption, which could cause nerve and sensation problems in your arms and legs.

To counter depletion: Take the medication with meals and eat foods high in potassium (such as bananas and raisins) and thiamine (such as pork and whole-grain bread). Zinc, magnesium and vitamin B_6 supplements also may be required.

ANTIBIOTICS

Antibiotics and antibacterial drugs, used for everything from small cuts to major infections, impinge on the body's absorption of calcium, Dr. Pinto says. Excretion of riboflavin in urine increases as well with tetracycline. Magnesium, zinc and iron also are poorly utilized with this drug, and vitamin K and folate can be depleted. Neomycin blocks vitamin B_{12} absorption.

To counter depletion: Take antibiotics and antibacterial drugs on an empty stomach several hours before or after eating mineral-rich foods or dairy products.

ANTIDEPRESSANTS

Tricyclic compounds like chlorpromazine used to treat depression can devastate the body's stores of riboflavin, according to Dr. Pinto. In one study, urinary excretion of riboflavin rose markedly soon after treatment with chlorpromazine and continued for several days after drug use ceased. "A clinically significant riboflavin deficiency may result from the use of these agents," Dr. Pinto says, "despite a diet adequate in the vitamin."

MAKING MEDICINE MORE EFFECTIVE

Some medications can cause significant disruptions in the body's vitamin and mineral balance. Conversely, some foods can interfere with the effectiveness of drugs. But the two aren't always antagonists. In fact, depending on what you eat and when you eat it, food sometimes can enhance the power of medications to make you feel better faster.

Generally, when a doctor instructs you to take your medicine with food, eat a meal high in carbohydrates, says John Pinto, Ph.D., of Memorial Sloan-Kettering Cancer Center in New York City. A high-carbohydrate meal will help the drug get into your system more quickly. A high-protein meal will reduce the effectiveness of the medication.

For example, in a study of children with asthma who were taking theophylline, Dr. Pinto says, bouts of wheezing were reduced when a high-carbohydrate (78 percent of calories from carbs), low-protein diet was eaten. The drug's power to control wheezing diminished when the kids began to eat high-protein, low-carbohydrate meals.

A low-protein diet also helps people with Parkinson's disease who are being treated with levodopa. The amino acids in protein compete with the drug for entry into the brain, Dr. Pinto says.

For treatment of urinary tract infections with the drug methenamine, therapy is much more effective if people increase the acidity of their urine by eating or drinking foods high in vitamin C—citrus juice, strawberries or broccoli, for example—two hours before taking the drug, Dr. Pinto says.

WHEN NUTRIENTS COLLIDE

Vitamin E helps vitamin A, but too much E harms A. Too much zinc tarnishes iron; too much iron puts a chink in zinc. Too much protein muscles calcium out of the body, so you drink more milk to replenish your calcium stores. But milk is high in protein, which . . .

"What a bag of worms," sighs John Milner, Ph.D., of Pennsylvania State University in University Park when talking about how more of one nutrient can promote the body's use of another at the same time it creates a deficiency in still another.

Take vitamin C, for example. But not too much. Vitamin C aids the body in utilizing iron, especially as you age and stomach acidity decreases. But excessive levels of C inhibit absorption of copper. "And when you're talking copper, you're also talking about iron and zinc, because they're all interconnected," Dr. Milner says. "Excesses or deficiencies of one invariably lead to problems with the other two."

Here's a quick rundown of how some key nutrients may be affected by the status of another.

Vitamin A. Too little protein in the diet lessens absorption of vitamin A. Fat in the diet helps the body absorb beta-carotene, the vitamin A precursor. Except if it's polyunsaturated fat; that limits beta-carotene absorption. Vitamin E supplements raise blood levels of A in those with deficiencies of A, but too much E can decrease the amount of A in the blood.

To counter depletion: Eat foods rich in riboflavin, such as low-fat milk and yogurt, liver, broccoli and asparagus.

Calcium. Some proteins may increase absorption but at the same time increase excretion of this bone-building mineral. Fat, so useful in helping the body absorb beta-carotene, decreases calcium absorption. If calcium intake is low, zinc supplements slow calcium absorption, causing an even greater deficiency. But no effect is seen if calcium levels are normal. Salty diets also cause an increase in calcium excretion.

Vitamin B_6. Too much protein leads to more excretion of B_6 and lower levels of the vitamin in the blood.

Iron. Zinc supplements decrease iron absorption, and in a combined zinc/iron pill, the higher the ratio of zinc, the lower the utilization of iron.

Zinc. Virtually no zinc is absorbed from mineral supplements with high concentrations of iron. But heme iron, from animal foods, doesn't deter zinc absorption. However, nonheme iron, from plants, can interfere with zinc absorption. Calcium also inhibits zinc absorption. Animal protein helps the body use zinc, but unsupplemented soy protein causes a deficiency.

Confused? It's no wonder. But you really face no more of a disadvantage than the experts, who also have to sift through this nutritional morass. "I suppose what this shows is that you can't be overzealous with any of these nutrients, because what enhances one area may inhibit another," Dr. Milner says. "And it underlines the importance of a varied type of diet. By eating a wide variety of foods, you minimize the risk of imbalances and give yourself a greater chance of meeting *all* your nutrient needs."

ANTACIDS

Plop, plop, fizz, fizz, oh, what a nutritional nuisance it is. If you can't believe you ate the whole thing, you won't believe the possible complications of your antacid cure for indigestion and heartburn. Over-the-counter antacids with ingredients such as aluminum hydroxide, sodium bicarbonate and magnesium trisilicate deprive the body of phosphorus. Mild phosphate depletion weakens muscles, and a more serious lack leads to a vitamin D deficiency. Extended use or high doses of antacids also destroys thiamine and skews absorption of the fat-soluble vitamins, particularly vitamin A. Iron absorption also is impeded.

To counter depletion: Don't eat the whole thing. Try to rely less on antacids, or take them only under your doctor's supervision.

CHOLESTEROL-LOWERING DRUGS

Cholesterol-reducing medications, such as cholestyramine, don't sound like a lot of fun. They cause belching, bloating, flatulence and constipation, among other side effects. But because they work by interfering with fat absorption, they also interfere with the absorption of fat-soluble vitamins A, D, E and K. Deficiencies of folate also may result.

To counter depletion: Ask your doctor about water-soluble vitamin A and D supplements and about the need for supplementary vitamin K and folate.

WATCH OUT FOR THE ANTINUTRIENTS

They've been targeted as the bad guys, antinutrient chemicals in some otherwise exceedingly healthful plant foods that can rip you off nutritionally. But oxalate, phytin and tannins, while they deserve their nasty reputations, aren't as bad as once thought.

OXALATE

The classic example always has been spinach, high in iron but in a form not absorbed easily by the body. The reason, researchers said, was the chemical oxalate in the plant. But newer studies suggest that all of the iron *naturally* occurring in spinach may, in fact, be available.

Because of how it's grown, spinach can show a misleadingly high iron content when analyzed, says William House, Ph.D., a research physiologist with the U.S. Department of Agriculture's (USDA) Plant, Soil and Nutrition Laboratory at Cornell University. Wind and rain splash spinach leaves with additional iron from the soil in which the plants are grown, Dr. House says. That dirt-derived mineral enters the leaves and drives up the measured iron content. But *that iron* cannot be absorbed by the body.

The assumption all these years was that oxalate in spinach inhibited iron absorption, Dr. House says. But when the USDA researchers grew spinach that didn't contain external iron from soil on its leaves in the laboratory, the plant turned out to be a fine source of iron for the body.

Oxalate, also found in rhubarb, "does appear to affect calcium utilization, though, by creating a calcium salt that's not soluble," says Dr. House.

PHYTIN

A substance that facilitates storage of minerals in seeds also interferes with the body's absorption of at least one of those nutrients, zinc. Phytin is found in almost all plant seeds, Dr. House says, and is especially high in legumes and cereal grains, such as wheat. "If you eat a lot of foods high in phytin, zinc availability will be depressed," he says, "but we don't think it's that important in most situations." People who suddenly switch from an omnivorous to vegetarian diet "may become a little zinc deficient temporarily, but studies do show that vegetarians still get enough zinc."

TANNINS

For people at risk of iron deficiency—menstruating women, young children and adolescents—tannins remain a concern, Dr. House says. These chemicals are found not only in coffee and tea but also in the hulls of some beans and in red wine. Rats fed bean hulls high in tannins show very little impairment of iron absorption, Dr. House says, but when the chemical is extracted and given to the rodents, "they show a small depression of iron absorption that is statistically significant."

Acquiring anemia from ingesting tannins probably isn't a major health concern, Dr. House says, but people should nevertheless try to get adequate iron in their diets.

CHAPTER 6

Special Nutrient Needs

Fine-Tuning Your Intake

So you think you're an average kind of person. Average height, average weight, average number of kids, average number of cars in the driveway. You have an average-looking dog in an average-looking yard, an average-looking cat napping on an averagely stuffed chair.

Well, your life may seem a lot like everyone else's, but there's a good chance your nutrient needs aren't. Your requirement for vitamins and minerals can change, depending on your personal habits, your activity level, even your age. Here's a closer look at some factors that may separate you or someone you know from the nutritional pack.

DIETING

Few dieters follow rational rules of repast as they attempt to lose weight. A significant cutback in calories or a fad diet with an unnatural reliance on one or two foods may hurl your body off its nutrient peak into the depths of deficiency.

"This business of periodically starving for calorie control or drastically reducing calories and not making appropriate adjustments in vitamin intake is risky," according to C. E. Butterworth, Jr., M.D., professor of nutrition sciences at the University of Alabama at Birmingham. But if you follow a few guidelines, losing weight doesn't have to be a nutritional bungee jump from a perilous precipice.

Don't void the vitamins. "Quality of the diet remains important," says Mindy Hermann, R.D., a spokesperson for the American Dietetic Association and a nutritional consultant in Mount Kisco, New York. "The main problem arises when a diet falls below 1,200 calories a day or if it's not well planned."

Most weight-loss programs do recommend taking some sort of supplement to meet the Recommended Dietary Allowances (RDAs) while curtailing caloric intake, she says.

The reason is that in cutting calories, "dieters cut the vitamins and minerals associated with those calories," according to Dr. Butterworth. "Unless they take supplements, they run the risk of getting transient vitamin deficiencies. They should be very careful."

Replenish the turnover. Of central concern are all the water-soluble vitamins, especially vitamin C and folate, that have a rapid turnover in the body. You're not getting enough of them because you've cut your meals, but your body continues to excrete them at a pretty good clip. Fat-soluble vitamins like vitamins A and E fade from the body more slowly, so no imminent deficiency danger exists, Dr. Butterworth says. But you still need to replace them over time.

Be nutritiously dense. In her classes at East Carolina University in Greenville, North Carolina, Kathryn Kolasa, Ph.D., head of the Nutrition Section in the Department of Family Medicine, likes to display a slide of a 450-pound woman. "The woman almost died of malnutrition," Dr. Kolasa says. "It always strikes people as odd to hear that, but it's true."

The slide-show subject was deficient in the whole array

of vitamins and minerals as well as protein. What did she eat that caused malnutrition? Biscuits, snack crackers and other high-fat foods that are not nutrient-dense, Dr. Kolasa recalls. "She ate a lot of fatty meats and didn't eat vegetables."

The success of a weight-loss plan—to lose the flab forever and to remain healthy from a nutritional standpoint—depends on a diet teeming with nutrient-dense dishes— foods high in vitamins and minerals but relatively low in calories and fat. Examples include low-fat dairy products, whole-grain breads and cereals, beans, fruits and dark green vegetables.

Spice your life with variety. The days of single-food fad diets—eat nothing but grapefruit and lose pounds fast, for example—have fallen by the wayside. Which is good, because that's where they belong—in a ditch. An unnatural preponderance of a single food can easily create deficiencies of nutrients lacking in that food. "Whenever you do that," Dr. Butterworth says, "you're inevitably going to miss something you'd get in a mixed, varied diet of fruits and vegetables."

SMOKING

Smokers hit themselves with a nutritional double whammy, for compared to their cigarette-free peers, they typically ingest fewer of the very vitamins that nicotine destroys in their bodies.

Because of their habit and their diets, smokers may need more—but generally consume less—beta-carotene and vitamin C, the antioxidants that may provide some protection against smoke's cancerous effects, according to Linda C. Harlan, Ph.D., a National Cancer Institute researcher and co-author of a study that examined the dietary habits of more than 11,000 smokers and nonsmokers.

Rise above the C-level. The most pronounced nutritional difference between smokers and nonsmokers is in vitamin C. Tobacco-users' bodies process C at a higher rate, either because smoke destroys it or because it is expended to counteract the carcinogens in smoke. While puffers seem to meet the RDA for C in their diets, "this level may not be high enough to counteract the increased vitamin C turnover resulting from their smoking habit," Dr. Harlan's study concluded.

And that's too bad, because not only does vitamin C help prevent carcinogens from forming and fight certain ones that do manifest themselves, it enhances the ability of vitamin E to combat cancer-causing agents—a two-pronged dose of protection.

In addition to the antioxidants, smokers also have a greater need for folate and vitamin B_{12}, according to Dr. Butterworth. Folate, essential for proper lung function, is damaged by smoke, he says.

Don't let meals go up in smoke. Blatantly bad eating habits compound smokers' nutritional nightmares. Compared to nonsmokers, they generally eat less, skip breakfast more, consume fewer nutritional supplements and drink more coffee and alcohol. They eat less poultry and fish, drink less skim milk and rely more heavily on luncheon meats.

As a result, they're shortchanging themselves even more on essential nutrients, such as beta-carotene, which has anticancer properties. "Our results," Dr. Harlan reports, "show that smokers, who may gain some protection from lung cancer by high carotenoid intake, are less likely than non-smokers to be consuming carotenoid-dense food," such as yellow, orange and dark green leafy vegetables.

Get juiced up. Smokers' eating habits may change because tobacco can alter their predilections for certain foods. "It changes taste preferences," Dr. Harlan says. "Smokers don't, for example, like fruit and juices," all high in vitamin C. They generally don't like sweet things, and fruits tend to be sweet. If you find your sweet tooth souring a little, make it a special point to drink some juice at breakfast or as a thirst quencher at other times during the day.

DRINKING

Alcohol does to drinkers what cigarettes do to smokers: It robs them of vitamins and minerals. And the poor dietary habits common in a booze-based lifestyle are likely to compound the damage.

"Drinking does destroy some nutrients," says Charles H. Halsted, M.D., professor of medicine and chief of the Division of Clinical Nutrition and Metabolism at the University of California, Davis, School of Medicine. It also interferes with the absorption of vitamins and minerals, he says.

Be careful with the B vitamins. Moderate and heavy drinkers typically suffer from deficiencies of three major nutrients—folate, which is important for blood formation and digestion; thiamine, which plays a significant role in brain and neurological function; and vitamin B_6, which also helps form healthy blood.

A thiamine deficiency is especially insidious because it could cause brain damage even before physical signs appear, some researchers assert. Diets fortified with thiamine and supplements can reverse the damage in its early stage, but once the harm advances, they don't have much effect.

Blood levels of riboflavin and C, as well as zinc, phosphate and magnesium, also may be depleted in moderate drinkers. Excessive consumers of alcohol, who are at risk from liver disease, may also ail from a "substantial" lack of vitamin A, according to Dr. Halsted.

Eat—don't drink—your meals. Alcohol essentially is a high-calorie, high-carbohydrate substance—"liquid bread is what some people call it," Dr. Kolasa says. But this is a barren loaf, for alcohol is almost devoid of vitamins and minerals.

In addition to what they guzzle from the bottle, drinkers may or may not consume an adequate number of nutrient-dense calories from food to make up for the vitamins and

---

KEEP THE BEAST IN THE BOTTLE WITH GOOD NUTRITION

Recovering alcoholics are less likely to fall off the wagon if their carts are loaded with vitamin-rich vegetables and other complex carbohydrates, and unburdened of sugar and caffeine.

When the traditional Alcoholics Anonymous 12-step recovery program is supplemented with nutritional therapy that homes in on good eating practices, participants are more likely to resist the temptation to revert to the rye, according to researchers at Bowling Green State University in Ohio.

Two groups of new AA members were studied—one following the conventional 12-step program only, the other adding to that a comprehensive nutrition program that included menu planning, individualized nutrition counseling, weight management, shopping, label-reading and dining-out tips. They were put on a diet of high-complex-carbohydrate, low-sugar, no-caffeine meals. Vegetables, beans, grains and whole cereals all are high in complex carbohydrates.

"We just had them follow normal dietary guidelines," says Elsa A. McMullen, Ph.D., a professor in the Depart-

---

minerals destroyed by alcohol. If they don't eat right, "tying one on" could refer to the nutritional noose they're slipping over their heads. Dr. Kolasa says, "If there are problems, it often is because of how drinkers have changed their diets, or rather how they've *let* their diets change."

Know your limit—and stop well short. Although not generally recommended, nonpregnant women probably can have up to three drinks a day and men up to six (a drink

ment of Applied Human Ecology at Bowling Green State University. "We made sure they were eating foods high in fiber and low in simple sugars. And we made sure they ate those kinds of foods for snacks and desserts, too."

Four months into the programs, members of the nutrition therapy group reported no alcohol intake, less craving for a drink and less sugar consumption than those in the traditional group. Desire for alcohol seemed to relate directly to eating sugar: The cravings for alcohol decreased from 80 percent before treatment to only 17 percent among the newly nutritionally conscious, while cravings in the standard group actually increased, from 50 to 80 percent. The reduction in the ache for alcohol also seemed to be correlated to replenishing the body's supply of thiamine (vitamin B_1) and folate.

Diets lacking in nutrients but high in sugar and caffeine may stimulate a thirst for alcohol, the Bowling Green researchers theorize. And they point to other tests in which thiamine-deprived animals increased their drinking of alcohol. Diets lacking in the amino acid tryptophan, whose levels in the brain can be regulated by upping complex carbohydrate consumption, diminish the body's supply of serotonin, a brain neurotransmitter. Low levels of serotonin frequently are found within the brains of alcoholics.

being defined as 12 ounces of beer or one shot of liquor) without risk of developing liver disease, provided their diets otherwise are nourishing, Dr. Halsted says. "Beyond that amount, risks for nutrient deficiencies and alcohol-related diseases increase, and they're setting themselves up for problems." Pregnant women should not drink at all, because we do not know the minimum level of alcohol consumption that is safe for the developing fetus.

EXERCISING

So you don't smoke. You don't drink. You don't chew tobacco, and you don't linger longer at the candy counter than you do in the produce section. In fact, you exercise. You walk, job, bounce about in aerobics classes and lift weights. Supremely healthy and no chance of a dietary shortfall, right?

Actually, for a couple of reasons, physically active people have greater nutrient demands than their sedentary, couch-bound counterparts, according to John Milner, Ph.D., head of the Department of Nutrition at Pennsylvania State University in University Park. Whether it's walking or weight lifting, exercise stimulates the metabolism, burning calories and enhancing the turnover of nutrients. It also contributes to the generation inside your body of destructive, ravenous oxygen molecules.

Get enough food to burn. "If you don't consume enough food and you exercise, you'll end up in a malnourished state," Dr. Milner says. The body will burn not only food and fat but muscle, too. It'll begin to feed on itself to provide the energy you demand. Complex carbohydrates from breads, grains and vegetables can provide the fuel required to get you through your workouts.

But don't curb protein intake for those additional carbohydrates, Dr. Milner warns, for "there might really be a problem." You need more protein to maintain the lean muscle mass you have and to grow more muscle. "If you're physically active, protein is required in a little higher quantity than you typically take in for muscle maintenance and repair." And to properly metabolize the amino acids in protein, to break them down and make them available for use by the body, you need additional vitamin B_6, Dr. Milner says.

Calm free radicals with antioxidants. Every time you take a breath, a small portion of the oxygen generates highly unstable molecules, called free radicals. Free radicals can attack certain vital components in your body, damaging cells and turning fats rancid. The more you breathe, the more free radicals you generate. Huffing and puffing exercisers process much more oxygen and generate many more free radicals than your average couch potato. They also suck in more air pollutants with each breath, which gives birth to even more reactive molecules.

And if that isn't enough to make you rip up your gym membership card and stash your StairMaster in the attic, consider this: When you work out, blood is redirected to the working muscles at the expense of other organs. Free radicals are generated in these exercising muscles. Once the workout is over and oxygen-rich blood returns to the deprived organs, still more free radicals are generated.

Before ditching your dumbbells with the thought that you may be healthier if you don't exercise, try taking some antioxidant vitamins. Repeated studies show that beta-carotene, vitamin C and vitamin E protect the body against what's called the oxidative stress of working out.

Two weeks of vitamin E supplementation "significantly decreased" the oxidation of fats seen in people riding stationary bicycles. Another study using vitamin E, vitamin C and beta-carotene reduced oxidation during exercise and at rest.

AVOIDING MEAT

You shun fatty meats, eggs and dairy products. You also eat a lot of low-calorie, high-vitamin vegetables and fruits. And you consume a variety of high-fiber, complex carbohydrate foods. If you are a vegetarian, you may think you're following the perfect prescription for nutritional health. And you are—to a large extent. But especially if you are a vegan, a strictest-of-the-strict vegetarian who doesn't eat eggs or dairy foods, your diet may be lacking a few nutrients you cannot do without.

Don't forget the B_{12}. The most conspicuous concern for a true-blue vegan is vitamin B_{12}, which can be obtained only from animal foods, such as meat or dairy products. The bacteria from some fermented plant products—such as soybean-based tempeh—do produce a form of B_{12}, and it may even be labeled as such on the package. But debate exists over whether that B_{12}-like substance can be absorbed to meet the body's needs; B_{12} in supplement form is the best insurance.

Squeeze metal from a plant. Iron also may be deficient in an otherwise sound vegetarian diet. Meat, fish and poultry contain easily absorbable iron (the heme form), but plants possess a form not so readily utilized (called nonheme iron). In addition, plants contain fiber and chemicals called phytates that may interfere with absorption of the nutrient. Eating iron-fortified cereals might help balance the equation. Vegetarians also should eat more foods containing vitamin C, which facilitates the absorption of nonheme iron from plants.

Zone in on bone. Calcium is another nutrient that may be lacking. Oxalic acid and phytates in plants inhibit absorption of this bone-building mineral. Vegetarians should make a point of buying and eating foods fortified with calcium, such as certain brands of orange juice, Dr. Kolasa says.

PREGNANCY

When you're pregnant, you literally are eating for two—well, maybe one and a half. Requirements for many nutrients increase dramatically, and some more than double, to ensure proper fetal growth and the mother's needs.

Since you're in the expecting mode anyway, you should expect to gain between 25 and 30 pounds, and only a small portion of that, of course, will be your bouncing baby. The key to a healthy pregnancy, Hermann says, is ensuring that those extra calories come from nutrient-dense foods—vegetables, grains and legumes—not from ice cream and pickles or some other fanciful food cravings.

When you multiply, add vitamins. To supplement or not to supplement during pregnancy? "Theoretically, when you're pregnant you can get everything you need just from food," Hermann says. "In practice, it's much different," not just because of food aversions but because the nutrient demand is so great. Many doctors recommend taking multivitamins and multimineral supplements throughout the stages of pregnancy. If you want to take supplements during your pregnancy, however, you should do so only with the consent of your obstetrician.

High doses of one B vitamin, folate, Hermann says, have been shown to reduce incidence of neural tube defects, the most common of all birth defects, in which the baby's spinal cord closes improperly.

Lower risks of birth defects in general have been associated with regular multivitamin supplementation near the time of conception (at least three times a week before conception through at least the first trimester), according to Centers for Disease Control (CDC) researchers. In one study, they found that those women who reported using multivitamins from at least one month prior to conception through the first trimester were 60 percent less likely to give birth to a baby with brain or spinal defects.

In several cases, you have to double up. "The demand for vitamin D doubles," Hermann says, "and folate requirements more than double." Women also need much more vitamin E and C and all the B vitamins for their gestating sons or daughters. Among the minerals, extra calcium is critical. Iron demands double, and more zinc and magnesium are required, she says.

Keep sickness at bay. An aversion to certain foods is "one of the biggest problems during pregnancy," Hermann says. "I know there was not a lot I could eat when I was pregnant. Granted, I may have been in the minority, but nausea and indigestion from certain foods is a constant concern that could lead to deficiencies."

Severe nausea and vomiting during pregnancy apparently can be countered with supplemental doses of vitamin B_6, according to a group of researchers from the Obstetrics and Gynecology Department of the University of Iowa College of Medicine. A 25-milligram B_6 supplement taken every eight hours significantly improved symptoms of severe nausea in a study group of pregnant women but did little to alleviate mild or moderate nausea. B_6 at such high dosage levels should be taken only under a doctor's supervision.

INFANCY

Following birth, you're cradling a well-nourished baby. But the nutritional challenge isn't over yet. "A baby is like a growing puppy," Dr. Butterworth says. "Its nutritional needs are a lot greater and different from an adult's."

Make it mother's milk. Complete nutrition for those crying, cuddling, whining, wetting bundles of joy can best be provided by one food: mother's milk. While human and formula milk are comparable in many respects, healthy breast milk does have several nutritional advantages.

Early breast milk contains substances that bolster a baby's immune system to help fight off allergies and infections. Commercial formulas cannot reproduce these early protective effects but are very helpful after the first few weeks. Breast milk also is abundant in choline, a nutrient whose importance may not reveal itself until baby is old and gray. Some animal studies showed that rats exhibited less memory deterioration in later life if, when first born, their diets were high in choline. Infant formulas vary in choline content.

Infants should be fed breast milk or formula for the entire first year of their lives, with pureed solid foods offered only as a supplement, according to Pat Harper, R.D., a spokesper-

NUTRITION FOR NURSING

Even after the additional nutrient demands of pregnancy, a woman's vitamin requirements remain quite high after giving birth if she feeds her baby naturally.

"You still need more of many nutrients," says Kathryn Dewey, Ph.D., a professor in the Department of Nutrition at the University of California, Davis. A lactating woman should consume an extra 500 calories a day to get those nutrients and to compensate for the energy her body expends in producing breast milk.

Five nutrients—calcium, zinc, magnesium, vitamin B_6 and folate—are especially important, Dr. Dewey says, "not just because they're needed in higher amounts but because the diets of American women are particularly low in them." The needs for protein, vitamins A and D and fluids also are quite high during lactation. In fact, the level of vitamin D in breast milk is directly related to the amount of D in the mother's diet. If she eats a D-deficient diet or she is not often exposed to direct sunlight (which stimulates the body's own production of the vitamin), the American Dietetic Association recommends supplementation.

The requirements for vitamins A and D and fluids, however, can be fulfilled if the mother drinks two or three glasses of milk a day in addition to the two glasses a day that are normally recommended, according to Pat Harper, R.D., of the American Dietetic Association.

son for the American Dietetic Association and a dietitian in Pittsburgh. The exceptions are pre-term babies or those with low birth weights, whose nutritional needs may be significantly higher than what mother's milk can provide at that point. According to American Dietetic Association recommendations, pre-term babies can be breastfed but may require special supplementation.

Don't cut out the fat—yet. Upon switching to commercial cow's milk, use whole, not skim or 2 percent, for the child's next year. "Babies need the extra calories, fat and cholesterol," Harper says. "It's the only time of their lives they need that." Their bodies are growing at an incredibly rapid rate, and the fat and cholesterol is vital for proper formation of cell walls and brain development.

THE TEEN YEARS

The teen scene is a time of revelry and rebellion, fast cars and fast food, growth spurts and the hormonal changes of puberty. The physiological growth spurt alone creates a greater nutrient demand, but the nutritional haphazardness of adolescence compounds the need. What's a teenager to do?

Bone up at a young age. While the requirement for almost all nutrients increases during the teenage years, calcium assumes a "critical importance," Harper says, especially for girls. Both young women and young men need at least the recommended 1,200 milligrams of the mineral. "In the teenage years and young adulthood, women build their maximum bone density and need extra calcium during that time. Strengthening their bones when young may help prevent osteoporosis later in life."

Turn on the iron. Both pubescent boys and girls need extra iron because their bodies are becoming bigger. For females that need continues: From age 11 through menopause, they require 50 percent more of the mineral (15 milligrams as opposed to 10 milligrams) than postpubescent males.

AGING

Eventually, time takes its toll on the body. It becomes harder to chew, harder to digest food, harder to absorb some of the nutrients—all of which means you have to work harder to ensure that your nutritional needs are met to keep you as healthy as possible.

Boost brain and body with B$_{12}$. At least one out of every five people older than 60 may need supplemental vitamin B$_{12}$. "It's one of the more important nutrients affected by aging," says Robert M. Russell, M.D., a professor of medicine and nutrition at Tufts University in Boston. Extra B$_{12}$ in the diets of senior citizens may help reverse senility-like lapses in memory and other neurological problems that disrupt muscle coordination and balance. Such symptoms often develop before the most apparent consequence of B$_{12}$ deficiency, pernicious anemia.

Many older people won't need frequent visits to a doctor for B$_{12}$ injections. B$_{12}$ pills should do the job, Dr. Russell says.

As you age, your stomach may no longer secrete enough acid to separate B$_{12}$ from protein. Or too much bacteria caused by the acid lack may interfere with absorption, a condition known as mild atrophic gastritis, says Dr. Russell, who also heads the gastrointestinal and micronutrient lab at the U.S. Department of Agriculture's Human Nutrition Research Center on Aging at Tufts.

"With mild atrophic gastritis, you can eat more foods containing B$_{12}$ to get more B$_{12}$ into your system," Dr. Russell says. Or you can take oral supplements which contain a crystalline (pure) form of the vitamin whose absorption is not impeded by a mild lack of stomach acids.

In severe cases of atrophic gastritis, though, no stomach acids at all are secreted, which means the body cannot produce another important absorptive aid called intrinsic factor. "No matter how much these people eat or take orally, it won't help them absorb vitamin B$_{12}$," Dr. Russell says. "These people would need injections of the vitamin."

Even though most older people with absorption problems

can take B_{12} supplements, Dr. Russell advises that they take them only in consultation with a physician, who will be able to monitor blood levels of the nutrient and assess any deficiency damage.

Be selective about calcium supplements. Atrophic gastritis and other stomach difficulties can retard the absorption of the bone mineral calcium from its most common supplemental form, calcium carbonate. Older people should look for supplements made from calcium citrate, Dr. Russell advises, and they should take the pills with their meals.

Let B_6 help you get more out of a meal. A marginal deficiency of vitamin B_6 is commonly found in older people, compared to younger adults. This nutrient is needed for healthy blood and for proper functioning of the nervous system. It also seems to play a role in strengthening the immune system.

Vitamin B_6 also contributes significantly to metabolizing proteins. Based on studies analyzing vitamin B_6 and protein intakes, vitamin B_6 levels in the blood and excretion of vitamin B_6 metabolites in urine, a research team at Tufts University found that the minimum vitamin B_6 requirements of elderly men and women are about 1.96 and 1.90 milligrams per day, respectively. The current RDAs for elderly men and women are 2.0 and 1.6 milligrams per day, respectively. Since the RDAs are intended to "meet the nutrient needs of practically all healthy persons," the research team concluded that the current RDAs for B_6 are insufficient and should be reevaluated. Rich sources of B_6 include bananas, poultry and kidney beans.

Don't forget fluids. Many people worry about bladder control as they age, Dr. Kolasa says, and their thirst sensations diminish. For both these reasons, they may drink less fluids than they need. The result can be dehydration.

"Especially in the summer in the cities, elderly people die from dehydration," Dr. Russell says. "First they become confused; and if the dehydration persists, they slip into a coma."

Despite the extra danger, fluid requirements for older people don't differ drastically from those for younger adults. Everyone, Dr. Russell says, should be drinking between eight and ten glasses of fluid a day.

Ally yourself with the antioxidants. Because of evidence that the antioxidant vitamins help protect the body from age-related diseases and other health problems, Dr. Milner says, elderly people should make sure they're getting enough beta-carotene and vitamins E and C. In addition, they also need to boost their intake of iron, calcium, folate and the trace element selenium, he says.

Overcome reasons not to eat. For a number of reasons, elderly people are less likely to eat adequately, Harper says. They lose teeth and coordination. Their senses of taste and smell fade. They're generally weaker and may even find it uncomfortable to swallow. Many of them live alone and, thus, eat alone, either out of the house or at home with simple "meals" like tea and toast. "They're not concerned with the impact of decreasing nutrient intake, and if they are, they don't know what to do about it," Harper says.

"Simply because of the change in eating patterns," Dr. Milner emphasizes, "the demand for some nutrients is magnified." And if they or their loved ones don't ensure that they're getting enough of the right foods, the demand may not be met.

PART 2

THE TOP DIETARY ISSUES

CHAPTER 7

Fiber

More for What Ails Us

You can almost picture a snake-oil salesman selling this stuff from the back of a horse-drawn wagon, waving little brown bottles and shouting to the crowd: "Miracle substance! Cures just about any ailment! Easy to use!"

Instead of a traveling salesman, we have TV advertisers pitching the benefits of their fiber-containing products, plus magazines and newspapers that sometimes seem to have latched onto fiber as the cure-all of the decade. High cholesterol? Diabetes? Constipation? Overweight? Fiber has been touted as fixing them all.

But fiber *does* help with all these woes, and more. Studies indicate that fiber may also help with gastrointestinal problems, gallstones and ulcers. And it appears to help prevent colon and breast cancer. "We had never thought a food ingredient such as fiber could have the marked influence on diseases it does," says Sharon Fleming, Ph.D., associate professor in the Department of Nutrition Sciences at the University of California in Berkeley.

FINDING FIBER IN FAST FOODS

So you try to work fiber into your diet—you really do—
but somehow more and more often you find yourself at
Wendy's or McDonald's or Taco Bell, gazing up at the
neon-lit menu and trying to pick out something that's not
too fattening or unhealthy.

Is there any fiber in fast food? Yes, but it's not always
easy to find, says Marion J. Franz, of the International Diabetes Center in Minneapolis and author of *Fast Food
Facts.* Most fast foods have so little fiber it's not even
listed on those little nutritional sheets many restaurants
provide. (You can forget about counting those few shreds
of lettuce on your Jumbo Burger—lettuce is not a particularly good source of fiber.)

Where *can* you find fast-food fiber? In beans in chili,
tacos or other Mexican foods, in vegetables at salad bars
or atop pizzas, in whole-wheat rolls or buns and in baked
potatoes (skin and all).

The salad bar is a sure bet, if you help yourself to a variety of vegetables and not just a pile of lettuce with a
meager sprinkling of carrots and tomato. "In general, by

WHY ALL THE HULLABALOO?

What happened? Fifty years ago you didn't see people
shaking bran flakes onto their cornflakes, or headlines popping off newspaper and magazine pages telling you about
the amazing properties of oat bran.

But 50 years ago people also weren't filling up on fiber-
impoverished fast food and refined white-flour products, points
out Dr. Fleming. They were much more likely to sit down to
meals loaded with fiber: fresh or home-canned vegetables and
fruit, whole-grain breads and a variety of grains and beans.

the time people get through a salad bar, they've gotten two to three grams of fiber in all the raw vegetables," says Franz. A great way to add still more fiber to your salad is to add garbanzos, those little round, tan legumes also known as chickpeas.

Baked potatoes are another good choice at burger barns: A large potato, including the skin, offers about 4 grams of fiber. Beans in chili or Mexican fare usually will provide 3 to 4 grams, and corn on the cob, if you can find it, has between 2 and 3 grams. Choosing a wheat roll for your foot-long turkey sub at Subway will add 1½ grams of fiber to your meal, bringing it to nearly 6½ grams total. And two slices of a medium Pizza Hut pizza offer from 4 to 7 grams of fiber, depending on your toppings and the type of crust (the thin crust has less fiber). If you opt for an individual-size pizza heaped with vegetables, you get 8 to 9 grams of fiber.

So it's not *impossible* to get a reasonable amount of fiber from your fast-food meal. You can choose salad and chili, baked potato and a sandwich on a whole-wheat bun, a couple of bean burritos or two slices of pizza—all combinations that will give you seven to eight grams of fiber.

"As people became more affluent, a status factor came into play," says Dr. Fleming. People abandoned basic foods such as whole-meal bread and beans in favor of fluffy white bread, cakes, pastries, meat and highly processed foods. These days, hectic lifestyles have also taken their toll: "If you're eating TV dinners and fast foods rather than freshly prepared meals, you don't have much chance of getting enough fiber," says Dr. Fleming.

Today it's estimated that the fiber content of the typical U.S. diet ranges from 11.1 to 23.3 grams per day, down from around 40.0 grams a century ago. Fiber has no nutritive value, so at first no one thought taking it out of foods would hurt anything. But along with the drop in fiber intake came an increase in the incidence of chronic diseases.

The idea that there might be a *connection* between how much fiber we ate and these diseases came from British surgeon Denis Burkitt, M.D., and his landmark studies published in the 1970s. Dr. Burkitt pointed out that in places such as Africa, where the diet is heavy on cereals, legumes and root vegetables and includes 50 to 100 grams of fiber per day, there were fewer cases of colon and rectal cancer, intestinal diseases, hemorrhoids, gallstones and heart disease. In contrast, in Westernized countries with less fiber consumption, these diseases were increasing.

THE MIRACLE INGREDIENT

Despite the seemingly miraculous qualities of fiber, you can't just swig a fiber-containing drink or munch on a bran muffin and assume you're protected from disease. To reap the benefits fiber can offer, nutritionists recommend you get your fiber from a variety of foods and at several meals instead of one sitting.

Nor does fiber make up for eating *unhealthy* foods. "People tend to say to themselves, 'Gee, I've sprinkled bran on three things today, so I can eat these candy bars, these french fries and this deep-fried chicken,'" says Dr. Fleming.

What *is* great about fiber is that it requires no prescription and doesn't cost a lot—you can find it in many foods in your grocery store, many of them quite inexpensive.

Dietary fiber is the part of plants that resists digestion, so it passes through the system basically without being broken down. There are two types of fiber, soluble and insoluble. Many foods contain both kinds of fiber, but some foods contain more of one type than the other.

OAT BRAN: FACT OR FANTASY?

Oat bran: The wonder food, right? No, wait, that's the stuff that doesn't work, right?

It's no wonder that consumers are confused. First came a highly publicized study about 19 percent drops in cholesterol levels from eating oat bran. Then in 1990 came a study in the *New England Journal of Medicine* that concluded that oat bran had little effect on cholesterol.

So what's the word on oats? "The general feeling is that it's a good food, but it was put too high on the agenda in terms of expectations," says David Jenkins, M.D., Ph.D., of the University of Toronto in Ontario. "The trouble with the oat bran story is that it was pushed too many miles," he says.

"Oat bran is no better than other kinds of bran," says Barbara Harland, R.D., Ph.D., of Howard University in Washington, D.C. "It's ridiculous to limit your diet to one source of fiber."

In some cases you have to take closer looks at the studies. In the 19-percent-drop study, cholesterol was lowered by eating a bowl of oatmeal and five oat bran muffins daily *in combination with* a low-fat, low-cholesterol diet. And the study debunking fiber used inconsistent methods of comparing diets, and the subjects were all slender young women with normal cholesterol levels.

The bottom line, says Dr. Jenkins, is that oat bran is a fine food, with a definite effect on cholesterol—maybe not as large as first believed, but it's there, and it's valuable.

Insoluble fibers—which include cellulose, lignin and some hemicelluloses—are linked to colon cancer protection and the prevention or alleviation of some digestive disorders. They also delay glucose absorption. You'll find insoluble fibers in wheat bran and whole grains and on the outside of legumes, fruits and seeds. Insoluble fiber is like a sponge, increasing the bulk of your stool and speeding it on its way through your intestinal tract.

Soluble fibers lower blood cholesterol and slow down how fast glucose gets into your bloodstream. Instead of hastening food's movement through you, soluble fibers decrease the pace. They're found in vegetables, fruits, brown rice, barley, oats and oat and rice bran, and include pectin, gums and some hemicelluloses.

A Multitude of Benefits

What exactly *does* this miracle substance accomplish? Although the jury is still out on some fronts, there is some consensus of opinion.

"The scientific community agrees that dietary fiber lowers cholesterol, relieves constipation, possibly reduces blood glucose response and may have a positive function in weight reduction," says David Jenkins, M.D., Ph.D., professor of medicine and nutritional sciences in the Department of Nutritional Sciences at the University of Toronto in Ontario. Dietary fiber can also help with gastrointestinal, gallbladder and gastric problems, according to the American Dietetic Association.

A diet high in fiber is often lower in fat and calories than one that is low in fiber, and some people argue that many of fiber's benefits can be attributed to the decrease in fat or calories. "The other factors may enhance the fiber effect," agrees Dr. Jenkins, "but that's not a bad thing."

Cutting Cholesterol

The link between cholesterol and fiber has gotten much media attention. Cholesterol is reduced primarily by soluble fiber, as in oat bran and psyllium, a seed used in laxative products such as Metamucil. According to some studies, fiber lowers harmful LDL (low-density lipoprotein) cholesterol without lowering good HDL (high-density lipoprotein) levels.

James W. Anderson, M.D., a pioneer in fiber research and professor of medicine and clinical nutrition at the University of Kentucky College of Medicine in Lexington, studied 105 men and women with elevated cholesterol levels. After taking psyllium for eight weeks, their LDL cholesterol had dropped nearly 9 percent more than while just eating a special cholesterol-lowering diet. In another study, a low-fat diet plus oat cereal lowered cholesterol 10 percent, while the same diet plus 13 grams of psyllium caused a *16 percent* drop.

Other studies confirm the cholesterol-lowering effect with other foods. In one study, a group of 41 men lowered their LDL cholesterol by eating 12 prunes daily (roughly six grams of fiber). In another study by Dr. Anderson, patients with high cholesterol experienced drops of more than 10 percent after three weeks of eating eight ounces of canned beans daily.

CURING CONSTIPATION

This is no laughing matter for the many people who suffer from it. The Western world's low fiber intake is the clear culprit here, say many doctors. Fortunately, fiber almost always provides relief. Fiber ranks high among *Prevention* magazine readers: 86 percent of respondents in a survey said bran and high-fiber cereal gave good results in relieving irregularity.

Insoluble fiber plus water forms a larger, softer stool that can pass easily and quickly. And when bacteria begin to break down the fiber, chemicals form that help things start moving.

If you're eating bran for a laxative effect, stick to coarse bran rather than finely ground bran, advises Jay Kenney, R.D., Ph.D., nutrition research specialist at the Pritikin Longevity Center in Santa Monica, California. "Finely ground bran has much less of an effect on constipation," he says. The laxative effect of wheat bran may also be reduced by cooking.

TO SUPPLEMENT OR NOT TO SUPPLEMENT

Adding fiber to your diet *does* require some time and planning, so you may be tempted to look for a quick-and-easy answer—such as fiber pills.

Most professionals urge caution when it comes to these pills. "Fiber pills are a disaster," says Sharon Fleming, Ph.D., of the University of California at Berkeley. "They're expensive, and, to a large degree, ineffective."

One problem is that fiber squeezed into a pill may not work the same as fiber in food. "The physical properties have been altered tremendously, and this can reduce the effectiveness of the fiber, gram for gram," explains Dr. Fleming. And you'd have to take a lot of pills to get substantial fiber. Five pills supply only about 2½ grams of fiber, about what you'd get in a small apple.

Even using bran as a supplement can be a mistake if you overdo it, says Dr. Fleming. "I would guard against sprinkling bran on everything," she says. Bran, whether in pills or the loose form, absorbs a lot of water, and without adequate liquid intake, Dr. Fleming points out, you're running the risk of impaction. If you like bran, don't eat it dry: Stir it into something wet, such as a bowl of oatmeal or a batter. Also use plenty of milk with high-fiber cereals, says Dr. Fleming.

Finally, if you're eating fiber only in concentrated forms, you're not getting the nutrients and minerals that generally accompany fiber when you eat it in foods. And because fiber *can* interfere with the absorption of minerals and vitamins, if you're increasing your fiber intake without increasing your nutrient intake—which is what happens when you pop bran pills or eat plain bran—you could put yourself at risk for deficiency.

Fiber can also help prevent hemorrhoids by eliminating constipation, which contributes to their formation. It can also make passing stools less painful when you do have hemorrhoids.

PREVENTING CANCER

Native Japanese, who eat less fat and more fiber than Westerners, have only about one-fifth our rate of breast cancer and colon cancer—but when Japanese immigrate to the United States and alter their diets, rates rise dramatically.

In colon cancer, fiber seems the most important factor. In Finland, where people eat as much fat as we do but also eat lots of whole grains and high-fiber foods, the rates of colon cancer are *one-third* of ours. And among the Hindu population in India, which eats a high-fiber diet, there's very little colon cancer. The Parsi community in Bombay, however, has a more Westernized diet—*and* colon cancer rates almost equal to those of Western countries. Closer to home, the Mormon population in Utah has a lower risk of colon cancer than the rest of the population: This group eats normally high American levels of fat but also eats cereal and breads made from stone-ground whole-grain flour.

How does fiber affect cancer risk? When we eat fat, some of the bile acids produced to process these fats develop into carcinogenic forms. Fiber can help by causing the stool to be bigger—which decreases carcinogen concentration in the stool—or it can bond with the carcinogens and carry them off. The oxygen produced in fiber fermentation may keep the bile acids from changing into their carcinogenic forms. Finally, fiber speeds the stool on its way, so if carcinogens *are* present, they'll spend less time in contact with the colon wall.

Insoluble fiber may lower estrogen levels in premenopausal women, which may help prevent breast cancer. In one study, 62 women ate wheat, oat or corn bran muffins, doubling their daily fiber intake to 30 grams. After two months, only the women eating wheat bran had significantly lower levels of circulating estrogen.

Effects have been seen in mammals of the four-legged variety. In a study of rats exposed to a carcinogen to induce mammary tumors, 90 percent of the animals eating a high-fat, low-fiber diet developed tumors, while only 66 percent of those eating a high-fat, high-fiber diet did.

Conclusion? "The most important thing the public can do is increase their overall dietary fiber intake from a variety of natural food sources," advises Bruce Trock, Ph.D., a cancer epidemiologist at Fox Chase Cancer Center in Philadelphia.

BATTLING THE BULGE

One reason fiber is successful in helping weight loss is simple: It fills you up. High-fiber foods make you feel full and tend to take longer to eat. They also tend to be low in fat.

Another benefit involves soluble fibers and insulin, the hormone that stimulates appetite and promotes fat storage. "The good news is that food fiber slows the body's insulin response," says Dr. Kenney.

DEALING WITH DIABETES

Diabetes, which is increasing annually by about 500,000 cases, according to Dr. Anderson, can be managed effectively by a high-carbohydrate, high-fiber diet. In some cases this regimen can alleviate the need for insulin: "Many diabetics don't need insulin. They need a diet program," says Dr. Anderson. Eating fiber also facilitates weight loss, which can help *avoid* diabetes.

Fiber can reduce glucose and insulin concentrations after meals, as seen in a study at the University of Virginia, where people with non-insulin-dependent diabetes received two 3.4-gram doses of psyllium fiber before breakfast and dinner. Their glucose levels were lower after those meals, and their serum insulin concentrations were reduced after breakfast and even after lunch.

Soluble fibers, such as those found in oat and rice bran, legumes and fruit and vegetables, seem to be the ticket. "The water-soluble fibers found in legumes, oats, barley and fruit, when eaten in a low-fat diet, have been shown to lower blood-fat levels," says Marion J. Franz, vice president of nutrition and publications at the International Diabetes Center in Minneapolis. Those fibers may also cause the sugar in your food to be absorbed more slowly, which gives your insulin a chance to keep your blood sugar on a more even keel.

TREATING INTESTINAL ILLS

In diverticulosis, fairly common in adults 50 and older, small pouches form in the wall of the colon because of intestinal pressure. When the pouches trap feces, they can become inflamed. Some studies suggest that fiber may help *prevent* diverticulosis, and it may also help by reducing intestinal pressure and helping clear out existing pouches.

Fiber can be used to treat constipation problems in irritable bowel syndrome and has been used to treat some cases of duodenal ulcers. Crohn's disease involves inflammatory lesions in the intestines; after symptoms have subsided, small amounts of fiber can be added to the diet, according to the American Dietetic Association. Once the disease is under control, fiber can help keep it from recurring.

GALLING GALLSTONES

Fiber may help prevent gallstones by stimulating bile flow and preventing reabsorption of bile. It's also possible that gallstones *result* from low-fiber diets and that fiber can prevent their formation.

FIBER CONTENT OF FOODS

Breads, fruits, vegetables and beans are generally your best fiber sources, but there are fairly large differences among individual foods, as this table shows.

Food	Portion	Fiber (g.)
BREADS		
Whole-wheat bread	1 slice	2.1
Pumpernickel bread	1 slice	1.9
English muffin	1	1.6
Rye bread	1 slice	1.6
Bagel	1	1.2
Waffle	1	0.8
White bread	1 slice	0.5
FRUITS		
Strawberries, fresh	1 cup	3.9
Dates, dried	5 med.	3.5
Orange	1	3.1
Apple	1	3.0
Applesauce	½ cup	1.9
Pineapple, canned	1 cup	1.9
Banana	1	1.8
Prunes, dried	3 med.	1.8

GUARDING THOSE GUMS

Chewing large volumes of fibrous foods helps massage gums and remove plaque, according to one study. All that chewing also stimulates the production of saliva, which helps clean teeth as well.

FITTING IN FIBER

Okay, you're committed. You *want* to increase the amount of fiber in your diet. Where do you start?

Food	Portion	Fiber (g.)
Cantaloupe	1 cup cubes	1.3
Grapes	1 cup	1.1
Orange juice	½ cup	0.1
VEGETABLES		
Brussels sprouts, cooked	½ cup	3.4
Peas, frozen	½ cup	2.4
Carrot, raw 7½" long	1	2.3
Broccoli, cooked	½ cup	2.0
Green beans, frozen	½ cup	1.8
Mushrooms, boiled	½ cup	1.7
Tomato, fresh	1 med.	1.6
Beets, canned	½ cup	1.4
Iceberg lettuce, shredded	1 cup	1.4
Corn, canned	½ cup	1.2
Celery, raw, chopped	½ cup	1.0
BEANS		
Black-eyed peas, boiled	½ cup	8.3
Kidney beans, canned	½ cup	7.9
Chick-peas, canned	½ cup	7.0
Pork and beans, canned	½ can	6.9
Lentils, dried, cooked	½ cup	5.2
Pinto beans, boiled	½ cup	3.4

"First, a trip to the grocery store," says dietitian and nutritionist Barbara Harland, R.D., Ph.D., associate professor of nutrition in the Department of Nutritional Sciences at Howard University in Washington, D.C. Pause before you toss the Froot Loops or white Wonder bread into your shopping cart.

Go whole grain. You want to select whole-grain breads, crackers and muffins, advises Dr. Harland. This also means checking labels: Just because a loaf of bread is brown and labeled "wheat" doesn't mean it's whole grain. (Refined white flour is wheat, too.) Check the list of ingredients or choose items labeled "whole wheat."

Select your cereal. In the cereal aisle you'll find many cereals that will add to your fiber intake. Again, check the labels for the number of grams of fiber per serving.

Favor this food group. Stock up on fresh, frozen and canned fruits and vegetables.

Peruse the packaged goods. Instead of reaching for white rice, choose brown rice or another whole grain such as barley, bulgur or millet. Buy whole-grain pasta instead of the refined variety. You can also stock up on whole-wheat flour, which you can substitute for white flour in many recipes.

Bring on the beans. "A food high in fiber that people often neglect is legumes: dried beans, lentils, peas," says Dr. Jenkins, who supplements his diet with barley and beans. You can buy these canned or in soups, but dried is cheaper.

A PAINLESS PATH TO HIGH FIBER

The next step, of course, comes in the kitchen and at the dining room table. The first problem is lack of time. Say you come home from work tired and hungry. You're not likely to reach for raw vegetables and spend an hour preparing them before you can eat—you're going to reach for a fast and easy food that quickly satisfies your hunger.

Have a plan. "Working fiber into your diet does take some effort," says Dr. Fleming. "It means planning ahead. It may mean cutting up your vegetables one night so you can have them the next night. It may mean eating at restaurants that offer salad bars with vegetables. It may mean making an effort—but it means taking care of ourselves."

Aim high. The American Dietetic Association recommends 20 to 35 grams of fiber daily (40 to 50 grams a day—or 25 grams per 1,000 calories—for people with diabetes).

Don't, however, double your fiber intake overnight. Introduce fiber into your diet *gradually*. And if you have diabetes, always be sure to check with your doctor before making any dietary changes.

Pay attention to basics. These tips can help you increase your daily fiber intake.

THE LOWDOWN ON BREAKFAST CEREALS

Counting on your breakfast cereal to provide a chunk of your dietary fiber requirements? Here's the number of grams of fiber per serving.

CEREAL	PORTION*	FIBER (g.)
All-Bran	1/3 cup	9.0
All-Bran with Extra Fiber	1/2 cup	14.0
Bran Buds	1/3 cup	11.0
Cherrios	1 1/4 cups	2.5
Common Sense Oat Bran	3/4 cup	3.0
Fiber One	1/2 cup	13.0
Fiberwise	2/3 cup	5.0
Frosted Bran	2/3 cup	3.0
Grape-Nuts	1/4 cup	2.8
Nutri-Grain Wheat	2/3 cup	3.0
Product 19	1 cup	1.2
Puffed Rice	1 cup	1.2
Raisin Bran	3/4 cup	5.0
Rice Krispies	1 cup	0.3
Spoon-Size Shredded Wheat	2/3 cup	3.0
Special K	1 cup	1.0
Total (wheat)	1 cup	2.0
Wheaties	1 cup	3.0

*Though serving sizes vary widely, all provide approximately 1 ounce.

MORE FIBER, LESS EFFORT

So you think fitting fiber into your diet means a complete revamping of how you eat? Changing your diet doesn't have to be tedious or difficult—sometimes small changes can make a big difference. Here's an example of how you can painlessly shift your menu to include more fiber in your diet. (The fiber values in the table are based on standard servings.)

FIBER IN YOUR OLD MENU . . . AND IN THE NEW

FOOD	FIBER (g.)	FOOD	FIBER (g.)
BREAKFAST		*BREAKFAST*	
Orange juice	0.1	Whole orange	3.1
Corn flakes	0.5	High-fiber cereal	9.0
Doughnut	negligible	Whole-wheat toast	2.1
LUNCH		*LUNCH*	
Hamburger on white bun	0.7	Chili	4.6
Fries	3.1	Baked sweet potato	3.4
Milk shake	negligible	Milk shake	negligible
DINNER		*DINNER*	
Lettuce salad	1.4	Lettuce salad with chick-peas, broccoli and mushrooms	6.1
Chicken	negligible	Chicken	negligible
White rice	0.2	Brown rice	1.7
SNACKS		*SNACKS*	
Apple	3.0	Pear	4.3
Potato chips	1.0	Popcorn (3 cups)	2.7
DAILY TOTAL:	10.0		37.0

- Eat whole fruit instead of drinking juice.
- Eat the skins of fruits and vegetables.
- Eat fruit with edible seeds such as kiwis, figs and blueberries.
- When preparing vegetable such as broccoli and asparagus, include more of the stem.
- Peel grapefruit and eat it like an orange instead of eating it with a spoon.
- Make your own bread crumbs or croutons from stale, whole-grain bread.
- Add beans, peas and lentils to soups, stews and salads.
- Scrub vegetables instead of peeling them.
- Add grated vegetables to meat loaf, casseroles and sauces.
- Use pureed vegetables instead of cream to thicken soups.

Resort to a super source. Still having trouble getting enough fiber? Try adding one of the following "supplements" per day—each offers four to five extra grams of fiber.

- Three dried figs
- One large pear
- Three medium plums
- Two medium peaches
- $1/2$ cup cooked legumes (such as chick-peas, kidney beans or lentils)
- $1/3$ to $1/2$ cup bran cereal
- One tablespoon corn bran, three tablespoons wheat bran or four tablespoons rice bran, stirred into cereal, fruit or yogurt
- $1 1/2$ rounded teaspoons psyllium or 2 teaspoons soy fiber mixed with a beverage. (You should be aware that some people are allergic to psyllium: Stop using it if you experience rapid heartbeat or rapid breathing, swollen face or tight throat.)

THE UNPLEASANT SIDE OF FIBER

Okay, we never said *everything* about fiber is great. In some people there are . . . well, certain unpleasant side effects. High-fiber foods can tend to be gas-producing, which at times can make you wonder if all that fiber is really worth the bother.

Don't despair! Even if previous forays into the world of high-fiber foods proved disastrous, there are ways to decrease your distress.

The first trick is to introduce fiber *gradually* into your diet, according to George L. Blackburn, M.D., Ph.D., associate professor of surgery at Harvard Medical School and chief of the Nutrition/Metabolism Laboratory at the Cancer Research Institute of New England Deaconess Hospital in Boston. Too much, too soon can result in gas and a bloated feeling. So if you're only eating 10 grams of fiber a day, don't rocket up to 25 grams a day all at once. Dr. Blackburn recommends adding fiber in 5-gram increments: Add 5 extra grams per day, and after five or six weeks, add another 5 grams, and so on.

Another simple trick is to soak beans before cooking,

ENOUGH . . . OR TOO MUCH?

How concerned should you be about how much of your fiber is insoluble and how much is soluble? "What you should be concerned with is that you're eating the right foods," says Dr. Jenkins. If you eat a variety of fiber-containing foods, don't worry about how much of each type you're getting.

You may also wonder how to know if you're getting enough total fiber. Let's face it, few of us are going to keep track of how many grams of fiber we eat, day after day. A quick way to determine if you're getting enough fiber is by your stools,

then pour off the water, and cook them in fresh water. This helps break down the sugars that cause the gas problem. Chewing thoroughly can also help.

And for those folks for whom all else fails, there's a secret weapon: a product called Beano. Much of the gas produced by high-fiber foods comes from hard-to-digest sugars, explains Luanne Hughes, R.D., manager of public relations for Beano. "When those sugars sit in your intestine undigested, bacteria feed on them." The results of this bacterial feast? Gas.

This is where Beano comes in. This bottled enzyme breaks down these sugars and substantially reduces the gas produced. Although it's named after the food that gives many of us trouble, the manufacturer claims it works on foods as diverse as flour, bran, brussels sprouts, squash, granola, peanut butter, tofu and more.

All you do is add drops of Beano to your first mouthful of gas-producing foods. Because not *all* the gas from fibrous foods comes from these sugars, Beano may not completely eliminate the problem, says Hughes, but it should substantially reduce it.

says Dr. Harland. "They shouldn't be very dark and hard to pass," she says. "A normal stool should be pale tan and soft."

If some fiber is good, a lot is better, you think as you heap bran on your oatmeal, pop fiber pills with lunch and snack on popcorn after dinner.

Hold it right there. Too much fiber, particularly in the form of bran or pills, can actually *clog you up*, says Dr. Fleming. Fiber absorbs a lot of liquid, and if you're eating fiber in a concentrated form and not taking in enough liquid, the fiber can literally form a plug inside you.

The second reason for not overdosing on fiber is that fiber binds some vitamins and minerals, decreasing their availability. For most of us, this isn't a problem. "If you're getting your fiber in foods, by increasing fiber, you're automatically increasing the nutrients," says Dr. Harland.

Who's in danger? People who take their fiber in forms such as fiber pills or fiber drinks, thereby adding fiber *without* adding nutrients; elderly people who exist on tea and toast; and some vegetarians, says Dr. Harland. Children who aren't eating a lot of calories may also be at risk, cautions the American Academy of Pediatrics.

Most of us, however, don't have to worry—as long as we're getting our fiber from a variety of foods. The "consumption of a complex, balanced diet from a variety of food sources should not lead to overt vitamin/mineral deficiencies," states the American Dietetic Association.

Health professionals agree that it all comes down to a very simple formula: Eat a wide variety of fiber-containing foods.

High-Nutrition Recipes

CHILI-TOPPED POTATOES

Beans are a treasure trove of fiber, so they deserve to make frequent appearances on your table. This simple entrée is equally good for lunch or dinner. You can vary it by substituting other beans and also by serving the chili over quick-cooking brown rice rather than potatoes.

4 **large baking potatoes**	1 **can (28 ounces) whole**
4 **teaspoons olive oil**	**tomatoes**
1½ **cups diced onions**	1 **cup defatted chicken**

1 cup diced sweet red peppers	stock
1 cup diced carrots	¾ cup mild or medium salsa
1 clove garlic, minced	1 can (19 ounces) red kidney beans, rinsed well and drained
1 tablespoon chili powder	
1 teaspoon ground cumin	
⅛ teaspoon ground red pepper	1 cup corn kernels

Pierce the potatoes all over with a fork. Place a paper towel directly on the floor of the microwave. Arrange the potatoes on it in a square pattern. Microwave on high for 5 minutes. Flip and rearrange the potatoes. Microwave on high for 5 to 7 minutes more, or until easily pierced with a fork. Cover with foil and let stand for at least 5 minutes.

Meanwhile, heat the oil in a 3-quart saucepan over medium-high heat. Add the onions, sweet red peppers, carrots and garlic. Sauté for 5 minutes, or until the vegetables are tender.

Stir in the chili powder, cumin and ground red pepper. Sauté for 1 minute, stirring constantly.

Drain the tomatoes, reserving ½ cup of the juice. Add the juice to the pan. Chop the tomatoes and add. Stir in the stock and salsa. Bring to a boil.

Reduce the heat to medium low and simmer for 10 minutes, stirring occasionally, until the mixture thickens slightly. Add the beans and corn. Simmer for 5 minutes.

Split the potatoes and lightly fluff the flesh with a fork. Serve topped with the chili.

Serves 4
Per serving: *352 calories, 5.8 g. fat (13% of calories), 12.3 g. dietary fiber, 0 mg. cholesterol, 578 mg. sodium*

ORANGE-RAISIN MUFFINS

Getting the recommended 20 to 35 grams of fiber a day into your diet can be a challenge. That's why you need to stock up at every meal, including breakfast. Muffins are always a welcome addition to the morning meal. And they're portable, so those who don't have time for a sit-down meal can take them along to work or school. These muffins are especially good spread with apple butter, which contains both soluble and insoluble fiber.

2 cups shredded bran cereal, such as All-Bran or Fiber One	¼ cup fat-free egg substitute
¾ cup boiling water	1 tablespoon grated orange rind
½ cup buttermilk	¾ cup golden raisins
½ cup orange juice	¾ cup unbleached flour
¼ cup oil	½ cup whole-wheat flour
¼ cup honey	1½ teaspoons baking soda

In a large bowl, combine the cereal and water. Let stand for 5 minutes, or until the bran softens.

In a medium bowl, whisk together the buttermilk, orange juice, oil, honey, egg and orange rind. Stir into the bran mixture. Add the raisins and mix well.

In a small bowl, stir together the unbleached flour, whole-wheat flour and baking soda. Pour over the bran mixture. Stir just until the flour is moistened; do not overmix.

Coat 12 muffin cups with no-stick spray. Divide the batter among the cups. Bake at 400° for 18 minutes, or until lightly browned.

Makes 12

Tip: *These muffins are best served warm. To reheat them easily, slice in half, wrap in a damp paper towel and microwave one muffin at a time on high for 25 to 30 seconds. They'll be moist and soft, with just-baked flavor.*

Per muffin: *180 calories, 5.2 g. fat (23% of calories), 5.1 g. dietary fiber, <1 mg. cholesterol, 148 mg. sodium*

CHICKEN AND RICE CASSEROLE

One good way to increase your fiber intake is by using brown rice instead of white. Another is to up your consumption of high-fiber cereal. This delicious casserole combines both techniques to produce a nutty-tasting main dish. Serve with three-bean salad and whole-grain bread for even more fiber.

12 ounces boneless, skinless chicken breast, cut into 1" cubes

1 cup diced onions

¾ cup diced mushrooms

2 teaspoons olive oil

1¼ cups quick-cooking brown rice

½ teaspoon dried thyme

½ teaspoon ground black pepper

2½ cups defatted chicken stock

1 box (10 ounces) frozen peas, partially thawed

1 cup shredded bran cereal, such as All-Bran or Fiber One

¼ cup wheat germ or bread crumbs

2 tablespoons grated Parmesan cheese

1 cup nonfat yogurt or nonfat sour cream

2 tablespoons minced fresh parsley

⅛ teaspoon hot-pepper sauce

Spread the chicken on a large, flat plate or in a 9" glass pie plate in as even a layer as possible. Cover with wax paper and microwave on high for 3 minutes. Stir, cover and microwave on high for 2 minutes, or until no longer pink. Set aside.

Meanwhile, in a large no-stick frying pan or Dutch oven over medium heat, sauté the onions and mushrooms in 1 teaspoon of the oil for 5 minutes, or until wilted. Stir in rice, thyme and black pepper. Add 2 cups of the stock and bring to a boil. Cover and simmer over medium-low heat for 10 minutes. Stir in the peas, cereal, chicken and the remaining ½ cup stock.

Coat a 7" × 11" baking dish with no-stick spray. Spoon the chicken mixture into the dish. In a cup, combine the wheat germ or bread crumbs, Parmesan and the remaining 1 teaspoon oil. Sprinkle over the casserole. Bake at 350° for 15 minutes, or until the crumbs are lightly browned.

In a small bowl, stir together the yogurt or sour cream, parsley and hot-pepper sauce. Serve with the casserole.

Serves 4

Tip: *If you don't have a microwave, brown the chicken in a large no-stick frying pan that you've coated with no-stick spray. Also, if your frying pan or Dutch oven is ovenproof, you may simply sprinkle the crumbs over the chicken mixture and bake the casserole right in the pan—you'll have fewer dishes to clean up!*

Per serving: *400 calories, 6.7 g. fat (14% of calories), 13.2 g. dietary fiber, 53 mg. cholesterol, 531 mg. sodium*

SPICED FRUIT COMPOTE

Dried figs and prunes are especially high in dietary fiber. You can snack on them, or you can turn them into a delicious compote to serve over cooked cereal at breakfast or over nonfat frozen yogurt after dinner. Another idea is to mix fresh blueberries or raspberries into chilled compote, then top the mixture with nonfat vanilla yogurt and granola.

1 cup water	¼ teaspoon grated nutmeg
1 tea bag (preferably Earl Grey)	12 dried figs, halved
	12 bite-size pitted prunes
1½ cups cranberry juice cocktail	6 dried apricot halves, cut in half
½ teaspoon vanilla	¼ cup dried cranberries or currants
½ teaspoon ground cinnamon	

In a 2-quart saucepan over medium heat, bring the water to a boil. Remove from the heat, add the tea bag and let steep for 10 minutes. Remove the bag, pressing to extract the water.

Stir in the cocktail, vanilla, cinnamon and nutmeg. Bring to a boil. Add the figs, prunes, apricots and cranberries or currants. Cover and simmer over medium-low heat for 15 minutes, or until the fruit is plumped and soft. Serve warm or chilled.

Serves 6

Per serving: *221 calories. 0.6 g. fat (2% of calories), 5.6 g. dietary fiber, 0 mg. cholesterol, 10 mg. sodium*

CHAPTER 8

Low-Fat Eating

For All the Right Reasons

The last time was a charm for William J. Fanizzi. After surgeons inserted a balloon catheter into his chest to unclog his coronary arteries for a fourth time, Fanizzi finally vowed to get serious about cutting the fat out of his diet.

The 67-year-old former pediatrician was never what you'd call a high-fat fiend—his wife, Lucy, saw to that. But certain delicacies come with the territory when you're Italian: spicy sausages, pepperoni pizza, homemade meat and cheese lasagna and crispy garlic bread smothered with butter. Add to years of nutritional no-nos a family history of heart problems, and—Mama mia—you have the makings of a sick man.

Fanizzi's not alone. Many experts rate eating too much fat second only to smoking as the greatest threat to our health. More than 68 million Americans—over one in four—suffer some form of cardiovascular disease. As many as 34 million Americans are overweight—a condition linked to, among other conditions, arthritis, diabetes, gallstones, high blood pressure, high cholesterol and breathing ailments. Half a million Americans each year suffer a stroke. Roughly one in nine American women develops breast cancer. And *all* these diseases have been linked to fat.

But here's an offer you shouldn't refuse: Low-fat eating can dramatically improve your health—from lopping off excess pounds to actually lengthening your life. In fact, one study suggests that the number of Americans killed by heart disease could be cut by as much as 42,000 a year—if they reduced their fat intake a mere 7 percent. For most people, that's a goal that could be met (or even exceeded) by simply cutting out that daily doughnut.

"Most Americans who have health problems would not have them if they ate a low-fat diet," says William P. Castelli, M.D., director of the famed Framingham Heart Study.

THE TALE OF THE TARAHUMARA

For proof of the devastating—and rapid—effects of a high-fat diet, look no further than this unique study involving the superfit Tarahumara Indians of Mexico. World famous for their running ability, the Tarahumara—which literally means "fleet of foot"—are virtually untouched by fat-related diseases like heart disease. In fact, they're in such great shape, their favorite sport is a form of kickball that makes pro soccer look like a grade-school drill: The game covers no less than 100 to 150 miles. Their average meal is also a little different from ours: lots of complex carbohydrates like pinto beans and thick corn tortillas. If it's a holiday, they might also eat some meat.

A few years ago, researchers from Oregon Health Sciences University decided to see what would happen if the Tarahumaras ate some old-fashioned diner food. Of course, they don't have diners, so the food had to be specially provided: high-fat goodies like cheese, butter, lard and egg yolks. "In short, the same foods eaten by many Americans," says Martha P. McMurray, R.D., who spent two months with the Indians on the project.

FAT ON FILE

To plan your healthy eating strategy, you need to know what is low in fat and what is high. This chart can help you get started.

FOOD	PORTION	TOTAL FAT (g.)
Cornflakes	1 cup	0.0
Rice cakes	1	0.2
White rice	1 cup	0.4
Low-fat (1%) cottage cheese	1/4 cup	0.6
Pretzel	1	0.7
Spaghetti, cooked	1 cup	0.9
Bagel (egg or water)	1	1.4
Half-and-half	1 Tbsp.	1.7
Pancake, from mix	1	2.0
Buttermilk	1 cup	2.2
Chocolate-chip cookie	1 small	2.2
Low-fat (1%) milk	1 cup	2.6
Turkey breast, roasted, without skin	3 oz.	2.7
Chicken breast, roasted, without skin	3 oz.	3.1
Low-fat yogurt	1 cup	3.5
Toaster pastry	1	5.7

In just five weeks, these formerly sleek, svelte Indians had gained an average of about 8.5 pounds. What's worse, their LDL (bad) cholesterol levels jumped an average of 31 percent—a danger sign for heart disease.

Food	Portion	Total Fat (g.)
Leg of lamb, trimmed, roasted	3 oz.	6.6
French toast, homemade	1 slice	6.7
Egg scrambled with milk and butter	1	7.3
Blue cheese dressing, regular	1 Tbsp.	8.0
Monterey Jack cheese	1 oz.	8.5
Instant chocolate-flavored breakfast drink	1 cup	8.8
Cream of mushroom soup, condensed, made with water	1 cup	9.0
Chocolate-covered peanuts	1 oz.	11.6
Beef frankfurter	1	12.8
Apple pie, homemade	4 oz.	13.1
Turkey sandwich on whole-wheat bread	1	13.1
Roast beef sandwich on rye bread	1	13.8
Ground beef, up to 30% fat	3 oz.	14.0
Almonds, dry-roasted	1 oz.	14.8
Chicken breast, batter-fried	1 piece	14.8
Pork sausage, smoked	1 link	21.6
Ham and cheese sandwich on rye bread	1	27.5
Chef salad with dressing	average	30.3

Fat Facts

Why does life-threatening heart disease follow high cholesterol? Simply put, "a major determinant of one's cardiovascular health is diet," says Dean Ornish, M.D., author of *Dr. Dean Ornish's Program for Reversing Heart Disease* and director of the Preventive Medicine Research Institute in Sausalito, California.

Consider: Animal products like beef, milk and cheese, and tropical oils like coconut oil, contain saturated fat—the most dangerous kind, according to the American Heart Association (AHA).

Corn oil and other vegetable oils like sunflower, safflower and soybean oil contain polyunsaturated fat. Canola and olive oils are high in monounsaturated fat. But, unlike saturated fat, both help reduce LDL cholesterol.

Your body does need some fat—it plays an important role in making up the membranes or coatings that protect your cells. But it doesn't need much. As a result, loading up on high-fat foods is the equivalent of a sludge spill in your cardiovascular system.

Fat and cholesterol from the meal is dumped into the bloodstream. The waxy mixture then circulates in the blood until an injury to the wall of an artery—caused by factors such as smoking or high blood pressure—causes some of it to collect.

As the cholesterol piles up over the years, the flow of blood is gradually reduced, narrowing and sometimes hardening the artery. This process is called atherosclerosis. The reduced blood flow forces the heart to work even harder, causing another common ailment: high blood pressure.

If the buildup severely slows or stops blood flow to the brain, a stroke occurs. If blood is cut off to the heart, the victim suffers a heart attack.

THE ORNISH APPROACH

At one time, it was thought that the devastating effects of heart disease, were, unlike love, forever: That is, unless surgery could undo the damage. But in fact, research by several doctors, including Dr. Ornish, shows that eating the right foods can not only stop heart disease in its greasy tracks but can actually reverse it.

To prove Dr. Ornish's theory, a group of patients with severely clogged arteries were divided into two groups. Those in the first group were directed to follow a commonly prescribed method of fighting heart disease—eat less red meat, more fish and chicken, margarine instead of butter and no more than three eggs a week; exercise moderately and quit smoking.

The rest were put on the ultimate low-fat diet, a strict vegetarian plan designed by Dr. Ornish that's 70 to 75 percent complex carbohydrates (rice, pasta, grains, beans, fruit and vegetables), 15 to 20 percent protein and no more than 10 percent of calories from fat. That meant no oils or animal foods, except egg whites and nonfat dairy products like skim milk. Even avocados, nuts and seeds were off-limits because of their high fat content. Caffeine and alcohol were also forbidden under the program.

The men who participated in the study were tested and then retested a year later. The results, confirmed by a special artery-viewing technique called angiography: In 82 percent of the men in the extreme low fat group, coronary artery blockages had diminished. No such reversal was evident in the other treatment group.

It's no surprise, then, that Dr. Ornish urges his patients not only to exercise, give up smoking and reduce stress but also to cut fat from their diets.

LOW FAT, LOW CANCER

Cutting fat may do more than just keep your heart healthy. An extraordinary study of 6,500 mainland Chinese suggests that it may also help keep you cancer-free.

In 1983, a group of researchers headed by T. Colin Campbell, Ph.D., of Cornell University in Ithaca, New York, in conjunction with the Chinese Academy of Preventative

Medicine and Medical Sciences and the University of Oxford, began exploring the link between food, environment, social practices and diseases.

Although the study is expected to continue through the 1990s, early results, when contrasted by Dr. Campbell with disease data from the United States, shed new light on a likely fat/cancer connection.

While the Chinese actually average more calories daily (Them: 2,636, Us: 2,360), our diet is three times higher in calories from fat. Is it any coincidence that Americans have roughly five times the incidence of breast cancer? Not to Dr. Campbell. "Based on what we've found so far, a diet low in fat and animal foods is a diet that I would consider optimal for long-term health," he says.

An American study of 80,000 nurses failed to show a link between fat intake and breast cancer—at least between women consuming 38 percent of their calories from fat and those whose intake of fat was 29 percent of total calories. But that may be because the "low" fat levels weren't low enough. Many experts believe that protective benefits don't kick in until fat falls below 20 percent of total calories.

Another convincing piece of evidence on the fat/cancer connection comes from George L. Blackburn, M.D., Ph.D., associate professor of surgery at Harvard Medical School and chief of the Nutrition/Metabolism Laboratory at the Cancer Research Institute of New England Deaconess Hospital in Boston.

Dr. Blackburn says that the Japanese eat roughly half as much fat as we do, and their postmenopausal breast cancer rate is half ours.

His conclusion: "Studies that compare different cultures have found that people whose diets are the lowest in fat have the lowest breast cancer rates."

Researchers are also moving ever closer to linking fat with colon and rectal cancer. A Harvard study comparing the eating habits of 7,284 men found that those who ate low-fat, high-fiber diets were 3.7 times less likely to develop polyps in the colon and rectum polyps—tiny growths of tissue that can turn into cancer. However, men who regularly ate red meat instead of less-fatty chicken and fish had an 80 percent greater risk of developing polyps, the study shows.

Although more research needs to be done, cancer of the colon may just be another example of cell growth gone haywire from too much fat. Excess polyunsaturated fat (greater than 6 percent of daily calories) actually forces the colon cells to grow faster. Combine this with the lack of fiber commonly found in a high-fat diet, and the environment is right for the growth of potentially cancerous polyps, says Dr. Blackburn.

OBESITY: BIGGER, NOT BETTER

It's no secret that a high-fat diet will also make you a bigger (but not necessarily better) person.

What's less well known is that obesity itself is a killer. If you're 35 percent overweight, for example, your chances of premature death are 50 percent higher than normal. People who are 100 percent overweight are as much as 600 percent more likely to die prematurely.

What makes you pack on the pounds? Eating more calories than you burn. Here's the math: one gram of carbohydrate or protein is equal to four calories. One gram of dietary fat is equal to more than double that—over nine calories. Translation: A gram of fat takes twice as much effort to burn off as a gram of carbohydrate or protein.

Your body is also a tightwad as far as dietary fat is concerned; it would rather save (store) the fat than spend (burn) it. When it comes to storing fat, almost none of the fat you eat is burned in the conversion process from food to ready energy. By contrast, approximately 20 percent of complex carbohydrates disappear during the same transformation.

THESE HEALTHIER FOODS PASS THE TASTE TEST

In the interest of science—and healthy eating, of course—the editors of *Prevention* magazine put their taste buds on the line to determine just how good those newly marketed nonfat versions of traditionally fatty foods really are.

The good news: You don't have to sacrifice satisfaction for security. Nonfat sour cream tastes great on a baked potato and has the same "mouthfeel" as the real thing. A fat-free, three bean vegetarian chili with only 90 calories per serving proved zesty. A potato salad made with nonfat mayonnaise stumped half the staff when they were forced to choose between the nonfat version and one made with regular mayo. Nine out of ten preferred tuna salad made with water-packed tuna and nonfat mayo over the traditional version. Nonfat frozen yogurt, waffles and even pound cake all scored big on taste without the fat.

In checking out the "lite" fare at the local grocery, be aware that not all lite foods are low in fat. Lite potato chips may have less fat than regular brands but may still be high in fat. Lite bread can be the same old loaf—just sliced thinner.

To cut through the clutter, simply study the label. Many reduced-fat-and-calorie food labels list nutrient information for both that product and their full-fat regular version. If not, you'll have to look for the full-fat version on the shelf and compare. In any case, calorie and fat amounts for the lite version should be reduced to about 25 percent of the original. Also important: Any food that delivers three grams of fat or less per 100 calories is a good choice, whether you see "lite" on the label or not.

But your body *will* burn fat, provided you reduce the amount of fat you're eating, according to a Cornell University study. In fact, researchers found that women fed low-fat foods for 5½ months lost about ½ pound a week.

And no one was counting the calories of the food they were eating—feasts included special low-fat versions of ice cream, cookies and pizza. But they were counting fat. All of the foods contained less than 25 percent fat as a percentage of total calories.

"The weight loss is relatively slow, but it's persistent and should result in a 10 percent loss of body weight per year," says David Levitsky, Ph.D., professor of nutrition and psychology at Cornell.

THE DIABETES CONNECTION

Life-threatening weight gain may seem bad enough, but unfortunately, obesity can also create another health hazard—diabetes. In fact, diabetes has been so closely linked to obesity that the American Diabetes Association coined the term "diabesity" to describe the connection, according to W. Stephen Pray, Ph.D., a professor of pharmaceutics at the School of Pharmacy at Southwestern Oklahoma State University, who's written extensively on the topic.

About 10 percent of diabetics are born with the disease, which can lead to blindness, kidney failure, even death. But most cases are caused by overeating, says Dr. Pray.

When you constantly eat too much—a common problem associated with a high-fat diet—your pancreas gets a workout. This large insulin-producing gland is treated like a factory that's added extra shifts to keep up. After years of overproduction, your pancreas may simply shut down, unable to produce the insulin your body needs to turn your food into energy, says Dr. Pray.

To get production in the insulin factory back in gear, says Dr. Pray, many people need only stop overeating. The pancreas may soon return to normal, eliminating the need for

shots, pills, or other medication, he says. (If you have diabetes, always check with your doctor before making any
changes in diet or medication.)

KNOWLEDGE IS POWER

By now you're probably convinced that eating a low-fat
diet could be the best thing since shop-at-home television.
But perhaps you're wondering if you can develop a low-fat
eating plan and make it stick.

Don't worry. A landmark study for the National Cancer
Institute shows that you can—if you're willing to apply your
new-found nutritional knowledge.

Researchers divided 303 women into two groups. One received detailed nutritional information—like the kind found
in this book. The other got no nutrition news.

Within six months, the amateur nutrition experts had slashed
their dietary fat from 39 percent to 21 percent—an astonishing reduction! They were still sticking to their low-fat guns
two years later. The no-nutritional-news crowd, however,
showed virtually no improvement in their high-fat ways.

What follows is a collection of fat-busting techniques.
Read them and select a particular diet or combine some of
the tips to create your own personalized low-fat eating plan.

Whatever your approach, give yourself a chance to suc-
ceed: Changing lifelong habits takes time. Just ask William
Fanizzi. "If I can stay away from Italian sausages, anyone
can cut the amount of fat they're eating," he says.

ARE YOU READY TO TAKE THESE STEPS?

Although Step One and Step Two diets sound like a
weight-loss program developed by Fred Astaire and Ginger
Rogers, they're actually the AHA's approach to progressively reducing the amount of fat you're eating.

But be warned: Because it's less austere than other diets,

some experts—like Dr. Dean Ornish—have criticized the AHA's approach. The AHA counters that many people are unable to make the dramatic dietary changes necessary to conform with harsh low-fat eating plans.

Before beginning either the Step One or Step Two diets, the AHA recommends that you have your cholesterol checked and then checked again, one to eight weeks after the first test.

Your cholesterol level is considered desirable if it's below 200. If it's between 200 and 239 milligrams, it's borderline high. If your cholesterol is above 240 milligrams, it's considered high.

STEP ONE

Under the Step One diet, total fat intake is set at less than 30 percent of calories. Saturated fat should be less than 10 percent of calories. Polyunsaturated fat should not exceed 10 percent of calories. Cholesterol intake should not exceed 300 milligrams a day. Carbohydrates should make up 50 percent or more of calories, with emphasis on complex carbohydrates. The rest of the calories should come from protein.

Within three months of starting the Step One diet, your cholesterol level should decline 10 to 15 percent.

A sample Step One diet supplying 1,600 calories a day includes:

Breakfast: Half a fresh grapefruit, 1 cup corn flakes, 1 nectarine, 1 cup 1 percent milk.

Lunch: 2 ounces broiled chicken thigh, one ear of corn on the cob with 1 teaspoon unsalted margarine, tossed salad (1 cup lettuce, 6 cucumber slices, Italian salad dressing), 5 slices melba toast, ½ cup strawberry frozen yogurt.

Dinner: 4 ounces round steak, ½ cup canned tomatoes, half a green pepper, 2 tablespoons diced onions, 3 steamed broccoli spears, carrot-raisin salad (made with ½ cup shredded carrots, 2 tablespoons raisins and 2 teaspoons mayonnaise), 1 whole-wheat dinner roll, 1 teaspoon unsalted margarine, 1 cup 1 percent milk, a small piece of angel food cake.

STEP TWO

If stronger dietary medicine is called for, the Step Two diet is designed to bring your saturated fat consumption to a new low, reducing it to less than 7 percent of total calories. Meanwhile, cholesterol is cut back to 200 milligrams a day. Depending on the specific foods chosen, total fat intake may also decline.

A sample Step Two, 1,600-calorie-a-day diet includes:

Breakfast: 1 cup cantaloupe cubes, 1 cup corn flakes, 1¼ cups strawberries, 1 cup skim milk, 1 slice whole-wheat toast, 1 teaspoon unsalted margarine.

Lunch: A turkey sandwich (made with 3 ounces turkey breast, 2 slices whole-wheat bread, 2 teaspoons mayonnaise, 1 lettuce leaf, 2 slices tomato), a tossed salad (made with 1 cup lettuce, 1 sliced tomato and 2 tablespoons French dressing), 1 apple.

Dinner: 3 ounces roast beef, ½ cup new potatoes, 1 teaspoon unsalted margarine, ½ cup steamed green beans, ½ cup steamed carrots, tossed salad (made with 1 cup romaine lettuce, 1 sliced tomato and vinegar), 1 cup skim milk, ⅔ cup orange sherbet.

THE PRITIKIN PLAN

To the late Nathan Pritikin—creator of the Pritikin Plan—fat and cholesterol were tantamount to arsenic. So it's no surprise that his program advocates one of the leanest diets around, allowing no more than 10 percent of calories from fat. Complex carbohydrates—like rice, pasta or beans—are supposed to take up a whopping 75 to 80 percent of the entire diet, while protein makes up 10 to 15 percent, according to Monroe Rosenthal, M.D., medical director of the Ocean

View Medical Group at the Pritikin Longevity Center in Santa Monica, California.

The goal: to achieve a total cholesterol level of 100 plus your age, with 160 the maximum. "There's no question that the data is out there to support the dramatic benefits of a low-fat, low-cholesterol diet such as we advocate," says Dr. Rosenthal.

In the Pritikin Plan, foods are assigned to three categories: go, caution and stop, according to Dr. Rosenthal.

Go foods. These include fresh fruits, vegetables, whole grains, nonfat dairy products, legumes, fish and lean fowl or lean red meat, he says.

Caution foods. These foods, which should be eaten in moderation, include sweeteners like honey and molasses, decaffeinated coffee, tea, low-sodium soy sauce, low-fat dairy products, monounsaturated and polyunsaturated oils, unsalted nuts, avocados and olives.

Stop foods. These are forbidden because they significantly raise the risk of heart disease, he says. They include animal fats, butter, tropical oils, mayonnaise, fatty meats, whole dairy products, salt, coconuts and macadamia nuts, egg yolks and fried foods.

Daily allowances under the plan include two servings of nonfat yogurt or skim milk, six to eight servings of vegetables, three whole fruits, four to five servings of unrefined carbohydrates like whole-grain bread, pasta, rice, beans, peas or potatoes, and one 3½-ounce serving of lean meat, poultry or fish, Dr. Rosenthal says.

"The average participant gets a 23 percent reduction in total cholesterol in a period of three weeks. In the first week alone they usually get a 17 percent reduction. We frequently see people come in with high blood pressure and adult-onset diabetes who leave the center in a few weeks with normal blood pressure, normal blood sugar, no symptoms and no need for medication," he says.

FIGURING YOUR FAT

Now that you've passed your own personal (your name here) Fat Reduction Act, you need to know how much fat you're putting in your mouth on a day-to-day basis.

There are two ways of keeping track. To figure the percentage of fat calories in any food, check the label for both grams of fat and calories per serving, then plug them into this formula: grams of fat × 9 ÷ total calories = percent of calories from fat.

For example: The label on a bag of potato chips indicates that each 160-calorie serving has ten grams of fat. Simply multiply those ten grams by nine (90), then divide by total calories (160), which gives you 0.56 or 56 percent fat.

If you're not a math whiz, you can keep track of the amount of fat in your diet by simply adding up the grams of fat you eat during the day. Most foods list the grams of fat per serving on the label.

To help you set your daily fat goals, we've done the calculations for you. They're based on 25 percent of your usual caloric intake. On average, nondieting women take in about 2,000 calories per day and men eat about 2,700.

If you find you're running over your fat budget at any time, simply cut back on the amount of fat you eat during the rest of the day in snacks and meals. Or if you've blown it for the day, cut back the following day.

CALORIE INTAKE	FAT (g.)
1,200	33
1,400	39
1,600	44
1,800	50
2,000	56
2,200	61
2,400	67
2,600	72
2,800	78

Fat-Fighting Tips

No matter what diet you choose, you can boost your chances of success by making low-fat choices at the supermarket or restaurant and in the kitchen by using these tips, suggested by the American Cancer Society, the American Heart Association and other experts.

Shopping

Make a map. Plan your trip to the supermarket by writing down the items you need on a list. Avoid impulse purchases.

Fill 'er up before you go. Never shop on an empty stomach.

Read the label, set a better table. Ingredients are listed in order of quantity—if you see fat or oil in the top four, be wary.

Get lean. When buying beef, choose either USDA Choice or Select for the leanest cuts. Because they have more marbeling, USDA Prime meats contain more fat.

Avoid organ and lunch meats. Brains, heart, kidney, liver and sweetbreads are high in fat. Ditto for bologna, hot dogs and sausages.

Dining Out

Drop a quarter. If a restaurant is unfamiliar to you, call and ask about their menu and cooking techniques.

Belly up to the bar. The salad bar, that is. Stay away from mayonnaise-based items and fatty dressings or condiments such as cheese, bacon bits and croutons.

Have it your way. Don't be afraid to special order entrées (broiled instead of fried) or substitute (salad instead of fries). Airlines also offer low-fat meals if you order ahead.

Bag it. Take home the remainder of a large portion of meat in a doggie bag and save it for another meal.

Say (no) cheese. Bag the cheese (and mayo) the next time you order a burger. Or get a chicken sandwich instead—just make sure it's not deep-fried.

Go topless. If an entrée is served with breading, topping or sauce, remove it before eating.

Be a crust-buster. If a fruit pie is served, avoid fat by eating the filling and leaving the crust.

REVISING RECIPES

Swap your sour cream. Puree low-fat or nonfat cottage cheese or light ricotta cheese. Mix in an equal amount of nonfat yogurt and a squeeze of lemon.

Substitute your white sauce. Puree low-fat or nonfat cottage cheese, thin with skim milk and mix with sautéed onions and garlic plus basil.

Banish eggs and oil. Buttermilk works just as well in Caesar salad dressing.

Quit putting cream in creamy soups. Cook your choice of vegetables with cubed potatoes or precooked white beans and defatted stock.

Discover herbs. Fresh cilantro, dill, garlic, parsley and chives are tasty replacements for those old, unhealthy standbys like oil and salt.

Stock up on chicken stock. Defatted chicken stock (scoop fat off the top after leaving in the refrigerator overnight) can be strained through cheesecloth and frozen in an ice cube tray for later use.

Whip up some (no-fat) whipped cream. Pour ⅓ cup skim milk into a small stainless steel or copper bowl. Set it in the freezer until ice crystals just begin to form (15 to 20 minutes). Thicken with a hand-held electric mixer by beating in ⅓ cup instant nonfat dry milk. Continue to beat on high until soft peaks form (about 2 minutes). If you like the cream sweetened, add 1 tablespoon honey and beat until stiff peaks form, about 2 minutes more. Use within 20 minutes.

Cooking Meat

Start lean. After browning meat, make sure to pour off the fat. Ground meat is generally higher in fat than unground meat.

Make your burgers lose weight. To get really lean burgers, pick a piece of beef and then have your butcher trim the fat before grinding. Or put the piece of meat in the freezer briefly when you get home—even hidden fat turns white when chilled. Then trim it yourself and grind in a food processor.

Deal the right serving. Limit beef, pork and lamb servings to about 3½ ounces (a little larger than a deck of playing cards).

Marinate for your plate. Lean cuts don't have to be tough—marinate them in citrus juice and herbs, low-sodium soy sauce, vinegar or even yogurt. The acid in these marinades will help tenderize the meat and make it more tasty.

Rub it in. Basting meats with low-sodium broth, pineapple juice or low-sodium soy sauce will eliminate the need for added fat for cooking.

Do some stovetop grilling. Allow fat to drain during cooking by using a stovetop grill pan.

Broil (without oil). Position the pan so the meat is three to five inches from the heat, and use a broiling rack and drip pan.

Make the most of your roast. Larger, tougher cuts of meat undergo a change for more flavor in dry, 350° oven heat.

Don't brood—braise. Also good for tough, lean cuts. Braised meat is browned and then simmered in liquid for an hour or more.

Make clay. A clay cooker is a mini-oven in an oven, slowly roasting while sealing in moisture. The cooker and lid must be submerged in water before use. Don't preheat the oven—it could cause the cooker to crack. Allow the cooker to cool overnight before washing. Also, don't use soap during cleaning. The cooker may absorb the soap and then release it into food.

Wok this way. Stir-frying gives tough lean meat a second chance. Marinate before using.

Cut and fan. Slice meat thinly and then fan slices so it looks like you have an even larger serving.

Add crumbs. Adding one part fine bread crumbs for every two parts seasoned ground beef will cut down on the amount of fat you receive from each serving.

Cool it. After making stew or soup containing meat, refrigerate until the fat congeals and then scoop it off.

Favor chicken. Most poultry is lower in fat than red meat.

Add fish to your dish. Replace red meat with fish, which is lower in total fat. Among the best: cod, catfish, flounder, shark, haddock, perch and grouper.

Go meatless. Dry beans, peas, lentils and tofu are good alternate sources of protein if combined with low-fat dairy products.

CUTTING BACK ON OIL

Divide and conquer. Use half the amount of oil called for in a recipe. Most of the time it won't change the way the dish turns out.

Paint fat away. Instead of pouring cooking oil into a pan, apply it with a brush or paper towel. All you need to do is add a thin coating to prevent sticking.

Get serious about sautéing. Watch your technique when sautéing or stir-frying. If you keep the heat high and stir constantly, you will need little or no oil to keep food from sticking. Or simply use a nonstick skillet.

Hit the switch. Instead of using oil, sauté with broth, juice or water.

Bake the nonstick way. Coat muffin tins or cookie sheets with a no-stick spray instead of oil, or use no-stick baking pans.

Mix and match. In recipes that call for a very flavorful fat—like bacon fat—use one-quarter the required amount. Make up the rest of the measure by using one-quarter unsaturated vegetable oil like canola, and for the remaining half substitute water, vinegar or stock.

Pick a new flavor. Experiment with darker, less refined oils such as walnut, grapeseed or fruity olive oil in place of the blander, highly refined ones. You can use less of them because they have a definite flavor.

Get off the stick. Liquid margarine has less hydrogenated oil—a source of saturated fat—than stick margarine. And because you don't have to wait for it to melt on toast, you use less.

Don't get creamed. Cream substitutes like nondairy creamers, sour cream substitutes and whipped toppings are high in saturated fat, according to the AHA, because they often contain coconut, palm or palm-kernel oil. Avoid them.

Pop off. No oil is needed to cook popcorn when you use an air popper. Simply follow the manufacturer's directions.

High-Nutrition Recipes

LIGHTLY BREADED HALIBUT

Fish should be a staple in the low-fat kitchen. If one of the ways you enjoy it is breaded and fried, you'll like this version, which gives the same crisp results with only a fraction of the fat. Serve the fish with corn on the cob, roasted or baked potatoes and coleslaw made using nonfat mayonnaise or nonfat yogurt.

1	pound haddock fillet	½	cup dry bread crumbs
2	tablespoons unbleached flour	½	teaspoon dried oregano
1	egg white	¼	teaspoon paprika
1	tablespoon water	¼	teaspoon ground black pepper

Rinse the fish and pat it dry. Cut it into 8 equal pieces. Dredge the pieces in the flour.

In a shallow bowl, whisk together the egg white and water until well mixed but not frothy.

On a sheet of wax paper, combine the bread crumbs, oregano, paprika and pepper.

Dip each piece of fish into the egg white, letting the excess drip off. Then dredge in the bread crumbs, coating the piece thoroughly.

Coat a no-stick baking sheet with no-stick spray. Add the fish, leaving space between the pieces. Lightly coat the top of the fish with no-stick spray. Bake at 375° for 10 to 12 minutes, or until the fish is crisp and flakes easily with a fork.

Serves 4
Per serving: *192 calories, 3.3 g. fat (16% of calories), 0.6 g. dietary fiber, 36 mg. cholesterol, 168 mg. sodium*

GRILLED PORK MEDALLIONS WITH BRAISED BEANS

You might think pork has no place in a low-fat diet, but many cuts are quite lean. The tenderloin, in particular, is very low in fat and makes an elegant dinner. This recipe was created by master chef Victor Gielisse for the American Cancer Society's educational program, the Great American Food Fight Against Cancer. The flageolets called for are tender French kidney beans that range in color from pale green to creamy white. They're available dried in many specialty stores. If you can't find them, substitute white beans, such as pea beans, haricots or canellinis.

1	pound dried flageolet beans, soaked overnight	2¼	cups defatted chicken stock
1	tablespoon canola oil	4	tomatoes, peeled, seeded and diced
1	leek, white part only, cleaned and chopped		
1	tablespoon sherry extract (optional)	1	pork tenderloin (about 20 ounces), trimmed of all visible fat
1	teaspoon dried tarragon	2	zucchini, julienned
1½	tablespoons chopped fresh parsley	2	yellow summer squash, julienned
¼	teaspoon ground black pepper		

Drain the beans and place in a 4-quart pot. Add cold water to cover. Bring to a boil, then simmer over medium-low heat for 1 hour, or until almost tender. Drain and set aside.

In a 2-quart saucepan over medium heat, warm the oil. Add the leeks and sauté for 1 minute. Add the sherry extract, if desired, and cook for 1 minute. Add the tarragon, parsley, pepper and 2 cups of the stock. Bring to a boil.

Add the beans. Reduce the heat to low and simmer for 20 minutes, stirring occasionally. Add the tomatoes and heat through; keep warm.

Meanwhile, cut the pork into 6 equal medallions. Grill or broil until just cooked through, about 4 minutes per side. Keep warm.

In a large no-stick frying pan over medium-high heat, warm the remaining ¼ cup stock. Add the zucchini and squash. Sauté for 3 to 5 minutes, or until crisp-tender.

To serve, arrange the zucchini mixture in a circle around the outer edges of dinner plates. Use a slotted spoon to ladle the bean mixture in the center. Top with the pork.

Serves 6
Per serving: *440 calories, 6.5 g. fat (13% of calories), 7.8 g. dietary fiber, 62 mg. cholesterol, 99 mg. sodium*

LEAN BEEF STROGANOFF

Beef stroganoff has a reputation for being high in fat, largely because of the rich sour cream it contains and the well-marbled cuts of beef used. This version uses ground top round, which is very lean, and a light sauce made with evaporated skim milk. If buying ready-ground meat, choose beef labeled 92% fat-free. This recipe was created by Houston chef Raymond Potter for the American Cancer Society.

12 ounces ground lean top round	1 cup evaporated skim milk
2 cups thinly sliced mushrooms	½ cup water
1 cup diced sweet red peppers	¼ cup cornstarch
1 cup sliced scallions	½ teaspoon cracked black pepper
¼ cup diced onions	12 ounces medium no-yolk egg noodles
1 tablespoon olive oil	¼ cup minced fresh parsley

In a large no-stick frying pan over medium-high heat, brown the meat, breaking up the pieces. Line a platter with a triple layer of paper towels. Spoon the beef onto the paper so any excess fat can be absorbed.

Wipe out the frying pan with a paper towel. Place the pan over medium-high heat, sauté the mushrooms, peppers, scallions and onions in the oil for 10 minutes, or until nicely browned. Add the drained meat to the pan. Pour in the milk and bring to a simmer over medium heat.

In a cup, combine the water and cornstarch until dissolved. Pour into the pan. Stir until the mixture thickens. Season with the pepper.

Meanwhile, cook the noodles in a large pot of boiling water until just tender. Drain and stir into the beef mixture. Sprinkle with the parsley.

Serves 4

Per serving: *490 calories, 9.6 g. fat (18% of calories), 4 g. dietary fiber, 67 mg. cholesterol, 164 mg. sodium*

CREAMY PASTA SHELLS

Most pasta sauces, such as Alfredo and béchamel, are loaded with fat from butter, cream and large amounts of cheese. This light sauce has a surprise ingredient: cauliflower, which has a mild taste and smooth texture when cooked and pureed.

12 ounces cauliflower florets	¼ teaspoon dried basil
1 large onion, sliced into thin wedges	¼ teaspoon ground black pepper
½ cup thinly sliced green peppers	⅛ teaspoon grated nutmeg
1 teaspoon olive oil	1⅓ cups low-fat milk
12 sun-dried tomatoes, thinly sliced	1 tablespoon lemon juice
1 cup sliced pimientos	¼ cup grated Parmesan cheese
½ teaspoon dried oregano	8 ounces medium pasta shells

Steam the cauliflower for 15 minutes, or until very tender.

Meanwhile, in a large no-stick frying pan over medium-high heat, sauté the onions and peppers in the oil for 5 minutes. Add the tomatoes and cook for 5 minutes. Stir in the pimientos, oregano, basil, pepper and nutmeg. Cover and keep warm over low heat.

Transfer the cauliflower to a blender. Add the milk and lemon juice. Blend until smooth. Transfer to a 2-quart saucepan and warm over medium heat. Stir in the Parmesan. Pour over the vegetables.

In a large pot of boiling water, cook the shells until just tender. Drain. Serve topped with the vegetable mixture.

Serves 4
Per serving: *361 calories, 5.9 g. fat (11% of calories), 5 g. dietary fiber, 11 mg. cholesterol, 192 mg. sodium*

CHAPTER 9

Cholesterol

A Dietary Troublemaker

The media howls about it. Your doctor warns you about it and your daughter tells you she watches for it as intently as if it were a mysterious stranger prowling the neighborhood.

In fact, it's pretty hard to find someone who *isn't* talking about their cholesterol. But what are we really doing about it? Apparently not as much as we should. While Americans are seemingly obsessed about this strange-sounding substance swimming around in their arteries, far too many of us are running around with cholesterol levels higher than 200—the number doctors agree is the safe limit for cholesterol in the blood.

And it's really not all that surprising, say some experts, considering the fact that cholesterol—while plenty talked about—is still one of the most misunderstood hot topics in health. After all, it's not easy to avoid something you can't even see. And then there's all that talk about good cholesterol and bad cholesterol. And about fat and cholesterol. Or wait, could it be that fat *is* cholesterol?

CHOLESTEROL DOES MAKE A DIFFERENCE

It's time to be in the dark no longer. We're about to set you on the strong and healthy path to cholesterol knowledge.

First, the hard truth. Eating too many foods rich in cholesterol, such as meat (especially organ meats), eggs and whole-milk dairy products, is a major contributor to heart disease, says Richard Shekelle, Ph.D., professor of epidemiology at the University of Texas Health Science Center in Houston.

And the evidence is spread far and wide.

In a classic 19-year follow-up study of 1,900 middle-aged men working at a Western Electric plant in Chicago, Dr. Shekelle and his colleagues linked dietary cholesterol to increased risk of fatal heart attacks. They found, for example, that if a man who was consuming 2,500 calories daily ate an additional 500 milligrams of cholesterol a day—the amount in two large egg yolks—he was 90 percent more likely to die of a heart attack than a man who didn't eat that extra cholesterol.

In addition, the researchers estimated that men who ate the lower amount of cholesterol had a life expectancy that was nearly 3½ years longer on average than that of men who regularly ate the higher amount of cholesterol.

"Our study and several other studies have found that dietary cholesterol does make a difference in the risk of developing a heart attack," Dr. Shekelle says.

In yet another major study, researchers followed the dietary habits of more than 8,000 Japanese-American men living in Honolulu. After ten years, the researchers concluded that, in addition to eating more protein, fat and saturated fat, the men who developed heart disease ate more cholesterol-rich foods than the men who didn't.

And, in a 20-year comparison study of men living in Ireland and Irish-Americans living in Boston, researchers found that those who died of heart disease were more likely to have consumed high amounts of saturated fat and cholesterol.

Overall, these studies indicate for every additional 200 milligrams of cholesterol you regularly consume per 1,000 calories, you increase your risk of heart disease by 30 percent, according to Jeremiah Stamler, M.D., a professor emeritus at the Northwestern University Medical School in Chicago.

THE GOOD, THE BAD AND THE DIFFERENCE

Now you know you were right all along—you *should* be concerned about your cholesterol. But what exactly is it that makes it such a menace to the body? After all, you do remember learning in biology class that cholesterol is an essential component of life. And it's true. Your body needs cholesterol to make cell membranes, hormones and bile acids. But your body makes all the cholesterol it will ever need on its own. The rest—meaning the cholesterol in the food that you eat—is pure excess. Here's what happens.

Cholesterol gets around in your bloodstream wrapped in substances called lipoproteins—packages of protein molecules and triglycerides (a type of fat). Low-density lipoprotein, commonly called LDL cholesterol, is the bad kind of cholesterol you've been hearing about. Unfortunately, it typically makes up about 70 percent of the cholesterol in the body. It's the one responsible for forming the plaque that builds up on artery walls, creating dangerous blockages that may choke off the blood supply and cause a heart attack.

But, yes, there is a good cholesterol. It goes by the name high-density lipoprotein, or HDL cholesterol. As HDL circulates through your blood it heads for the liver. There it is converted into bile acids or excreted from the body. On its journey it picks up LDL cholesterol—but only as much as it can handle—and takes it along out of the body. That's what's so good about it. And that's why, researchers have found, that the more HDL you have, the better off you will be. In fact, doctors now feel that the individual values of your HDL and LDL are a better indicator of heart health than total cholesterol. An HDL level of 70 or higher is considered protective against heart disease.

"Eating cholesterol raises cholesterol in your body. There's no question about that," says Daniel Eisenberg, M.D., a Los Angeles cardiologist and assistant clinical professor at the University of Southern California School of Medicine. And American cholesterol levels are typically too high because we eat too much cholesterol—an average of 400 to 500 milligrams per day in meats and animal products such as ice cream, cheese and butter. And the excess ends up exactly where we don't want it: on our artery walls. Experts estimate that for every 100 milligrams of dietary cholesterol consumed per 1,000 calories on a regular basis, blood cholesterol rises by about ten points.

THE FAT CONNECTION

Of course it's foolish to think that we can totally avoid cholesterol. But we can limit it. According to both the American Heart Association and the National Cholesterol Education Program, the safe limit for cholesterol consumption is less than 300 milligrams a day. And the easiest way to reach that goal is to restrict your intake of saturated fat. For saturated fat raises blood cholesterol even more than dietary cholesterol does. And both saturated fat and cholesterol are usually found in the same foods.

Studies show that adhering to a low-fat eating program has helped many people lower their cholesterol by 10 to 15 percent and reduce their estimated risk of coronary heart disease by 20 to 30 percent.

If you have any excess cholesterol in your body, it's safe to assume that two-thirds of it started out as saturated fat on your plate, says William P. Castelli, M.D., director of the Framingham Heart Study.

HOW FOODS MEASURE UP

You can't see it, smell it or taste it. So how do you know when you're eating something that contains cholesterol? Well, here's a big clue: Cholesterol is found in any food of animal origin—including beef, chicken, fish, milk and eggs. The key is to limit the amount of those foods you eat and consume those that have the least amount of cholesterol and saturated fat. The following table ranks the cholesterol and saturated fat content of some common foods.

FOOD	PORTION	CHOLESTEROL (mg.)	SATURATED FAT(g.)
Pork kidney	3 oz.	408	1.3
Beef liver	3 oz.	331	1.6
Beef kidney	3 oz.	329	0.9
Quiche Lorraine	1 slice	285	23.2
Egg	1	212	1.6
French vanilla ice cream, soft serve	1 cup	153	13.5
Veal cutlet	3 oz.	115	1.6
Waffle	1 (7")	102	4.0
Bearnaise sauce	½ cup	99	20.9
Hollandaise sauce	½ cup	94	20.9
Liverwurst	3 oz.	90	6.0
Chuck roast	3 oz.	86	2.7
Turkey bologna	3 slices	84	4.4
Corned beef	3 oz.	83	5.4
Lamb loin chop	3 oz.	81	2.9
Duck, without skin	3 oz.	76	3.6
Salmon	3 oz.	74	1.6
Chicken breast, roasted	3 oz.	73	0.9
Extra-lean ground beef	3 oz.	71	5.5
T-bone steak	3 oz.	68	3.5
Haddock	3 oz.	63	0.1

FOOD	PORTION	CHOLESTEROL (mg.)	SATURATED FAT(g.)
Rainbow trout	3 oz.	62	0.7
Vanilla ice cream, regular	1 cup	59	8.9
Beef, eye of round, lean	3 oz.	59	1.5
Turkey breast	3 oz.	59	0.9
Whole-milk ricotta cheese	1/2 cup	58	9.4
Salami	3 oz.	55	7.7
Egg noodles	1 cup	53	0.5
Cod	3 oz.	47	0.1
Bran muffin, homemade	1	41	1.2
Snapper	3 oz.	40	0.3
Whole milk	1 cup	35	5.6
Halibut	3 oz.	35	0.4
Yellow layer cake w/icing	1 slice	33	2.8
Fig bars	4	27	0.9
Butter	2 tsp.	21	4.8
2% milk	1 cup	18	2.9
Cottage cheese, creamed	$^1\!/_2$ cup	17	3.2
Mozzarella cheese	1 oz.	16	2.8
Sherbet	1 cup	14	2.4
Low-fat yogurt, plain	1 cup	14	2.3
Buttermilk	1 cup	9	1.3
Cream pie	1 slice	8	15.0
Skim milk	1 cup	4	0.3
Pudding pops	1	1	2.5
Corn chips	1 oz.	0	1.5
Margarine, stick	2 tsp.	0	1.5
Popcorn, air-popped	1 cup	0	trace
Gelatin	$^1\!/_2$ cup	0	0

"My bias is that saturated fat is as bad or even worse for blood cholesterol levels than dietary cholesterol is," says Carl Lavie, M.D., a co-director of cardiac rehabilitation and prevention at the Ochsner Medical Institution in New Orleans.

"Fortunately, most foods that are high in saturated fat are also high in cholesterol. So if you avoid one type of food because of saturated fat, you're probably leaving cholesterol out of your diet, too," says Alan Chait, M.D., past chairman of the American Heart Association Nutrition Committee.

But there are some foods that have high amounts of cholesterol *without* saturated fat. Seafood and eggs are the best example. Eggs are very low in fat but, ounce for ounce, contain more cholesterol than any other food.

How to Avoid Shell Shock

The fact that eggs are laden with cholesterol is hardly news to anyone anymore. Egg consumption in the United States has dropped more than 20 percent since 1967. Americans have gone from eating 316 eggs annually per person to 249. That still averages out to more than 20 dozen eggs a year per person. Yes, you probably eat more eggs than you think. For even if you don't break eggs into a pan for your morning breakfast, you can still get more than your share in baked goods and other prepared foods you eat every day.

And we're not just talking chickens here. Fish eggs such as roe or caviar also have large amounts of cholesterol.

Nature planned it that way. "Cholesterol is absolutely vital to creating and maintaining cell walls," says George Seperich, Ph.D., a food scientist and associate professor of agribusiness at Arizona State University in Tempe. "So when you eat the egg of any species, you're consuming something that is going to have a high amount of cholesterol.

"Egg consumption is something you need to be aware of

if you want to keep your cholesterol consumption in check," he says. Here's how.

Opt for a substitute. Some food manufacturers are marketing egg substitutes that are cholesterol-free and are lower in fat than whole eggs. They're all made with egg whites and have vitamins and minerals added to replace the nutrients of the yolk. Because these egg substitutes can be frozen, a package can be stored up to a year. They can be used in any dish requiring eggs, including casseroles, pancakes and desserts. Unfortunately, you have to be willing to pay: Egg substitutes can cost up to three times as much as regular eggs.

Try making your own. As an alternative, try making your own homemade substitutes, suggest William Connor, M.D., and his wife, Sonja Connor, R.D., authors of *The New American Diet System*. To do it, put six egg whites, ¼ cup powdered nonfat milk and one tablespoon oil in a mixing bowl and then blend until smooth. You can use the mixture for cooking and baking just as you would regular eggs. (About ¼ cup equals one whole egg.) You can store it in a jar in your refrigerator for up to one week, or freeze it.

Two halves are better than a whole. Another alternative when baking is to use two egg whites in place of each whole egg called for in the recipe. To replace some of the fat that would come from the yolk and may be needed for a successful outcome, add one teaspoon of vegetable oil for every yolk not used.

A healthier omelet. If you occasionally still want to use some whole eggs—to make scrambled eggs or omelets—then try using three egg whites with just one egg yolk.

KNOW THE HIDING PLACES

Once you get beyond eggs, knowing where to find the cholesterol in food tends to get a little difficult for most people, says Mary Felando, R.D., a cardiovascular nutrition

NIBBLE AWAY AT CHOLESTEROL

If you're serious about watching your cholesterol, then changing *how often* you eat may be as important as altering *what* you eat.

Small meals eaten frequently during the day may help keep your cholesterol under control and reduce your heart attack risk, according to researchers at the University of Toronto in Ontario.

In a preliminary study of seven men who each ate 17 meals totaling 2,500 to 3,000 calories a day, the researchers found that after two weeks total cholesterol levels dropped 9 percent and LDL cholesterol (the "bad" cholesterol) fell 14 percent.

The researchers believe that large meals cause the release of high levels of insulin. That, in turn, seems to stimulate cholesterol production by the liver. Eating frequent but smaller meals apparently short-circuits that process, says Thomas Wolever, M.D., Ph.D., a coauthor of the study and associate director of the Risk Factor Modification Center at St. Michael's Hospital in Toronto.

Of course, eating 17 meals a day isn't practical for most people—the men who did it ate prepackaged meals and carried alarm clocks to remind themselves when to eat. Moreover, Dr. Wolever thinks it would take discipline to avoid overeating. (In the study, a typical "meal" was either a couple of cookies, an apple or a half-sandwich.)

A later study of 2,000 people by researchers at the University of California at San Diego found drops in both total and LDL cholesterol in those eating four or more meals a day. "The key is taking whatever you're eating and spreading it out throughout the day. So eating five meals a day is probably better than eating less than three," Dr. Wolever says. "Many people tend to eat one big meal a day. I think that eating three evenly sized meals is fine. But if your three meals are a cup of coffee for breakfast, a muffin for lunch and a huge meal at dinner, that's the wrong way to go about it."

specialist in Los Angeles. But it's really quite easy. Just think animal. Cholesterol is only found in foods derived from animal sources—such as beef, lamb, pork, poultry, fish, shellfish, milk, butter, ice cream. You name it.

"But some people aren't aware of that connection," says Felando. "Many people who come to see me think that chicken doesn't have any cholesterol. So they're eating half a chicken every day for dinner," she says. "But in reality, chicken is a very high cholesterol food." The fat/cholesterol connection in food isn't so strong that you can automatically assume that the less fat, the less dietary cholesterol. It's not that simple.

A three-ounce piece of broiled chicken, for example, has 73 milligrams of cholesterol. But the same size portion of broiled T-bone steak has about 68 milligrams of cholesterol, even though it has more saturated fat.

Organ meats hit the top of the list as the foods containing the most cholesterol. Pork kidneys, for example, have more than 400 milligrams per three-ounce serving.

Shellfish, particularly shrimp, have always taken a bad rap for being a bad-for-you food because of all their cholesterol. In fact, shrimp's pretty high on the list at 166 milligrams for a three-ounce serving. And other fish, such as salmon and pollock, have about as much cholesterol as chicken. But these fish and shellfish have an advantage that meat doesn't: They are all low in saturated fat. And remember, saturated fat is the primary cholesterol elevator in the bloodstream.

In fact, there is another reason to favor fish and shellfish over other cholesterol-laden foods. They also contain fish oil, also known as omega-3 fatty acids, which have actually been shown to have a cholesterol-lowering effect in the body.

BE CHOLESTEROL CONSCIOUS

Unless you intend to become a strict vegetarian, it's almost impossible to avoid cholesterol entirely. But you can

TAKE THE SURF OVER THE TURF

If you feel guilty about eating shellfish because it's high in cholesterol, here's good news.

"You're better off eating shrimp, lobster and crab than you are eating Cheddar cheese, beef, pork or lamb," says William P. Castelli, M.D., director of the famed Framingham Heart Study. "And the other shellfish—oysters, clams and scallops—are the best 'meats' you could possibly eat because they're the vegetarians of the sea and are very low in saturated fat and cholesterol."

In fact, researchers at the University of Washington who fed 18 men six types of shellfish for 21 days in place of cheese, meat and eggs found that some shellfish had a positive influence on blood cholesterol. Among the men who ate crabs, clams, mussels and oysters, levels of harmful LDL cholesterol, dropped. Levels of good HDL cholesterol rose. Shrimp and squid didn't improve cholesterol levels, but they didn't harm them either. Overall, the researchers concluded that shellfish—especially when replacing fatty meats—are good for the heart.

And there's more good news for seafood lovers. Because of advances in testing methods, shellfish have been found to contain less cholesterol than was once believed.

Here's how the most popular varieties of shellfish stack up. For comparison, a three-ounce serving of lean ground beef has 74 milligrams of cholesterol and 6.2 grams of saturated fat.

SEAFOOD (3 OZ.)	CHOLESTEROL (mg.)	SATURATED FAT (g.)
Shrimp	166	0.25
Oysters	93	1.07
Crab, blue	85	0.19
Lobster	61	0.09
Clams	57	0.16
Mussels	48	0.72
Scallops	28	0.07

keep within healthy limits by becoming a savvy cholesterol watcher.

Cut back on meat. Of course, the most obvious way to beat dietary cholesterol is to eliminate meats from your diet entirely. Short of that, try eating less meat.

"If you want to include animal foods in your diet, you should limit them to three or four ounces a day. That's one serving about the size of a deck of cards," Felando says. "You should choose fish most often. I'd say eat it at least three times a week."

Concentrate on carbos. Eating lots of plant foods such as beans, oat bran, grains, fruits, vegetables and potatoes is a good dietary strategy because they contain no cholesterol unless they're prepared with dairy products such as milk, butter or cheese.

"If you're not eating a lot of starchy (carbohydrate) foods, you're not really following a low-fat, low-cholesterol diet. You should be having at least two to four servings of starches with every meal," Felando says. "I know it's hard for people to understand that because our mothers taught us to eat roast beef, but never to eat bread and mashed potatoes at the same meal. Even now, when my mother comes over and I serve corn and potatoes for dinner, she'll say, 'Isn't this two starches together?' But it's really okay because the people in nations that eat a lot of starches are the people who don't have problems with cholesterol."

And beans and oats add a special punch: Eating them has been shown to help bring cholesterol down.

Check out those label claims. When you're shopping, read food labels and be cautious about product claims, says Dr. Lavie. A product such as potato chips, for example, may be labeled cholesterol-free, but may contain significant amounts of saturated fat which you now know, raises the cholesterol level in your body.

TAKE THE CHOLESTEROL PLUNGE

If making a few dietary changes can lower your cholesterol a bit, what kind of effort does it take to send your cholesterol diving?

"The key factor is diet," says Monroe Rosenthal, M.D., medical director of the Ocean View Medical Group at the Pritikin Longevity Center in Santa Monica, California. "When you push dietary cholesterol and saturated fat way down below a certain threshold, you'll see a dramatic linear response in the blood."

Exactly what that threshold is, no one knows for sure. But Dr. Rosenthal believes that it's less than 100 milligrams of cholesterol a day—a level that's consistent with the Pritikin Eating Plan, containing less than 10 percent of calories from fat. (The average American eats about 500 milligrams of cholesterol a day in a diet that contains about 40 percent fat).

"We do know that if someone switches from a high-fat diet to a somewhat modified diet, the effect on blood cholesterol is usually minimal," Dr. Rosenthal says. "But if that person then goes from a moderately reduced-fat diet to the Pritikin Eating Plan, in which cholesterol and saturated fat are drastically cut, blood cholesterol could take a steep drop."

On the Pritikin Eating Plan, participants are advised to consume no more than one $3\frac{1}{2}$-ounce serving of lean meat, poultry, or fish and two cups nonfat dairy products per day. (Egg yolks and organ meats are not allowed.) Generally, the focus of the diet consists of fresh fruits and vegetables, whole grains, cereals, legumes and potatoes.

The result? The average cholesterol drop at the Pritikin Longevity Center in a 21-day period is a dramatic 23 percent. But many Pritikin participants do even better than that, Dr. Rosenthal says. In some cases, cholesterol levels have tumbled as much as 40 percent in three weeks.

"Only by being a skeptical and educated consumer can you cut through some of that. You need to be wary," says Karen Glanz, Ph.D., a professor of health education at Temple University in Philadelphia.

Be flexible. The secret is not to be too rigid about what you eat from day to day, suggests Karen Donato, R.D., coordinator of nutrition education and special initiatives for the National Heart, Lung, and Blood Institute in Bethesda, Maryland.

"It's not any one food, one meal or one day that's going to cause a high blood cholesterol problem," she says. "It's the cumulative effect that's the concern. In planning meals, you should try to average things out so that over a span of several days you're consuming less than 300 milligrams of dietary cholesterol daily. So if you have 600 milligrams one day, 200 the next, 250 the day after, and 150 the following day, it will still average out properly.

"That's the moral of the story here," she says. "We're not telling people that they can never eat eggs, cheese, meat or other foods that have saturated fat and cholesterol in them. We're not telling them that they have to totally revamp the way they eat. But there are some subtle dietary changes that they can make that will bring their cholesterol levels down."

High-Nutrition Recipes

CHICKEN AND AVOCADO

Avocados have such a rich, creamy texture that you'd swear they were loaded with cholesterol—but, of course, only animal products contain the substance. This very easy recipe pairs them with chicken breasts, capers and quick-cooking brown rice. One thing you should know about avocados, though, is they contain a fair amount of fat, so you should save them for special occasions.

1¼ cups defatted chicken stock	1 tablespoon olive oil
	½ cup chopped pimientos
1 cup quick-cooking brown rice	2 tablespoons capers, rinsed
4 boneless, skinless chicken breast halves (4 ounces each)	½ cup lemon juice
	¼ cup minced fresh parsley
1 tablespoon unbleached flour	½ avocado, thinly sliced

In a 2-quart saucepan over medium heat, bring the stock to a boil. Add the rice. Cover and cook over medium-low heat for 10 minutes, until all the stock has been absorbed. Fluff with a fork and keep warm.

Meanwhile, dredge the chicken in the flour. In a large no-stick frying pan over medium-high heat, warm the oil. Add the chicken and brown for about 5 minutes per side, or until cooked through. Transfer to a plate and set aside.

Add the pimientos and capers to the pan. Sauté for 2 minutes. Add the lemon juice and cook over medium heat for 2 minutes, scraping up browned bits from the bottom of the pan with a wooden spoon. Stir in the parsley. Return the chicken to the pan and cook for 1 minute.

Serve with the rice and avocado slices.

Serves 4
Per serving: *347 calories, 10.1 g. fat (21% of calories), 3.1 g. dietary fiber, 66 mg. cholesterol, 203 mg. sodium*

LEAN CALIFORNIA BURGERS

Using ground turkey is an excellent way to cut back on fat when making burgers. This recipe uses the type of ground turkey readily available in supermarkets. For even leaner burgers, buy boneless turkey breast and grind it yourself in a food processor.

1 **pound ground turkey**	¼ **cup fat-free egg**
½ **cup dry bread crumbs**	**substitute**
2 **tablespoons onion flakes**	4 **crusty hamburger buns**
2 **tablespoons dried parsley**	4 **thick tomato slices**
flakes	**Lettuce**
⅓ **cup tomato sauce**	

In a large bowl, mix the turkey, bread crumbs, onion flakes and parsley flakes. Add the tomato sauce and egg. Mix well and form into 4 large patties.

Coat a broiler rack with no-stick spray. Place the patties on the rack and broil until browned on both sides and cooked through.

Serve on the buns topped with tomatoes and lettuce.

Serves 4
Per serving: *377 calories, 6.7 g. fat (16% of calories), 2.6 g. dietary fiber, 74 mg. cholesterol, 641 mg. sodium*

ORIENTAL SEAFOOD AND RICE SALAD

Even though seafood, such as shrimp and scallops, does contain cholesterol, levels are lower than previously thought. More important, these foods are very low in saturated fat, which doctors believe to be more of a dietary culprit when it comes to raising serum cholesterol. Combining a modest amount of seafood with rice and vegetables, as in this salad, produces a hearty main course that's quite low in cholesterol.

6	ounces bay scallops	1	teaspoon sesame oil
4	ounces medium shrimp, peeled, deveined and halved lengthwise	2	tablespoons cider vinegar
1	cup frozen peas	1	tablespoon low-sodium soy sauce
2	cups cold cooked rice		
1	cup diced carrots	1	tablespoon grated fresh ginger
1	cup diced sweet red peppers	1	clove garlic, minced
½	cup thinly sliced scallions		Pinch of ground red pepper
1	tablespoon olive oil	2	tablespoons toasted sesame seeds

Bring about 1" of water to a boil in a large frying pan. Add the scallops and shrimp. Poach over medium heat for about 4 minutes, or until the shrimp is just beginning to turn pink; do not overcook. Stir in the peas, then drain immediately.

In a large bowl, toss together the rice, carrots, diced peppers and scallions. Add the seafood mixture and toss lightly.

In a small bowl, whisk together the olive oil, sesame oil, vinegar, soy sauce, ginger, garlic and ground pepper. Pour over the salad and toss well. Sprinkle with the sesame seeds. Serve immediately or chill.

Serves 4
Per serving: *318 calories, 8.2 g. fat (23 % of calories), 3.3 g. dietary fiber, 57 mg. cholesterol, 315 mg. sodium*

BEEF AND MUSHROOM LASAGNA

Finely chopped mushrooms have a meaty texture and taste, so you can substitute them for part of the ground beef in many recipes. This lasagna uses skim milk and nonfat ricotta, both of which have less cholesterol than their full-fat counterparts, to further lower the cholesterol count.

9	lasagna noodles	2	cups skim milk
8	ounces extra-lean ground beef	2	tablespoons cornstarch
2	cups minced mushrooms	1	cup nonfat ricotta cheese
1	cup finely chopped onions	¼	cup fat-free egg substitute
1	teaspoon dried basil	1¼	cups tomato sauce
¼	teaspoon ground black pepper	½	cup shredded part-skim mozzarella cheese

Cook the lasagna in a large pot of boiling water for 12 minutes, or until just tender. Drain, rinse with cold water and set aside.

In a large no-stick frying pan over medium-high heat, brown the beef, breaking up the pieces. Add the mushrooms and onions. Cover the pan, reduce the heat to medium and cook for 3 minutes, or until the mushrooms have given up their liquid. Remove the lid and cook, stirring often, until the mixture is very dry. Stir in the basil and pepper; set aside.

In a 1-quart saucepan, whisk together the milk and cornstarch. Cook over medium heat, whisking frequently, until the mixture comes to a boil and thickens. Remove from the heat and whisk in the ricotta and egg. Stir into the beef mixture.

Coat a 9" × 13" baking dish with no-stick spray. Spread about ½ cup of the tomato sauce in the dish. Top with 3 of the noodles in a single layer and half of the beef mixture. Repeat with another layer of noodles and beef. Top with the remaining 3 noodles and ¾ cup tomato sauce. Sprinkle with the mozzarella.

Bake at 350° for 25 minutes. Let stand 10 minutes before cutting.

Serves 9

Tip: *The easiest way to mince the mushrooms is in the food processor. Halve or quarter about 8 ounces of mushrooms, then transfer to a food processor and chop with on/off turns. You'll end up with about 2 cups (don't worry if there's more; mushrooms have no fat and practically no calories, so you can use all you want in this casserole).*

Per serving: *244 calories, 6.9 g. fat (26% of calories), 1.3 g. dietary fiber, 20 mg. cholesterol, 269 mg. sodium*

CHAPTER 10

Sodium

The Rewards of Moderation

Retired Pennsylvania steelworker Roy. E. Rogers was the kind of person who thinks food without added salt is like champagne without the bubbles. Without salt, Roy believed, food would taste a little less tantalizing, a little too flat. But then he swapped his surplus sodium for something worthy of a champagne celebration: a new lease on life.

"As soon as the plate was set down, I'd pick up the salt-shaker and go to town," Roy says. In the past, he wouldn't have dreamed of eating corn on the cob, a sirloin steak, a tomato salad or any other food on his plate without making it look like a snow-covered landscape.

But a super-high blood pressure reading and a strict warning from his doctor prompted Roy to mend his salty ways.

These days, Roy eats corn on the cob without a pinch of salt. He passes up mashed potatoes smothered in sauerkraut. Instead of salty sausage breakfasts at the fast-food restaurant, Roy has switched to whole-grain cereal. And when he feels the urge to toss a topping on his food, now it's more likely to be a sprinkling of herbs.

Roy's low-salt eating style has paid off. At his last checkup, his blood pressure had eased down an amazing 50 points, well within the normal, safe range. "I haven't had to take a single pill," he says.

A PRECAUTIONARY STEP

You don't have to wait until your blood pressure is sky-high to shake your salt habit and take a giant step toward better health.

There is mounting evidence to show that cutting back on dietary sodium may help keep your blood pressure in the safe zone and reduce your risk of heart attack and stroke.

That's the conclusion reached by three British researchers from the Medical College of St. Bartholomew's Hospital in London after analyzing published studies of blood pressure and sodium intake involving 47,000 people throughout the world.

After reviewing the data, the researchers made this stunning estimation: If all adults stopped eating highly salted processed food and adding salt at the table, the incidence of stroke could be reduced by 26 percent and heart disease by 15 percent.

"Few measures in preventive medicine are as simple and economical and yet can achieve so much," declared the researchers.

Does this mean we should confine ourselves to a menu of bland, boring food with as much flavor as a slice of cardboard? Are pretzels shimmering with white crystals never to cross our lips?

Let's not go overboard. "You should aim to limit *excessive* salt in your diet—not all salt," says Bonnie Liebman, a licensed nutritionist and director of nutrition for the Center for Science in the Public Interest in Washington, D.C.

Granted, there are some foods that aren't fit to eat without salt, she says. Cottage cheese containing no salt, for instance, is barely palatable. "The point is, once you've cut down on surplus salt by eating more foods with nonsalt seasonings, then there's room for some moderately salty foods."

A Little Salt Goes a Long Way

Salt wasn't always regarded as the sinister white mineral in the black hat. In earlier days, salt was highly prized as a preservative for keeping meat and fish from spoiling and as a flavorful seasoning to cover up the taste of half-rotten food. So great was its value that sources were often depleted—wars were waged and lives were lost for salt.

Ironically, many people today are risking their lives over salt for the opposite reason: because it's so abundant in the foods we consume.

That's not to say we don't need any salt. Table salt, technically called sodium chloride, is the most common source of dietary sodium, a mineral our bodies need. Sodium's primary function is to regulate the proper balance of vital fluids and chemicals in our system.

But we can get all the sodium we need from the sodium naturally occurring in food without adding a pinch of salt. The estimated requirement is less than 500 milligrams a day—the equivalent of about ¼ teaspoon.

The problem is that the average American ingests anywhere from 3,000 to 6,000 milligrams of sodium—the equivalent of 1½ to 3 teaspoons of salt a day. That's more than ten times what we need.

Sound excessive? Actually, it can happen almost before you realize it. Consider, for example, that if you have nothing more than a pastry and two slices of Canadian bacon for breakfast (that's 1,800 milligrams of sodium), a serving of New England clam chowder for lunch (1,900 milligrams) and fast-food chicken with fries for dinner (1,100 milligrams), you've taken in almost 5,000 milligrams of sodium. Add a dill pickle and you gain nearly 1,000 milligrams more.

DO YOU HAVE SALT WATER ON TAP?

You're careful about the foods you eat. Yet you may be getting more sodium than you'd find in a handful of corn chips each time you drink a glass of tap water.

Researchers have found that many U.S. communities exceed the 20 milligrams of sodium per liter limit for drinking water recommended by the American Heart Association for people on sodium-restricted diets. That could be a problem if you have high (or borderline high) blood pressure.

Scientists looking at drinking water in two communities showed that a higher level of sodium was related to higher blood pressure levels.

Keep in mind that sodium-rich drinking water doesn't always taste salty. To find out what your levels are, call your local health department. If your drinking water exceeds the recommended limit and you have high blood pressure, consult your physician. "The best advice for sodium-sensitive people may be to drink bottled water, which has no sodium," says Carolyn Hoffman, R.D., director of dietetics at Central Michigan University in Mount Pleasant.

You should also consider avoiding drinking water that has been softened by a home water softener. Water softeners replace calcium and magnesium (the minerals that make the water "hard") with sodium—a lot of sodium. Softening of water can increase the sodium content fivefold.

"If you use a water softener, you should run a separate pipe for your drinking water that bypasses the softening process," says Hoffman.

Many people seem to handle all that salt without any immediate detriment to their health. Their kidneys simply excrete the excess amount.

But for some people, the kidneys can't handle the overload. In these people, dubbed salt sensitive, the excess salt
remains in the system. The bloodstream absorbs extra water
to dilute the excess sodium, increasing the blood volume.
Because the heart must pump harder to move this extra
blood, pressure builds up in the arteries. Eventually, increased blood pressure (also called hypertension) can
harden the arteries, making them susceptible to blockage.
The result may be heart attack or stroke.

In this way, excess salt sets the stage for high blood pressure and possibly heart disease.

WHO IS SALT SENSITIVE?

Very specific medical tests are needed to accurately determine who is sodium sensitive and who isn't. But doctors
say you could get a clue about salt's effects on your system
from blood pressure measurements taken before and after
going on a low-salt diet for six to eight weeks.

Your blood pressure measurement is a ratio of pressure
that blood exerts against your arteries when the heart pumps
(the systolic blood pressure) and when it's at rest (the diastolic blood pressure). Optimal blood pressure is 120/80 or
less. High blood pressure is 140/90 or greater.

About half of the people with high blood pressure clearly
are salt sensitive, according to G. Gopal Krishna, M.D., associate professor of medicine at the University of Pennsylvania in Philadelphia. Yet, there's emerging evidence
showing that a lifetime of overdosing on salt could have unhealthy effects on most people's blood pressures.

To begin with, there's solid data showing that in salt-
loving societies such as ours, blood pressure rises as we
grow older. In a study called the Multiple Risk Factor Intervention Trial, for example, researchers measured blood
pressure and then checked on the mortality rates of more

than 350,000 men over a ten-year period. At the start, 80 percent of the men had above-optimal (greater than 120 systolic) blood pressure. And there were higher death rates for those who were above optimal—the higher the pressure, the higher the death rate.

In contrast, other studies reveal that in societies where very little salt is consumed, such as in remote parts of Brazil and parts of Africa, blood pressure does not rise significantly as people age. In fact, those populations rarely develop high blood pressure.

"Clearly, the evidence shows that an increase in blood pressure is not a natural phenomenon as we age," says Rose Stamler, professor of epidemiology and preventive medicine at Northwestern University Medical School in Chicago. "It's more likely that we're all genetically programmed—some more than others—to become 'salt sensitive' to today's high doses of salt."

This type of salt sensitivity, however, may not show up until our senior years, according to a lengthy study at the Indiana University School of Medicine's Hypertension Research Center in Indianapolis. In the study, people who had normal blood pressures did not show a sensitivity to salt until their sixth decade.

THE PRICE OF PLENTY

High blood pressure is the price many people pay for decades of ingesting 20 times more sodium than they need, says Stamler. For many, the kidneys and circulatory system just can't handle that kind of abuse.

In fact, says Stamler, "more than half of U.S. adults have high blood pressure by age 60." And while salt intake should certainly concern individuals with high blood pressure, she says, those with above-optimal (over 120/80) or borderline-high blood pressures also need to be careful. In one study,

20 percent of those people aged 30 to 44 who had high normal blood pressures and took no preventive measures moved up to definite hypertension in just five years.

The bottom line: "Most of us would benefit from reducing our salt intake, no matter what our current blood pressure," she says.

Other experts wholeheartedly agree. If your blood pressure is normal, cutting back on salt may keep it from rising, according to Norman Kaplan, M.D., professor of internal medicine at the University of Texas Southwestern Medical Center in Dallas. "Reducing sodium can't hurt; it may help and might even save your life," says Dr. Kaplan.

If your blood pressure is already high, most studies suggest that cutting your salt intake in half might lower your blood pressure several points, says Marvin Moser, M.D., clinical professor of medicine at Yale University School of Medicine.

If you're taking pills for high blood pressure, cutting back on salt might make it possible to go with less medication or none at all—though only your doctor can accurately advise you on this.

In the Hypertension Control Program study conducted jointly in Chicago and Minneapolis, patients with mild hypertension participated in nutritional therapy, including reduction of salt intake to not more than $4\frac{1}{2}$ grams (1,800 milligrams of sodium) a day. After four years on this regimen, 39 percent of the patients were able to control their blood pressures without medication. As for those people who still required medication, salt reduction meant fewer pills and less side effects.

WHAT TO AIM FOR

The National Academy of Sciences says that we should consume no more than 2,400 milligrams of sodium a day.

Ideally, we should aim for no more than 1,800 milligrams. That's the equivalent of just a smidgen less than a teaspoon of salt. (If you have high blood pressure, consult your doctor before making any dietary changes.)

To keep your salt intake at the one-teaspoon-a-day limit, you'll have to do more than swear off your saltshaker. Less than a quarter of our dietary sodium comes from salt sprinkled on food at the table and during cooking, studies show. More than three-fourths of our sodium intake comes from salt added by food manufacturers during processing.

Most convenience, or ready-to-eat, food is loaded with sodium, says Liebman. "Salt is a cheap way to add universally appealing flavor and sometimes increase shelf life," she says.

The more processing, the more sodium that's likely to be in the food. While 3½ ounces of raw potato contains just 7 milligrams of sodium, for example, the same amount of instant mashed potatoes dishes up 348 milligrams. And the same weight of potato chips contains a whopping 469 milligrams. Likewise, a ½-cup serving of fresh peas contains only about 2 milligrams of sodium, while an equal amount of canned peas contains almost 100 times that much. Sodium even finds its way into our desserts: There are 147 milligrams in a piece of ready-to-eat apple pie compared to just a trace in a fresh apple.

The rule is: "Eat as close to fresh and 'from scratch' as possible," says Dr. Krishna.

Your menu should be laden with fresh fruits and vegetables, he adds, not just because salt is less abundant in these foods but also because they're rich in potassium.

"Potassium helps your body get rid of excess sodium," says Dr. Krishna. For optimum blood pressure control, he says, try to maintain a balance of potassium to sodium in your daily diet.

SODIUM LURKS WHERE YOU LEAST EXPECT IT

Which has more sodium: one homemade waffle or a pretzel? Incredibly, the waffle has over five times more sodium than the pretzel.

If you guessed wrong, it's no wonder. The presence of sodium isn't always easy to detect. Three-quarters of our dietary sodium is hidden in prepared foods. Surprisingly, waffles, bread, cereals and other grain products, not snack foods, are the leading source of sodium. Moreover, many salt-laced foods, such as pudding or diet soda, for instance, may not taste a bit salty. Yet one cup of pudding has more than 250 milligrams of sodium. The soda contains about 35 milligrams.

Be on the lookout for these other sneaky sources of sodium.

FOOD	PORTION	SODIUM (mg.)
Chicken noodle soup	1 cup	1,106
Macaroni and cheese	1 cup	1,086
Low-fat (1%) cottage cheese	1 cup	918
Kidney beans, canned	1 cup	873
Tuna salad	1 cup	824
Roast beef sandwich	1	792
Turkey with gravy, frozen	5 oz.	787
Mushrooms, canned	1 cup	663
Tomato juice, canned	¾ cup	657
Potatoes au gratin, from mix	1 serving	601
Bologna	2 slices	578
Biscuits, from mix	1	350
Pizza with cheese	1 slice	336
Pancakes, from mix	2	322
Bacon	3 slices	303
Rice Krispies	1 cup	290
Beets, canned, cooked	½ cup slices	233
Nonfat yogurt	1 cup	174
Whole-wheat bread	1 slice	148
Shrimp, canned	3 oz.	144
Peanut butter	1 Tbsp.	76
Angel food cake	1 piece	58

MAKE CUTBACKS GRADUALLY

Don't try to cut back on salt cold turkey. If you rush into low-salt eating, your taste buds will rebel and you'll be hunting for salty foods like a bear hunts down honey.

You can gently win your taste buds over to an appreciation of this new low-salt way of eating by mixing some low-sodium foods with higher-sodium ones. For example, you may not care for the bland taste of low-sodium cheese eaten alone. But the difference is not so noticeable if you blend low-sodium Cheddar and regular Swiss for melting on your homemade pizza. Here's another ploy: Try unsalted peanut butter atop a regular, salted cracker (or vice versa).

After three or four weeks of gradually decreasing salt, experts say you can expect your taste buds to be reformed and your salt cravings to wane. In a few months, you might even prefer less salty foods, one study suggests. Researchers compared the salt taste preferences of people on a low-sodium diet with those of people eating a normal diet. After five months, the low-salt group overwhelmingly chose less salty crackers while the other group had unchanged tastes.

AT HOME

The easiest way to begin trimming the salt from your diet is to cease sprinkling at the table or during cooking. Refuse to be a saltshaker robot—taste your food before salting it. Then if you still think it needs "a little something," read on.

Transform your saltshaker. Make it into a spice or herb shaker. Try filling it with dill, paprika and dried parsley—a great combo that can zip up everything from baked potatoes to meat loaf.

Use substitutes sparingly. Commercial salt substitutes contain potassium chloride. Adding a small amount of salt substitute to foods will make the food taste "salted," says dietitian Mary Winston of the American Heart Association in

Dallas. But if you have high blood pressure and take medication, check with your doctor first. Potassium chloride can cause problems if you have kidney disease.

Be wary, too, of the so-called lite salts. The "lite" designation does not mean no sodium—just less of it.

Make friends with pepper. And pour on the garlic, onion and celery powders, too. (Just avoid the *salt* versions of these seasonings.)

Keep lemon juice handy. A drop or two from this perky fruit seems to have the same zesty effect on the taste buds as salt does, says Liebman. "Steamed broccoli dressed with lemon juice is delicious," she says.

Rinse canned goods. If you use canned foods, be sure to drain and rinse them. One study showed that rinsing canned green beans for one minute removed nearly half of their added sodium. Rinsing water-packed tuna for the same length of time reduces sodium by nearly 80 percent.

Switch to low-sodium baking ingredients. Cook and bake using unsalted margarine. Or use vegetable oil, which is salt-free. If a recipe calls for soup or bouillon, look for the low-salt variety. One regular instant bouillon cube contains 1,000 milligrams of sodium. That's almost half of the recommended quota for the day.

Experiment with homemade condiments. Most of those zippy commercial condiments can zap you with a heap of sodium. A single tablespoon of catsup or mustard has over 170 milligrams of sodium, for instance. A tablespoon of soy sauce has over 1,000 milligrams. One commercial chili seasoning for tacos has nearly 3,000 milligrams per one-ounce packet. A homemade version (made with paprika, crushed oregano, cumin, turmeric, garlic powder and ground red pepper) has virtually none.

When cooking from scratch, you can control the amount of sodium, says Winston. Here's how to give food zing without salt's sting.

HOW TO SEASON WITHOUT SURRENDERING FLAVOR

If you're wondering how to appease your taste buds without salt, you need not worry. "There are hundreds of alternatives to salt," says Mary Winston, dietitian and author of the *American Heart Association Low-Salt Cookbook*. "Start by borrowing from some exotic cuisines: use items like curry, sesame seeds and ginger to create the taste of foods from India and China, for example. Or use table wines to impart a European flavor."

With a little imagination, you'll soon come to think of salty foods, as, well, salty. Here's how to add more spice to your life.

• **Experiment with herbal and spice blends.** For beef dishes, herbs such as marjoram, bay leaf and rosemary are naturals. For chicken, try curry powder, sage or savory. Allspice and turmeric are terrific on fish, while anise brings out the best in beets.

• **Mix and match tastes and textures.** Sweet foods matched with robust meats are particularly delicious, says Winston. Try roasting cinnamon-topped apple slices with pork chops. Or use mandarin orange wedges in a roast beef marinade.

• **Use fresh herbs whenever possible.** Prepare at the last moment and add them for "fresher, more 'alive' taste," says Winston.

• **Be prepared to pulverize.** Pound garlic, chilies and fresh herbs and spices with a mortar and pestle to release their flavors. And use a food processor to grate fresh horseradish, which packs more punch than the salted, bottled kind.

• **Treat yourself to dried toppings.** Mushrooms, tomatoes, cherries, cranberries and currants impart a more intense flavor when dried than when fresh, says Winston.

• **Discover citrus zest.** The zest of lemon, lime or orange is the part of the peel without the white pith. It actually holds the most intense flavor, says Winston. Grate it with a flat grater, to give just the right "bite" to foods.

• Mix mustard powder with water to make "a very sharp condiment that's just as powerful as the salty commercial kind," says Winston.

• Try a dash of aromatic bitters when making gravies, sauces or salad dressings.

• Sprinkle paprika on your popcorn.

• Drizzle flavored vinegars on garden greens. Rosemary-laced vinegar perks up radicchio and red-leaf lettuce, for example, with no oil needed. Flavored vinegars also provide great bases for making savory marinades for meats. Try tarragon vinegar mixed with a drop of hot-pepper sauce or unsalted liquid smoke. Pour it on chicken as it grills.

WHEN SHOPPING

You've sworn off pickles, bacon and the other salty-tasting foods. That's the easy part. The fact is, most of our sodium is hidden in processed foods, commercial baked goods and fast foods. And often you can't rely on your tongue to steer you from these salt-laden foods; you must rely on your eyes.

Here's how to become a salt sleuth when you grocery shop.

Read labels with an eagle eye. Look for packaged products labeled "sodium-free" or "very low sodium." Under current Food and Drug Administration guidelines, products can only be called sodium-free if they contain less than 5 milligrams of sodium per serving; products labeled low sodium must not exceed 140 milligrams, and very low sodium cannot contain more than 35 milligrams of sodium per serving. On the other hand, a product labeled "one-third less" salt, such as Campbell's Healthy Request soup, for example, could still contain plenty of salt. In this case, one serving of chicken noodle has 420 milligrams less sodium than the regular version but still contains 460 milligrams.

Avoid products listing salt, or sodium chloride, or baking soda among the top five ingredients. In general, try to steer clear of items containing more than 150 milligrams of sodium per serving, suggests Stamler.

As far as avoiding foods containing other forms of sodium, such as monosodium glutamate, you don't have to be so careful, experts say. "Preliminary studies seem to indicate that sodium chloride is the sole troublemaker in high blood pressure," says Dr. Krishna. "Other nonsalt sodiums don't seem to affect blood pressure."

Check out low-fat products carefully. Diet margarine, for example, has more sodium than regular margarine, according to Winston.

Look for low-salt versions of your favorite foods. Hundreds of low-sodium products from soups to nuts allow you to prepare your favorite meals without excess salt. If your traditional spaghetti recipe calls for a cup of marinara sauce, for example, substituting the reduced-salt type for the salted variety erases over 850 milligrams of sodium from your family's meal.

Sometimes these products are hard to find. Low-salt salsas, for example, might be relegated to the dietetic section of your supermarket. But the hunt is worth it. Here are some tips to set you in the right direction.

• Make a detour around the deli. Most deli items from prepared salads and dips to cold cuts are heavily salted. When possible, look for low-salt varieties. Request fresh cooked turkey and lean roast beef instead of precooked meats, for example.

• Steer clear of salt-laden dehydrated mixes for soups, sauces, salad dressings and puddings.

• Look for unsalted canned or frozen vegetables. Avoid those with sauces added.

• Ferret out the natural cheeses. Processed cheese and cheese spreads have up to 900 milligrams per two-ounce serving, while natural cheeses may have half that amount. Low-sodium cheeses, such as Colby and Monterey Jack, are available.

• Buy low-salt crackers. While many varieties of rice cakes contain no sodium, for example, four saltine crackers contain 125 milligrams.

DINING OUT

If you eat out frequently, you may have a tough time keeping a lid on your salt levels. Still, it's not impossible. All it takes is a little low-salt savvy.

Dine in restaurants where food is cooked to order. This way, you will have some control over salt, whereas in restaurants that have food prepared ahead of time, you don't, says Winston. A cooked-to-order broiled hamburger patty, for example, contains about 70 milligrams of sodium. The ready-to-eat-fast-food version contains over twice that much.

Order sauces on the side. That goes for gravies and dressings, too. Be sure to ask for low-sodium dressings, or better yet, oil and vinegar—they're salt-free.

Hold the extras. A leading fast-food cheeseburger with "the works" has over 1,100 milligrams of sodium. You can cut the salt content in half if you tell the counter person to hold the cheese, mustard, catsup and relish.

Don't eat too many dinner rolls. Nearly 30 percent of our dietary sodium comes from bread and grain products. A single slice of enriched white bread or whole-wheat bread contains about 150 milligrams of sodium.

Remove fillings and breadings. If you order a fruit pie, remove the salty crust and eat only the filling. Ditto for breaded fish. Baked fish with breading gives you over 1,000 milligrams of sodium. With breading removed, it's 575 milligrams.

Steps like these may seem like deprivations at first. "But stick with it," Dr. Krishna says. "If you can follow your low-salt eating program for at lest three to four months until you've had time to adjust, you should be all set."

EXERCISE YOUR OPTIONS

With careful shopping, it's possible to choose many of your favorite foods in reduced-salt or no-salt varieties. Note the differences below.

FOOD	PORTION	SODIUM (mg.)
BUTTER		
Unsalted	1 Tbsp.	2
Salted	1 Tbsp.	117
CASHEWS		
Unsalted	1 cup	22
Salted	1 cup	877
CORN		
Fresh or frozen	1 cup	8
Canned	1 cup	646
CRACKERS		
Wheat	4	60
Saltines	4	125
GREEN BEANS		
Fresh	1 cup	4
Canned	1 cup	882
OATMEAL		
Cooked	1 cup	2
Instant	1 cup	285
PORK		
Pork chop	3 oz.	63
Canned ham	3 oz.	1,067
SWISS CHEESE		
Natural	1 oz.	74
Processed	1 oz.	390
TOMATO PASTE		
Unsalted	1 cup	170
Salted	1 cup	2,070

High-Nutrition Recipes

STUFFED CABBAGE

Tomato sauce can be a hidden source of sodium. Look for brands that are labeled either "low sodium" or "no added sodium." When cooking rice, as for these cabbage rolls, use either plain water or salt-free stock.

8	large cabbage leaves	½	teaspoon dried oregano
1	cup finely chopped onions	1½	cups cold cooked rice
2	teaspoons olive oil	1	egg white
8	ounces ground turkey	2	cups no-added-sodium
1	clove garlic, minced		tomato sauce
½	teaspoon dried thyme		

Blanch the cabbage leaves in boiling water for 1 minute. Drain and lay the leaves flat on a tray. Set aside.

In a large no-stick frying pan over medium heat, sauté the onions in the oil for 5 minutes, or until softened. Crumble the turkey into the pan and cook, breaking up the pieces, until browned. Stir in the garlic, thyme and oregano; cook for 1 minute.

Remove the pan from the heat. Stir in the rice, egg white and ½ cup of the tomato sauce. Let stand for a few minutes until cool enough to handle.

Divide the mixture among the cabbage leaves. Enclose the filling by tucking in the side edges and rolling up the leaves.

Coat a 9" × 13" glass baking dish with no-stick spray. Spread about ½ cup of the remaining tomato sauce in the bottom. Add the rolls, seam side down. Pour the remaining 1 cup tomato sauce over the top.

Cut a piece of wax paper to fit over the rolls. Then cover the pan tightly with foil. Bake at 350° for 30 minutes.

Serves 4
Per serving: *261 calories, 4.2 g. fat (15% of calories), 3.9 g. dietary fiber, 37 mg. cholesterol, 95 mg. sodium*

CHICKEN SAUSAGE LINKS

Besides being high in fat, regular sausage also contains lots of sodium. You can easily make lean, lower-sodium links or patties at home. These contain ground chicken and minced apples. You may also substitute ground turkey for a slightly different taste. (For the leanest patties, buy boneless, skinless chicken or turkey breast, cut it into cubes and finely chop in a food processor using on/off turns.) Serve with reduced-cholesterol scrambled eggs, homemade hash browns and low-sodium catsup for a special weekend brunch.

½ cup unsalted plain or seasoned dry bread crumbs	¼ teaspoon ground black pepper Pinch of ground red pepper
¾ cup minced apples	
½ teaspoon dried sage	1 egg white, lightly beaten
	8 ounces ground chicken

In a large bowl, combine the bread crumbs, apples, sage, black pepper and red pepper. Stir in the egg white. Add the chicken and mix well. Shape into 8 links measuring about 4½" × 1".

Coat a broiler pan with no-stick spray. Broil about 6" from the heat until lightly browned on the outside and cooked through, about 4 minutes per side. Drain on paper towels.

Serves 4
Per serving: *133 calories, 2.5 g. fat (17% of calories), 0.9 g. dietary fiber, 40 mg. cholesterol, 150 mg. sodium*

YAMS WITH HONEY TOPPING

This is a nice side dish that can double as a light lunch. Be sure to choose cottage cheese with no added sodium— regular types can easily contain over 450 milligrams per half cup. If you're in a real hurry, you may microwave the sweet potatoes—four take from 15 to 20 minutes.

4	medium sweet potatoes	⅛	teaspoon ground
1½	cups unsalted dry-curd		cinnamon
	cottage cheese	⅛	teaspoon grated nutmeg
2	tablespoons honey	1	tablespoon snipped
			chives

Bake the sweet potatoes at 375° for 1 hour and 15 minutes, or until easily pierced with a fork.

In a food processor, blend the cottage cheese until smooth, about 3 minutes. Add the honey, cinnamon and nutmeg. Mix well.

Halve the potatoes and fluff the flesh with a fork. Top with dollops of the cottage-cheese mixture. Sprinkle with the chives.

Serves 4
Per serving: *215 calories, 0.6 g. fat (3% of calories), 4 g. dietary fiber, 4 mg. cholesterol, 25 mg. sodium*

CREAMY CARROT SOUP

Soups can be a challenge on a low-salt diet because most store-bought types are loaded with sodium. And making your own doesn't guarantee a low-sodium potage if you start with bouillon cubes or salty canned stock. Instead, either make your own stock or buy a brand that contains no added salt.

1 onion, diced,	¼ teaspoon dried dill
2 teaspoons olive oil	Pinch of grated nutmeg
12 ounces carrots, thinly sliced	4 cups defatted low-sodium chicken stock
4 ounces parsnips, thinly sliced	2 cups cooked rice
½ teaspoon ground black pepper	¼ cup nonfat sour cream
	Dill sprigs

In a 3-quart saucepan over medium heat, sauté the onions in the oil for 5 minutes, or until lightly browned. Add the carrots and parsnips; cook for 5 minutes, stirring often.

Stir in the pepper, dill, nutmeg and 2 cups of the stock. Cover and simmer for 20 minutes, or until the vegetables are tender. Transfer to a blender and process until smooth. Return the mixture to the pan.

Stir in the rice and the remaining 2 cups stock. Heat through. Ladle into soup bowls and garnish each serving with a dollop of the sour cream and some dill.

Serves 6
Per serving: *182 calories, 2.8 g. fat (14% of calories), 3 g. dietary fiber, 0 mg. cholesterol, 84 mg. sodium*

CHAPTER 11

Calcium

For Healthy Bones and More

When you were a kid you never thought twice about calcium—but chances are you were gulping three or four glasses of milk a day and guzzling ice cream whenever your mom would let you. You were getting plenty of calcium without even trying.

But times have changed. You have changed, and eating habits have changed. Many of us, ever aware of middle-age spread and how much fat we're eating, steer clear of calcium-rich foods such as cheese and ice cream. And instead of the milk we used to drink, many of us—young and old alike—swill soft drinks as if *they* contain some essential nutrient.

But the evidence is clear that we need calcium *throughout* our lives. Yes, it's crucial that children get ample calcium to build strong bones and teeth, but calcium can help keep your bones healthy long after childhood. And it has many other roles as well. It's involved with the functioning of your heart, blood, muscles and nerves, and in some cases it can help control blood pressure. Studies indicate that calcium also can alleviate many premenstrual problems, significantly reduce chances of premature births and lower chances of colon cancer and possibly breast cancer.

Fine, you say, but you eat a healthy diet and couldn't possibly be calcium deficient. Think again. The American Dietetic Association says you need a minimum of 800 milligrams of calcium a day, while children, teens, young adults and pregnant and breastfeeding women should take in at least 1,200 milligrams daily. Some professionals suggest that postmenopausal women need to consume even more. Many of us, however, don't come close.

When Paul Saltman, Ph.D., a biology professor at the University of California in San Diego, studied the food intake of 137 postmenopausal women—all well educated and with middle-class incomes—he found they weren't eating as well as they thought they were. "These were all women who said they were taking good care of themselves," says Dr. Saltman. "But the fact was, over two years, their calcium intake from food averaged only about 560 milligrams a day."

Nationwide, the average for all women aged 45 to 54 is only 474 milligrams daily. And more important, girls and young women seldom meet the daily requirements in their bone-forming years. Calcium intake is less of a problem for men and boys, who eat more and thus come closer to meeting minimum levels.

A MINERAL YOUR BODY DEMANDS

Calcium is an essential mineral that comes tidily packaged with other nutrients in a variety of foods—such as dairy products, leafy greens and canned sardines and salmon (with bones). The bulk of the calcium in our bodies, about 99 percent, is in our bones, and the rest is split evenly between our teeth and blood. And although it's a relatively small amount, the calcium in our blood is important: It's involved with many vital functions, including regulating muscle contractions, heartbeat, blood clotting and nerve transmission.

The calcium in your bones acts like deposits in a bank: Your body "borrows" calcium daily from your bones for your blood to use. But it also *re-deposits* calcium regularly from the foods you eat. This means that even during adulthood new bone is continually being formed—a process known as remodeling, which affects 10 to 15 percent of our bone surface at one time.

The system can go haywire, however, when you aren't supplying enough calcium in your diet to replace the calcium being withdrawn from your bones. Regardless of whether you're getting enough dietary calcium, your body will continue to "draw out" calcium from your bones. And if you are pregnant or breastfeeding and low on calcium, your body will also withdraw bone calcium to meet the baby's needs.

In general, we begin to lose bone around age 40 to 44. And to make matters worse, as we get older, we begin to lose some of our ability to absorb calcium—just as our intake of calcium is likely falling off, too.

It doesn't take a medical degree to figure out that if you keep sapping calcium from your bones without replacing it, you're going to run into trouble. (Just like when you make more withdrawals from your bank account than deposits.) Although it may take years for the effects of a serious deficiency to become apparent, eventually your calcium-starved bones become weak, porous, fragile and prone to break easily. This condition is known as osteoporosis, and it's common in postmenopausal women and some elderly men.

Osteoporosis: The Bone Weakener

Remember when Grandma fell and broke her hip? Or more likely, broke her hip and fell? Chances are her bones had become thin and fragile because of osteoporosis, and her brittle hip shattered.

MILK: IT DOESN'T ALWAYS DO A BODY GOOD

Paul Wexler began experiencing puzzling symptoms soon after he was out of his teens: lethargy, bloating, diarrhea. He dragged himself from doctor to doctor while his symptoms worsened, and one doctor even suggested his problem was psychological. Finally a physician made a simple, quick, and accurate diagnosis: Wexler was lactose intolerant. He could not digest milk.

The story ended happily for Wexler, whose uncomfortable symptoms disappeared as soon as he cut out milk products. But for millions of Americans like him, milk spells distress with a capital *D*.

The culprit is lactose, the sugar in milk, which you normally break down with an enzyme called lactase. But if you don't produce enough lactase, you can't digest milk properly.

As babies, most of us produce plenty of lactase, but we produce less as we get older. And by the time we're adults, many of us—as many as 60 to 90 percent of Jews, Orientals, blacks, Mexican-Americans and native Americans—are lactose intolerant to some degree. The problem is less common among American whites, affecting only 5 to 20 percent.

So if milk turns your intestinal tract into a raging battle zone, how do you get enough calcium?

In people with osteoporosis, bones can break under their own weight. The complicating factor is that often the bone doesn't simply break—it shatters into pieces too small to be put back together. One-fourth of people over 55 who break their hips will not walk unaided again.

Osteoporosis affects primarily the hips, wrists and spine and results in about 1.3 million fractures a year. In many

Settle for less. Being lactose intolerant doesn't necessarily mean you can't *ever* consume dairy products, says Liz Diemand, R.D., of Thornton, Colorado, spokesperson for the American Dietetic Association. Not everyone is as intolerant as Wexler.

"Try consuming dairy products in smaller portions," says Diemand. "Try just four ounces of milk, in combination with other foods."

Take a dairy detour. You can also try yogurt or aged cheeses, such as extra-sharp Cheddar, which are lower in lactose. "Many lactose-intolerant people can tolerate yogurt, because the bacteria help the digestion of lactose," explains Diemand. (But not all yogurts have live bacteria cultures—check the label.)

Try something special. You can also buy reduced-lactose milk, which contains 70 percent less lactose than regular milk, or lactase supplements that contain the lactase enzymes you're missing. These come in a liquid you can add directly to milk, or as chewable tablets.

Go with the green. You can load up on calcium-rich nondairy foods, such as broccoli, kale and mustard greens. "But if this is your only source of calcium, it's difficult to get enough in your diet," says Diemand. If you're consuming no milk products, she recommends that you ask your doctor about a calcium supplement.

cases, vertebrae may compress and collapse. There are no early warning signs. The first indications may be a decrease in height or the formation of a "dowager's hump" as bone in the spine collapses.

Who gets osteoporosis? Many factors are involved, including how much bone mass you have to start with—which can be linked to race (black people, for instance, have more

CALCIUM AND ITS PALS

Calcium can't do its bone-building job without two companion nutrients—vitamin D and phosphorus.

Vitamin D. Generally the vitamin D you need comes from exposure to the sun, and most people make enough vitamin D in the sunny summer months to last through winter. But people who seldom or never get out of doors can be deficient in vitamin D—and this can be a problem for older people who may be housebound.

"It's increasingly my opinion that a major problem in the elderly—along with inadequate *calcium* intake—is insufficient vitamin D," says Lindsay Allen, R.D., Ph.D., professor of nutrition sciences at the University of Connecticut in Storrs. "Also, older people don't make vitamin D as well in their skin from sunlight as younger people." Studies support this: One study found that women who did not receive a vitamin D supplement lost more bone density than women who did get the supplement.

bone mass than Caucasians) or to how much calcium you consumed and how physically active you were during your bone-forming years.

Risk factors you can't do much about include being light-skinned, having a delicate frame, undergoing early menopause or having relatives who have had osteoporosis. Factors you *can* control include being underweight or sedentary, eating a low-calcium diet, smoking and drinking more than two drinks per day.

Women are particularly vulnerable to osteoporosis partly because of calcium losses that can occur during pregnancy and menopause. If you don't consume enough calcium dur-

Two cups of milk fortified with vitamin D, however, will give you the recommended daily allowance of 200 international units. You can also increase your vitamin D level by going outdoors without sunscreen and exposing your face, arms and hands to the sun for five to ten minutes in the morning or late afternoon three times a week, says Michael Holick, M.D., Ph.D., director of the Vitamin D and Bone Research Laboratory at the Boston University School of Medicine.

If you can't handle either sun or milk, take a multivitamin supplement with 200 to 400 international units of vitamin D, says Dr. Holick. Or eat foods that supply vitamin D, such as sardines, salmon, tuna and cheese.

Phosphorus. Getting adequate phosphorus is seldom a problem, as this mineral abounds in cola-type soft drinks, processed foods, meats, dairy foods and poultry. Too much phosphorus in the diet, however, can interfere with calcium absorption, so if you're an inveterate soda-guzzler, you may want to cut back on your intake.

ing pregnancy and nursing, it will be "robbed" from your bones. And drastic bone loss can occur during menopause when estrogen production falls off, because estrogen is necessary for bones to absorb calcium.

You can avoid this dramatic menopausal bone loss by hormone replacement therapy, which includes low doses of estrogen and progesterone. Women who have had breast cancer should not take estrogen, however. And those with diabetes, asthma or heart disease may also be advised not to take hormones. Is osteoporosis and significant bone loss inevitable, particularly if you aren't starting out with a lot of bone mass? Not necessarily.

THE LINK WITH WHAT YOU DRINK

You could be taking in even *more* than your required levels of calcium—and still not have adequate calcium available. What gives?

How much calcium is available to you may be related to what you drink, whether it's coffee, alcohol or soft drinks.

Coffee. One study showed that the risk of hip fracture in middle-aged women who drank more than 6 cups of coffee a day was nearly three times higher than that of women who drank less than 1½ cups a day. Caffeine may harm bones directly, or indirectly by prompting calcium losses through frequent urination.

Alcohol. Alcoholic beverages can interfere with your ability to absorb and use calcium. And because women's ovaries are sensitive to the effects of alcohol, it may alter the hormonal balance necessary to maintain strong bones. And as if that's not enough, it's possible that alcohol's diuretic qualities promote calcium losses through the urine.

CALCIUM TO THE RESCUE

While you shouldn't think of calcium as a cure-all or sure-fire preventive for bone problems or osteoporosis—most professionals agree that additional measures are usually needed to halt bone loss—calcium *can* help. Researchers disagree on how much it helps and how much of its effect is due to other factors, but the bottom line is that some studies show that calcium may reduce the amount of bone you lose, help fend off osteoporosis and help prevent fractures.

"In preventing fractures, the evidence for calcium is strong," says Robert Heaney, M.D., chairman of the Congressional Office of Technology Assessment's scientific advisory panel on osteoporosis.

High levels of alcohol may counteract any beneficial effect calcium has on blood pressure. When researchers at the University of California Medical Center in San Diego studied data on 7,000 middle-aged men of Japanese descent living in Hawaii, they found that in light drinkers, higher calcium intake helped keep blood pressure levels down. In heavier drinkers, however, the calcium had no effect.

Soft drinks. Some studies suggest that soft drinks—because of their citric and phosphoric acid content—can decrease utilization of calcium or cause increased excretion. One survey found that athletic women who drank carbonated drinks had 2.3 times as many fractures as those who did not. Researchers are not all in accord, however. "It's debatable," says Elwood Speckmann, Ph.D., director of research programs at Shriners Hospitals for Crippled Children in Tampa, "but generally you should avoid extremes of nutrient intake. Inadequate calcium and excessive phosphorus is going to cause problems, just as too much calcium and not enough phosphorus would."

One study showed that men and women past 60 who took in more than 765 milligrams of calcium a day had 60 percent fewer hip fractures than people getting less than 470 milligrams. Another study indicated that women with a lifetime calcium intake of 1,000 milligrams a day had 60 to 70 percent fewer hip fractures than women getting half that amount.

And a study at the University of Massachusetts Medical Center found that 30- to 40-year-old women who consumed 1,500 milligrams of the mineral a day from low-fat, calcium-rich foods had lost none of their bone mass over three years, while women consuming 800 milligrams a day had lost 3 percent.

WHO NEEDS CALCIUM SUPPLEMENTS?

So you need to take in more calcium. No problem, you decide, wheeling down the aisle and tossing a jumbo bottle of calcium supplements in your shopping cart.

What's wrong with this picture? A couple of things.

First, no one should *indiscriminately* take supplements, says Elwood Speckmann, Ph.D., director of research programs at Shriners Hospitals for Crippled Children in Tampa. Not everyone needs a supplement—you may be able to more effectively get your calcium from food—and people who do require supplements should pay careful attention to *how much* calcium is supplied and in what form.

Nutritionists believe the first approach to resolving a calcium deficiency should be to eat more foods containing calcium. "I don't like to see people rely on supplements and forget about what they're getting in their diets," says Liz Diemand, R.D., of Thornton, Colorado, a spokesperson for the American Dietetic Association. If at all possible, it's better to get your calcium along with other nutrients in a "package deal" in foods such as low-fat milk, yogurt, cheeses, broccoli and greens.

But in some cases you just can't take in enough calcium via food to meet your needs. Who's a candidate for supplements? People who can't digest milk or milk products; pregnant or nursing women, who have an increased need for calcium; and elderly people with limited appetites.

It's best to check with your doctor before adding a supplement, particularly if you have a family history of kid-

Optimally, of course, you build strong bones in childhood and young adulthood and consume plenty of calcium *before* menopause. "Women who get enough calcium all their lives appear to have much less risk of losing significant amounts of bone after menopause," says Bess Dawson-

ney stones. And always check the dosage of the supplement: Some people think if a little is good, a lot is better—but that's not always true. Calcium in excess of 2,500 milligrams a day can cause problems such as urinary stone formation and constipation and can interfere with absorption of iron, zinc and other minerals.

Another potential hazard of overdosing is hypercalcemia (excess calcium in the blood). Up to 2,500 milligrams of calcium a day won't cause a problem in healthy adults, but it *can* if you have a condition such as hyperparathyroidism or chronic kidney disease. And huge doses of calcium—four and more times the normal dose—can cause hypercalcemia in anyone.

Think you're getting your calcium from chewing antacids? You may be—but check those labels. Calcium-containing antacids such as Tums may have up to 500 milligrams of calcium, but antacids that contain aluminum and magnesium hydroxide can cause phosphate depletion and a *loss* of available calcium.

And don't assume that your calcium supplement is a fix-all for your bones. Calcium doesn't work alone: Vitamin D, lactose and protein all help calcium absorption, and regular weight-bearing exercise plays a crucial role in protecting bones.

Two final tips: If you're taking a calcium supplement, it's better to spread out the dosage throughout the day rather than taking it all at once, and to drink six to eight 8-ounce glasses of water a day.

Hughes, M.D., of the U.S. Department of Agriculture's (USDA) Nutrition Research Center on Aging at Tufts University in Boston. Studies suggest that calcium taken immediately after menopause is of no use in preventing bone loss.

BEST AND WORST CALCIUM SOURCES

Some of the top sources of this important nutrient are listed here as well as a couple that just don't deliver.

FOOD	PORTION	CALCIUM (mg.)
A+ SOURCES		
Nonfat yogurt	1 cup	452
Skim milk	1 cup	302
Buttermilk	1 cup	285
Part-skim mozzarella cheese	1 oz.	181

Dairy products are by far the richest in calcium, and that calcium is also easily absorbed by the body. Depend on them to achieve recommended calcium intake.

A SOURCES		
Sardines	6	275
Salmon, pink, canned (with bones)	3 oz.	181

Good supplementary calcium sources. They're high in calcium because of the tiny bones, but sardines can also be high in fat.

B+ SOURCES		
Pinto beans, cooked	½ cup	118
Kale, chopped, cooked	½ cup	86
Bok choy, shredded, cooked	½ cup	79

This doesn't mean, however, that you should *neglect* your calcium intake during this period: Better late than never. "Even if you don't start taking extra calcium until early menopause, it will help prevent bone loss later, even if the results don't show up for five or six years," says Dr. Dawson-Hughes.

For two years, Dr. Dawson-Hughes studied 301 healthy postmenopausal women, some of whom received an additional 500-milligram supplement of calcium per day. The

FOOD	PORTION	CALCIUM (mg.)
Mustard greens, chopped, cooked	½ cup	52
Kidney beans, cooked	½ cup	43
Broccoli, chopped, cooked	½ cup	36

Greens and beans are moderately high in calcium, and that calcium is available to the body. Unfortunately, you'd have to eat mounds of them to meet the daily calcium levels that experts recommend. Depend on them as supplementary calcium sources.

Figs, dried	6	161
Almonds, toasted, unblanched	1 oz.	76
Hazelnuts	1 oz.	55
Brazil nuts	1 oz.	50
Prunes, dried	5	22

Like greens and beans, nuts and dried fruits are good as a supplementary source of calcium, but you'd have to cover your plate with them to meet daily requirements. Also, nuts are high in fat, and dried fruits are loaded with calories.

F SOURCES

Spinach, cooked	½ cup	122
Ground beef, lean, cooked	3 oz.	8

Spinach is high in oxalate, which makes its calcium unavailable to the body. Meats have insignificant calcium content.

women who got less than 400 milligrams of total calcium per day lost 2 to 3 percent of their bone mass in the two years, while bone loss was greatly reduced in the women receiving supplements. The best results were found in women at least six years past menopause.

What about other therapies or additional strategies to avoid osteoporosis? Besides estrogen for menopausal women, vitamin D plays a vital role. And exercise is also crucial: All the calcium in the world won't stop or prevent bone loss if you don't exercise, says Dr. Heaney.

Helping High Blood Pressure

But calcium doesn't just affect bone health. Among other things, it may also help keep your blood pressure down.

A study by David McCarron, M.D., co-head of the Division of Nephrology at the Oregon Health Sciences University in Portland, indicates that people with mild high blood pressure may be able to decease their levels to normal by increasing their dietary calcium intake. Intake at or above 800 milligrams a day holds strong potential benefit for pregnant women and people who drink too much alcohol, according to Dr. McCarron.

And a 1991 study of 1,194 women in Argentina found that those in their twentieth week of pregnancy who took 2,000 milligrams of calcium a day had fewer problems with high blood pressure than did others who received a look-alike placebo with no calcium.

"Calcium is particularly good, it seems, in affecting normal age-related increases in blood pressure," says Jeffrey Blumberg, Ph.D., associate director of the USDA's Human Nutrition Research Center on Aging at Tufts University.

Easing Menstrual Problems

For women who suffer from the monthly miseries of premenstrual syndrome or other menstrual problems, studies suggesting that calcium can ease much of their discomfort may be the best news they've heard in a long time.

Dramatic results were found in a 5½-month study by the USDA's Agricultural Research Service in Grand Forks, North Dakota. For 78 days, five of the ten women received 1,300 milligrams of calcium daily and the other five received 600 milligrams. For another 78 days of the study, the groups were switched.

"Women with higher calcium intakes showed a really dramatic decrease in a variety of symptoms," says research psychologist James G. Penland, Ph.D. On the higher levels of calcium, nine of the ten reported fewer mood changes such as irritability, tension, loneliness, and depression, and seven of the ten reported fewer cramps and backaches during the menstrual phase of the cycle. The women also reported retaining less water during the premenstrual phase of their cycle.

At the lower levels, says Dr. Penland, the women showed poorer work efficiency and overall efficiency. "They also slept more, avoided social activities and had an increase in concentration problems, insomnia, forgetfulness and accidents," he says.

And in another study at the Metropolitan Hospital in New York City, women suffering from PMS symptoms found they had fewer mood swings and less water retention and pain when they took 1,000 milligrams of calcium daily in addition to their regular diets.

CUTTING CANCER RISKS

Calcium against cancer? Possibly. Evidence is mounting that calcium at levels of 1,200 milligrams or more per day may lower the risk of colon cancer and possibly breast cancer.

"There are tentative findings that link higher levels of calcium intake with lower colorectal cancer risk in humans," says Martin Lipkin, M.D., head of the Irving Weinstein Laboratory for Gastrointestinal Cancer Prevention at Memorial Sloan-Kettering Cancer Center in New York City.

The link between cancer and calcium was proposed in 1980 by brothers Cedric Garland, D.P.H., and Frank Garland, Ph.D., who found that colon and rectal cancer deaths were highest in areas with least sun, and later found a similar pattern with breast cancer. (Sunshine lets us make vitamin D, which in turn helps us absorb calcium.) They suggest that calcium intake levels of 1,800 milligrams per day for men and 1,500 milligrams per day for women are useful for reducing occurrences of colon cancer.

Although evidence linking calcium and breast cancer is far from conclusive, studies with rats suggest that low amounts of vitamin D and calcium and high levels of phosphate, increase the risk for mammary tumors when a high-fat diet is eaten.

How might calcium exert a protective effect? At least for colon cancer, a possible mechanism has been proposed: During the digestive process, bile acids that can be cancer-causing are produced in the colon. Calcium appears to bind with these acids and keep them from irritating the colon wall. One study found that calcium slows down the reproduction of immature cells taken from the colon wall, and helps make cancer cells "age" and die.

AND STILL MORE BENEFITS

A study at Johns Hopkins Adolescent Pregnancy Clinic found that calcium helped reduce the risk of premature births among pregnant teenagers. Only 7 percent of the teenaged mothers-to-be who received 2,000 milligrams of calcium daily from their fifth month on gave birth prematurely, while 21 percent of the group receiving a placebo had premature babies.

And of 2,000 respondents to a *Prevention* magazine survey, almost 74 percent reported that taking calcium helped reduce muscle cramps or spasms. "There may be a good physiologic basis for that," says Dr. Dawson-Hughes. "It is very well recognized that even slightly low potassium and low calcium levels cause muscle cramps." Seventy percent of readers also reported that calcium helped aching bones or joints, although there's no scientific evidence to back up this effect.

LOOKING OUT FOR YOUR NEEDS

Where do you get your calcium?

Head for the dairy case. "The best sources are milk and dairy products," says Bettye J. Nowlin, R.D., Los Angeles dietitian and a spokesperson for the American Dietetic Association. Dairy products aren't all high in fat: You can choose low-fat or nonfat cheese, yogurt, and milk. "You can sprinkle

---

TEN QUICK TIPS TO BOOST YOUR CALCIUM INTAKE

1. Choose frozen yogurt, ice milk or puddings made with low-fat or skim milk for dessert.

2. Sprinkle Parmesan or Romano cheese on soups, salads, vegetables and popcorn.

3. Use low-fat or skim milk instead of water in canned soups and oatmeal and during baking.

4. Use plain yogurt in place of mayonnaise in salad dressing and other recipes.

5. Add a slice of cheese to sandwiches, or melt some on toast, English muffins or bagels.

6. Add one or two tablespoons of nonfat dry milk to hot cereals, stews, casseroles, meat loaf or mashed potatoes.

7. Use farmer's cheese, ricotta cheese or cottage cheese as a sandwich or toast spread.

8. Try tofu in place of beef or chicken in stir-fry recipes, or add it to soups and salads.

9. Choose broccoli, collards, kale, bok choy or turnip greens.

10. Have low-fat milk shakes instead of soft drinks.

---

cheese on a salad; use low-fat grated cheese in casseroles; add nonfat dry milk to meat loaf," advised Nowlin.

Eat a fair share of fish and broccoli. Other good sources are canned salmon and sardines (if you eat the soft bones as well), calcium-fortified orange or grapefruit juice, and broccoli. You can also find calcium in leafy greens such as kale, collard greens and turnip greens. Tortillas that are lime-processed (check the package) contain calcium, as does tofu.

Strive for three to four servings a day. Each serving of calcium-rich foods provides about 300 milligrams, says Nowlin. So if you aim for three or four servings per day, you'll be getting 900 to 1,200 milligrams. It's also best to spread out your calcium intake throughout the day, as your body can more efficiently absorb it in small doses.

AMOUNTS THAT PROTECT BEST

For best results in preventing osteoporosis, the National Osteoporosis Foundation suggests these daily intakes of calcium.

AGE/CONDITION	CALCIUM (mg.)
1-10	800
11-24	1,200
25-50	1,000
Pregnant women	1,200
Lactating women	1,200
Premenopausal women	1,000
Postmenopausal women	
If taking hormone replacement therapy	1,000
If not taking hormone replacement therapy	1,500
51+	1,000

Your Daily Quota

Exactly how much is enough? There's no simple answer: The amount you need may vary according to your stage of life, and it can be different from person to person.

"Some women absorb only 15 percent of the calcium in their foods, while others absorb three times as much," says Dr. Heaney. People on high-fiber diets may absorb less, because fiber can bind calcium and make it less available. The rate also varies with age: As kids, we absorb about 75 percent of the calcium we take in. As adults, the amount typically drops to around 15 percent.

Calcium from a variety of foods is without a doubt your best bet. Generally, if you reach for three or four servings of calcium-rich foods a day—or five, if you're pregnant or nursing or in menopause—you'll be meeting your calcium needs.

High-Nutrition Recipes

Raspberries and Honey-Yogurt Cream

Low-fat dairy products are a best bet when you're looking to increase your intake of calcium. This smooth yogurt sauce is easy to prepare and goes with most any fresh fruit.

1 cup nonfat yogurt	½ teaspoon vanilla
¾ cup nonfat sour cream	4 cups red or black raspberries
2 tablespoons honey	
2 teaspoons grated orange rind	

Spoon the yogurt into a yogurt-cheese funnel or a small sieve lined with cheesecloth. Place over a bowl, cover and let drain at room temperature for 1 hour. Transfer to a medium bowl. Whisk in the sour cream, honey, orange rind and vanilla.

Divide the berries among 4 dessert bowls. Top with the yogurt cream.

Serves 4
Per serving: *166 calories, 0.8 g. fat (4% of calories), 5.5 g. dietary fiber, 1 mg. cholesterol, 84 mg. sodium, 141 mg. calcium*

LOUISIANA SALMON CAKES

Most brands of canned salmon contain small edible bones, which are a good source of calcium. This recipe gets an extra helping of calcium from the nonfat ricotta cheese that's also incorporated into the patties. Serve the cakes with rice, noodles or baked potatoes and coleslaw.

¼ cup minced onions	1 teaspoon Worcestershire sauce
1 tablespoon water	1 teaspoon Dijon mustard
1 can (15½ ounces) salmon, drained well and flaked	¼ teaspoon hot-pepper sauce
1 cup nonfat ricotta cheese	1 cup seasoned dry bread crumbs
¼ cup fat-free egg substitute	1 teaspoon olive oil
2 tablespoons minced fresh parsley	

Combine the onions and water in a custard cup; cover with vented plastic wrap. Microwave on high for 1 minute, or until the onions are softened.

Transfer to a large bowl. Add the salmon, ricotta, egg,

parsley, Worcestershire, mustard, hot-pepper sauce and ¾ cup of the bread crumbs. Mix well. Cover and refrigerate for at least 2 hours.

Form the mixture into 4 patties. Coat them with the remaining ¼ cup of the bread crumbs.

Heat the oil in a large no-stick frying pan over medium heat. Add the patties and brown on both sides.

Serves 4
Per serving: *261 calories, 7.5 g. fat (27% of calories), 1.2 g. dietary fiber, 46 mg. cholesterol, 747 mg. sodium, 214 mg. calcium*

KALE AND POTATO CASSEROLE

Many leafy greens, such as kale, contain good amounts of calcium. This easy kale and potato casserole gets extra calcium from buttermilk and low-fat cheese.

1½ pounds baking potatoes
¾ cup buttermilk
¼ cup fat-free egg substitute
½ teaspoon ground black pepper
¼ teaspoon dried dill
1 large onion, thinly sliced
1 teaspoon olive oil
1 pound kale, coarse stems removed
½ cup reduced-fat Cheddar cheese
¼ cup seasoned dry bread crumbs

Peel the potatoes and cut into 1" chunks. Place in a large saucepan with cold water to cover. Bring to a boil and cook for 15 minutes, or until the potatoes are tender. Drain and place in a large bowl. Mash with a potato masher.

Stir in the buttermilk, egg, pepper and dill. Set aside.

In a large frying pan over medium heat, sauté the onions in the oil for 5 minutes, or until softened.

Meanwhile, wash the kale in cold water and shake off the

excess. Halve large leaves lengthwise. Cut the kale into crosswise shreds about ¼" wide. Add to the frying pan with the water clinging to the leaves. Cover and cook for 10 minutes, or until wilted.

Stir into the potato mixture. Fold in the cheese.

Coat a 2-quart casserole with no-stick spray. Add the potato mixture. Sprinkle with the bread crumbs. Bake at 400° for 15 minutes, or until the crumbs are lightly browned and the casserole is heated through.

Serves 4
Per serving: *297 calories, 5.4 g. fat (15% of calories), 2.4 g. dietary fiber, 9 mg. cholesterol, 211 mg. sodium, 245 mg. calcium*

TANGY TOFU SALAD

This luncheon or dinner salad contains three nice sources of dietary calcium: tofu, broccoli and kidney beans. For even more, you could toss in a bit of low-fat cheese or serve the salad atop shredded leafy greens, such as bok choy or kale. Although the percent of calories from fat in this recipe is a little high, it's largely due to healthy unsaturated fat—most of it coming from the tofu.

2 cups broccoli florets, lightly steamed	½ cup thinly sliced scallions
1 can (15 ounces) kidney beans, rinsed and drained	2 tablespoons minced fresh basil
½ cup diced sweet red peppers	8 ounces firm tofu
	½ cup fat-free Italian dressing

In a large bowl, toss together the broccoli, beans, peppers, scallions and basil.

Drain the tofu and gently squeeze out excess moisture

using several thicknesses of paper towels. Cut the tofu into
$\frac{1}{2}$" or smaller cubes. Add to the bowl. Drizzle with the
dressing and toss lightly.

Serves 4
Per serving: *172 calories, 5.5 g. fat (26% of calories), 5.8
g. dietary fiber, 0 mg. cholesterol, 282 mg. sodium, 169 mg.
calcium*

CHAPTER 12

Iron

Don't Get Caught Short

"**It's** the fastest way to get iron in your diet," the sword swallower dryly jokes after sliding a two-foot-long saber out of his mouth. Having enough iron in the body is paramount to good health, but downing knives is hardly the way to get it. In fact, getting too much or too little iron is no joking matter.

Iron plays an absolutely vital role in every single cell of your body, says iron researcher Richard G. Stevens, Ph.D., an epidemiologist at Battelle Pacific Northwest Laboratories in Richland, Washington. It puts the red in red blood cells and makes it possible for those cells to deliver life-giving oxygen from the lungs to the rest of your body. Iron also helps the body release energy, grow and fight infections.

IRON AT WORK

Once iron enters the body, it tends to stay there for quite a while. When a bit of iron signs on with a red blood cell, it's guaranteed a job for the cell's entire working life, about four months. When the blood cell finally retires and breaks up, most of its liberated iron goes to the bone marrow. From there, most of it quickly becomes part of a new blood cell and goes back to work. The remaining iron goes either into storage or is used by other cell systems. If you're eating right, the amount of iron going into storage equals the amount of iron coming out. And, if you're eating right, you shouldn't come up short even if a little iron escapes, which it does. In fact, in women, a little iron is lost each month through menstrual bleeding.

"Usually, there's a balance between iron loss and absorption," says James D. Cook, M.D., professor of medicine and director of the Division of Hematology at the University of Kansas Medical Center in Kansas City. "When there's increased iron loss—through excess menstrual bleeding, for example—the body increases the rate of iron absorption."

Iron needs vary depending on a person's age and sex. In an average day, an average man needs to replace about 1 milligram of iron. Women in their childbearing years need to replace about 1½ milligrams per day.

The amount of iron that your body needs to replace every day is really small compared with Recommended Dietary Allowances (RDA). The RDA for women age 50 and under is a whopping 15 milligrams, for example. Why so much?

The answer lies in the difference between absorption and intake. When your body needs iron, it can absorb on average only about 10 percent of the iron you take in. Eat an iron-rich dinner that provides ten milligrams, and your body will absorb about one milligram, which is just about right—for many people.

DEFINING DEFICIENCY

It is fairly easy to get enough iron into your diet. But what happens if you don't? When a person doesn't eat enough iron-rich foods to replace iron losses, cells start double-dipping into stored iron, and deficiency begins.

Having "iron-poor, tired blood" (as TV ads used to call

iron deficiency) means there's just not enough oxygen oomph in the blood to fuel the body and meet its energy needs. "People with low-level deficiencies are just not up to snuff," says Connie Weaver, Ph.D., professor of foods and nutrition at Purdue University in West Lafayette, Indiana. "They feel tired, and it's harder to fight off infections."

If deficiency deepens until iron stores are almost gone—as in anemia—red blood cells shrink, making it difficult for the body's cells to get enough oxygen. This means the heart and lungs have to work a lot harder. The resulting strain can cause a person to look pale and feel weak and fatigued, says Dr. Weaver.

There are, medical experts say, three general causes of iron deficiency: high blood loss, low iron intake and rapid body growth. As luck would have it, women are much more likely than men to have problems on all these counts.

Iron is lost during menstruation and needs to be replaced, explains Dr. Weaver. "Adequate iron intake is something menstruating women should be especially conscientious about," she says.

Adolescent girls and women on weight-loss diets need to be doubly concerned, she says.

Men are not immune to iron deficiency, but *nutritional* iron deficiency in men is rare, says Dr. Cook. "When iron deficiency does occur in men over age 18, it almost always means there's been blood loss of some kind," he says. Slow, internal bleeding that goes undetected—from long-term aspirin use, for example, or certain digestive diseases—can deplete iron stores.

MINING IRON (WITH A FORK)

For most healthy adults, nutritionists say, maintaining sufficient iron supplies is a snap. All it takes is eating the right kinds of foods.

IRON IN THE LIFE CYCLE

Young, old and in between, people need iron every day. But the amounts we need vary over the years. Here's a rundown of the changing daily Recommended Dietary Allowances for iron and the reasons that our iron needs change through the years.

AGE/CONDITION	RDA (mg./day)		MAJOR FACTORS
	WOMEN	MEN	
0-6 months	6	6	At 0-3 months the infant is still drawing on iron stored up while in the womb.
6 months-10 years	10	10	Growth requires greater iron usage.
11-18 years	15	12	Rapid growth in adolescence increases iron needs. Onset of menstruation in girls further increases need for iron.
19-50 years	15	10	Iron needs in women remain high until menopause. Men require less iron and maintain higher body iron stores than women.
Pregnancy	30		Increased blood volume and developing fetus demand high iron intake.
Lactation	15		Iron demands return to pre-pregnancy level.
51+ years	10	10	After menopause women need less iron.

Meat me at the dinner table. "By far, the most concentrated, most absorbable source of iron is red meat," says Janet P. Hunt, Ph.D., a research scientist at the USDA Human Nutrition Research Center in Grand Forks, North Dakota. "And red meat has even more highly available iron than white meats from poultry or fish," she says.

What's all this about "absorbable" and "available" iron?

Iron comes in two forms: heme and nonheme. Heme iron is the kind your body can most readily absorb and comes only from animal sources—red meat, poultry and fish, for example. Nonheme iron, which comes mostly from plant sources, is the hardest for the body to absorb. Meat contains both heme and nonheme iron.

Supply the ironworks. There's no need to go overboard at the butcher shop, however.

"Generally, eating a small (3½-ounce) serving of lean, red meat two or three times a week, plus poultry and fish two or three times, should be adequate for maintaining iron stores," says Andrew J. Silver, M.D., of the St. Louis University School of Medicine and Veterans Affairs Medial Center in Missouri. And lean meat actually has more iron than its fatty cousins.

Forget the liver. While liver used to be prescribed as the best antidote for iron deficiency, doctors no longer recommend it because it is so high in cholesterol. The trade-off just isn't worth it.

Please pass the vegetables. All this does not let you off the hook as far as eating your vegetables is concerned. Plant products, including beans and grains, are rich sources of nonheme iron.

ABSORB MORE

But getting iron from vegetables, legumes and grains is not as simple as popping them in your mouth. Your body must first change it into an absorbable form. Here's how.

Please pass the meat *and* vegetables. Stir-fry thinly sliced beef with broccoli and snow peas, or serve chicken with bean burritos, and you reap a double iron reward: "Meat increases the amount of iron your body can absorb from other foods eaten at the same time," says Dr. Hunt. "There is some as-yet-unknown factor in both red and white meats that can double or triple iron absorption from vegetable sources."

Think C. Add a few sections of orange or tangerine to your green salad. Citrus fruits provide vitamin C (ascorbic acid), which can help make nonheme iron more absorbable. "Make sure you have a source of ascorbic acid in your diet, especially if your iron is in nonheme form," Dr. Hunt advises. "It can easily double iron absorption."

To be effective iron enhancers, vitamin C-rich foods should be eaten at the same meal as iron-rich foods. A few other vitamin C sources that can help you mine the iron from meat and vegetables dishes are broccoli, peppers, tomatoes and potatoes.

Have a tomato juice cocktail. Drink vegetable juices to get iron and vitamin C in one big gulp. "Tomato juice is especially good because it contains high levels of both iron and vitamin C to help your body absorb it," says Dr. Weaver.

End on a high-C note. Top off a high-iron meal with a vitamin C-rich dessert. Citrus fruits, such as oranges and grapefruit, will do the trick, as will strawberries, raspberries and cantaloupe.

ADDING TO YOUR SUPPLY

Your iron supplies are affected not only by what you eat but by how you prepare it as well. Here are a few kitchen tips to help you make sure that your iron supply doesn't run short.

Don't undress foods. Eat the jackets of baked potatoes and use whole, unpeeled fruits and vegetables to get the full iron punch they supply. Iron is often most concentrated in the skins.

Avoid overcooking. Eat raw vegetables when you can, or cook them for a short time in very little water. Recapture the iron that cooks out of vegetables by re-using cooking water in soups or sauces. (Note that heme iron from meat is less affected by cooking then nonheme iron.)

Cook in iron. Cook slow-simmering, acidic foods—like tomato sauce—in iron pots. Some foods absorb a small amount of iron from the pot. Researchers aren't sure how much iron your *body* will absorb from the food, says Dr. Cook, but there's apparently no harm in using iron cookware.

IRON OUT THE WRINKLES IN YOUR DIET

There are also a few foods that can throw your iron absorption system out of sync if you eat them at the wrong time. These are perfectly fine foods, but they contain chemical components that can interfere with the body's ability to use iron. But you don't have to cross them off your menu. Here are some simple steps you can take to keep your iron-absorbing machinery working in tip-top fashion.

Choose brews with iron in mind. "Tea and coffee inhibit iron absorption," says Dr. Cook. Tea and coffee can rob you of half or more of the iron in foods. You don't have to forgo your coffee altogether. Just take your coffee break an hour before or after meals.

Go easy on the fiber. It's important to get fiber in your diet, but if upping iron absorption is your goal, you should be aware that fiber can push food through the digestive system so fast that iron doesn't have a chance to be absorbed. Also, many high-fiber foods contain phytic acid, a substance that traps and binds iron, making it unabsorbable. If you're eating a high-fiber diet, make sure you have lean red meat on the menu a couple times a week. And discuss your diet with your doctor.

TAKING IT ALL IN: IRON-RICH FOODS

Planning menus that include high-iron foods will help you meet your daily iron needs, says Connie Weaver, Ph.D., of Purdue University in West Lafayette, Indiana. (Women 50 or younger need 15 milligrams of iron a day; older women and all men need 10 milligrams a day.) In general, iron from red meat, shellfish and fish is easiest for the body to use. But vegetables, dried beans, grains and iron-fortified cereals and breads are good sources of iron, too. The table below lists some of the best food sources to help you mine a bountiful supply of iron.

FOOD	PORTION	TOTAL IRON (mg.)
ANIMAL SOURCES		
Clams, cooked, moist heat	10 small	12.6
Oysters, cooked, moist heat	6 med.	5.6
Light tuna, canned in water	3 oz.	2.7
Top round beef, broiled	3 oz.	2.5
Pork tenderloin, roasted	3 oz.	1.3
Haddock, cooked, dry heat	3 oz.	1.2
Turkey, light meat, roasted, no skin	3 oz.	1.2
PLANT SOURCES		
Total cereal	1 oz.	18.0
Tofu, regular, raw	½ cup	6.2
Potato, baked	1	2.8
Kidney beans, cooked	½ cup	2.6
Blackstrap molasses	1 Tbsp.	1.3
Figs, dried	3	1.3
Oatmeal, cooked	1 cup	1.2
Raisins	¼ cup	0.8
Broccoli, cooked	½ cup	0.7

IRON OVERLOAD

Some bodies simply do not know when to say no to iron. Two or three people out of a thousand—mostly of northern European descent—inherit a disorder that allows their bodies to overload on iron.

Like mild iron deficiency, mild iron overload is virtually symptomless, says James D. Cook, M.D., of the University of Kansas Medical Center in Kansas City. This means that men with this condition would probably not know it before they're 40 years old. By then, they may have as much as 20 to 40 grams of iron in their bodies—ten times more than the average. Women who are prone to overloading usually don't know it until they are well past menopause.

But when symptoms of iron toxicity finally show up, they do so with a serious bang: "Liver disease, aching joints, darkening of the skin, early-onset diabetes, sexual dysfunction and heart problems are some of the signs of iron overload," says Dr. Cook.

The treatment? Surprisingly, it's not to consume less iron but actually to give blood. "After diagnosis, people give blood donations once or twice a week until the excess iron is removed. That can involve 50 to 200 donations in the first year or two of treatment. Thereafter, giving blood every two to three months is sufficient to take care of the amount of iron they absorb through diet," Dr. Cook says.

ENRICHED AND FORTIFIED FOOD

So far, we've discussed making the most of naturally occurring iron in foods. Yet, almost any cereal, pasta, bread or baked good you buy contains flour that is enriched or fortified with iron. You might well wonder whether all that extra iron isn't more than enough?

The answer is a simple yes and no. Nutrition experts say that enriching commonly eaten, inexpensive foods has been a real boon, especially for people who can't afford or have trouble eating enough iron-rich meats and vegetables. Anemia in infants and children, for example, has declined drastically in the last two decades or so, thanks, in large part, to fortified foods.

But, while eating enriched foods may prevent severe iron shortages, it's not a cure-all for iron deficiency. Dr Weaver explains why: "Not all the iron from fortified sources is well absorbed. Often, they use electrolytic iron, which is basically iron filings. Manufacturers use it because some of the more absorbable forms of iron give food an off-flavor or odor, or cause the product to become rancid sooner."

So go ahead, enjoy your morning cereal. But don't assume that a cereal label that boasts 100 percent of the RDA for iron per serving guarantees complete protection. It's important to season your diet with the spice of life: variety. It gives you a better chance to get all the nutrients you need, including plenty of absorbable iron.

TESTING ONE, TWO, THREE

If your doctor suspects you're running low on iron because of a poor diet, he or she may order a blood test. "There's a wide range of symptoms related to iron that affect body tissues," says Dr. Cook, "but simple signs, like paleness or fatigue, are not reliable indicators of iron levels."

If diet and blood tests point toward iron deficiency, and if you are in a high-risk group, your doctor may prescribe iron supplements. Adolescent girls, pregnant women and growing children are most likely candidates for supplements. "Their iron requirements are often higher than their diets can meet, and their doctors may recommend supplements," says Dr. Cook.

But aren't iron pills or multivitamins with iron safe for everyone? The answer is a qualified no. While over-the-counter iron supplements are *probably* safe for most people, a decision to take them should certainly be discussed with your physician. "People—particularly men, as well as women beyond childbearing age—shouldn't take iron supplements for long periods of time without a physician's recommendation and supervision as well as a laboratory test to make sure that have a reason to take iron," says Dr. Cook.

Some studies have even raised the possibility that excess iron stores might increase the risk of cancer for some people.

"It is not wise to take supplements for years on end without a physician's approval," Dr. Silver agrees. "It's possible for iron supplements to mask a condition—such as slow, internal blood loss—that needs a different treatment. Taking iron unnecessarily in large amounts can also cause other problems, such as liver damage or iron toxicity."

If your doctor does recommend over-the-counter iron supplements, ask your pharmacist for a supplement of *ferrous* iron, such as ferrous sulfate, to assure maximum absorption, Dr. Hunt suggests. It's more easily absorbed than other types of supplements.

High-Nutrition Recipes

APPLESAUCE CAKE

Blackstrap molasses contains lots of iron. One way to use it is in a moist spice cake, such as this one. If you really like blackstrap's flavor, you may use it exclusively instead of di-luting it with light molasses.

1½ cups unsweetened applesauce	1 teaspoon baking soda
½ cup blackstrap molasses	1 teaspoon ground cinnamon
½ cup light molasses	½ teaspoon powdered ginger
¼ cup canola oil	
¼ cup fat-free egg substitute	½ teaspoon ground allspice
½ cup whole-wheat flour	¼ teaspoon ground cloves
½ cup unbleached flour	

In a large bowl, whisk together the applesauce, molasses, oil and egg. Add the flours, baking soda, cinnamon, ginger, allspice and cloves. Mix well.

Coat a 9" × 9" baking dish with no-stick spray. Add the batter and smooth the top with a spatula. Bake at 325° for 45 minutes, or until the top center of the cake springs back when touched lightly. Cool before serving.

Serves 12
Per serving: *152 calories, 4.7 g. fat (27% of calories), 1.1 g. dietary fiber, 0 mg. cholesterol, 90 mg. sodium, 3.3 mg. iron*

HEARTY MEAT LOAF

Beef is an excellent source of dietary iron. But it can also contain lots of fat and cholesterol, so you don't want to eat too much. One way to strike a happy medium is to combine a modest amount of lean beef (such as ground top round) with plenty of vegetables and grains, as in this meat loaf.

1	cup finely chopped carrots	½	teaspoon dried basil
1	cup finely chopped onions	½	teaspoon dried
1	tablespoon water		marjoram
1	pound ground lean top	½	teaspoon ground black
	round		pepper
1	cup rolled oats	1	cup tomato juice
½	cup bran		
¼	cup fat-free egg		
	substitute		

Combine the carrots, onions and water in a 1-quart glass measure. Cover with vented plastic wrap. Microwave on high for 4 minutes, or until the vegetables are just softened.

Transfer to a large bowl. Crumble the beef into the bowl. Add the oats and bran. Toss together lightly but thoroughly.

In a small bowl, whisk together the egg, basil, marjoram, pepper and ¾ cup of the juice. Pour over the meat and mix well.

Coat an 8" × 8" pan with no-stick spray. Add the meat and pat gently into a loaf shape. Pour the remaining ¼ cup juice over the meat.

Bake at 350° for 45 to 50 minutes, or until cooked through. If the top begins to brown too much, cover with a piece of foil.

Serves 6
Per serving: *198 calories, 4.2 g. fat (19% of calories), 4 g. dietary fiber, 43 mg. cholesterol, 214 mg. sodium, 3.2 mg. iron*

GINGERED BEEF AND VEGETABLE STIR-FRY

Here's another beef recipe, this one using the stir-fry technique. Marinating the lean meat before cooking it enhances its flavor and helps to tenderize it a bit.

1	pound boneless top round steak	2	scallions, julienned
2	tablespoons low-sodium soy sauce	1/3	cup julienned celery
		1/4	cup plus 1 tablespoon water
1	tablespoon grated fresh ginger	1	cup snow peas
1	tablespoon minced garlic	1	teaspoon arrowroot or cornstarch
2	teaspoons sesame oil	3	cups hot cooked brown or basmati rice
1	cup julienned sweet red peppers		

Place the steak in the freezer until partially frozen, about 20 minutes. Trim off all visible fat. Slice the meat across the grain and on the diagonal to make thin (1/4") strips. Place in a medium bowl. Add the soy sauce, ginger, garlic and 1 teaspoon of the oil. Mix well and let marinate while you cook the vegetables.

In a wok or large frying pan over high heat, heat the remaining 1 teaspoon oil. Add the peppers, scallions and celery. Stir briskly to coat the vegetables with the oil. Add 1/4 cup water and cook for 2 minutes, stirring occasionally. Using a slotted spoon, transfer the vegetables to a plate.

Add the meat and its marinade to the wok. Cook, stirring frequently, for about 5 minutes, or until the meat browns slightly. Add the cooked vegetables and snow peas.

In a cup, combine the arrowroot or cornstarch and the remaining 1 tablespoon water. Add to the pan. Stir until the sauce thickens, about 1 minute. Serve over the rice.

Serves 4
Per serving: *372 calories, 8.6 g. fat (21% of calories), 4.1 g. dietary fiber, 65 mg. cholesterol, 379 mg. sodium, 4.2 mg. iron*

LINGUINE WITH CLAM SAUCE

Clams are a super source of iron. One classic way to enjoy them is over pasta. This recipe is an adaptation of one presented by heart researcher William P. Castelli, M.D., at a conference held by the American Diabetes Association. Each serving contains more than twice the Recommended Dietary Allowance for iron.

2 **medium onions, diced**	½ **teaspoon ground black pepper**
2 **cloves garlic, minced**	
1 **tablespoon olive oil**	¼ **cup chopped pimientos**
2 **cans (8 ounces each) minced clams**	8 **ounces linguine**
½ **cup apple cider or alcohol-free white wine**	¼ **cup chopped fresh parsley**
3 **tablespoons lemon juice**	¼ **cup chopped fresh basil**

In a large no-stick frying pan over medium heat, sauté the onions and garlic in the oil for 3 minutes, or until softened.

Drain the clams, saving the liquid. Set the clams aside. Add the liquid to the frying pan. Add the cider or wine. Bring to a boil and cook until the total volume is reduced by half, about 15 minutes. Stir in the lemon juice, pepper and reserved clams.

Cover the pan, reduce the heat to medium-low and simmer for 5 minutes. Stir in the pimientos.

Meanwhile, cook the linguine in a large pot of boiling water for about 8 minutes, or until just tender. Drain. Return the linguine to its pan. Add the clam mixture, parsley and basil. Toss to coat. Cover and cook over medium-low heat for 5 minutes.

Serves 4
Per serving: *453 calories, 6.7 g. fat (12% of calories), 0.5 g. dietary fiber, 76 mg. cholesterol, 138 mg. sodium, 35 mg. iron*

CHAPTER 13

Potassium

A Protector from Our Past

Dateline: The Stone Age. Grok, a typical cave dweller, is preparing food for the day.

For breakfast, he eats a juicy cantaloupe smashed open against a jagged rock. He places a banana, some nuts and a squash in a goatskin sack for lunch. Then he's off to scrounge groceries—a few figs here, some potatoes there—to haul back to the cave, dodging wild beasts along the way.

Few of us would want to trade our condos or Cuisinarts for Grok's crude lifestyle. But if we *were* to return to our dietary roots and adopt his menu of potassium-rich plant foods, experts say we might at least be more likely to stave off modern-day diseases such as stroke, heart disease, diabetes and even cancer.

A QUESTION OF BALANCE

Louis Tobian, M.D., professor of medicine and head of the Hypertension Department at the University of Minnesota in Minneapolis, is the leading advocate for a return to an ancestral diet.

According to Dr. Tobian, the prehistoric cuisine, consisting mostly of vegetables, fruits, nuts, roots and occasionally wild game, contained very little sodium but lots of potassium. Both these minerals—in the proper ratio—are essential to health. When dissolved in body fluids, they carry on a sort of unceasing tug-of-war across the walls of cells, which ultimately determines the water balance inside the body.

Because humankind evolved for thousands of years on a potassium-rich diet similar to Grok's, our bodies have become very efficient at getting rid of any excess potassium. And because sodium was normally in short supply, our bodies have become programmed to store it up.

Where we've gotten ourselves in trouble, says Dr. Tobian, is by starting to eat the reverse of the prehistoric diet—one that's incompatible with the way we are biologically programmed. Today's typical diet skimps on fresh plant food. Instead it is laden with salty "factory food" that has had much of the potassium squeezed out during processing. And the closest some come to fruit is the prune filling inside a Danish. As for vegetables, we may eat lots of potassium-rich potatoes, but too often they're the salty, fried-in-fat kind.

We pay a high price for eating this lopsided, "unnatural" diet that is out of sync with our bodies, according to Dr. Tobian. "There's strong evidence suggesting that a lifetime of eating a typical modern diet can lead to heart disease and stroke," he says.

For example, researchers found that people in Scotland, who eat mostly low-potassium foods, have a greater incidence of heart disease than people in southern England, who eat higher amounts of potassium-rich food. In the United States, blacks in the southeast who typically eat potassium-poor diets have a higher stroke risk than any other group in the country.

THE PICKS OF POTASSIUM

Choosing a variety of potassium-rich foods can help you meet your daily goal of at least 3,000 milligrams easily and deliciously.

FOOD	PORTION	POTASSIUM (mg.)
Avocado	1	1,204
Raisins	1 cup	1,089
Acorn squash, baked	1 cup	891
Potato, baked	1	844
Spinach, cooked	1 cup	838
Cauliflower florets, raw	1 cup	795
Navy beans, cooked	1 cup	719
Apricots, fresh	1 cup	628
Plain nonfat yogurt	1 cup	579
Orange juice	1 cup	496
Cantaloupe	1 cup cubes	494
Skim milk	1 cup	447
Chicken breast, broiler/ fryer	1	440
Sockeye salmon, fresh, cooked	3 oz.	319
Flounder, cooked	3 oz.	292
Ground beef, extra-lean	3 oz.	266
Turkey white meat	3 oz.	259
Turkey dark meat	3 oz.	247
Bran muffin	1	172
Pumpernickel bread	1 slice	145
Whole-wheat bread	1 slice	50

KEEPING THE LID ON BLOOD PRESSURE

Laboratory studies show convincingly that a diet short on potassium boosts blood pressure—a leading cause of heart disease and stroke.

In a small but impressive study conducted at the Temple University School of Medicine and the University of Pennsylvania in Philadelphia, researchers placed ten men with normal blood pressures on two experimental diets, one providing normal amounts of potassium and the other low in potassium. Nine days on the normal potassium diet showed no significant change in blood pressure readings. But after going on the low-potassium diet, their blood pressures went up. The men also retained more sodium and fluid.

Similar results were found in people with high blood pressures. "Our research shows that when we feed people with either high or normal blood pressures a low-potassium diet, their blood pressures will increase in less than two weeks," says G. Gopal Krishna, M.D., associate professor of medicine at the University of Pennsylvania. One reason is that a low-potassium diet causes people to retain more sodium. Over time, this high sodium level attracts water, increasing blood volume and raising blood pressure.

But the good news, says Dr. Krishna, is that when these same people were put on a high-potassium diet, their blood pressures went down. "A high-potassium diet counteracts sodium's harmful effects on blood pressure," says Dr. Krishna.

Potassium even appears to be helpful for people with high blood pressures who take medication. Researchers at the University of Naples in Italy put a group of people on blood pressure medication on a potassium-rich daily diet of beans, fruits or vegetables for a year. The result: They slashed their drug intake by more than 50 percent.

The combined evidence makes one thing clear: "When it comes to controlling blood pressure, the amount of potassium in your diet may be more important than how little salt you eat," says Dr. Krishna.

HOLDING SODIUM IN CHECK

Potassium performs many jobs in the body. It is responsible for maintaining proper fluid balance within the cells, and it helps nerves transmit messages and assures proper muscle functioning. But the secret to its protective power against high blood pressure is its ability to police the amount of sodium in the body.

Both potassium and sodium are electrolytes, substances that separate into electrically charged particles called ions. A high-salt, low-potassium diet disrupts the proper electrolyte balance, throwing the fluid balance out of whack. The result: Blood flow in the arteries slows down.

As surplus salt attracts water, blood volume expands, boosting pressure in the arteries. This high volume begins to take its toll on your arteries. Over many years, high blood pressure damages these vessels in various areas, like the heart, brain or kidneys. Eventually, a heart attack or stroke can occur.

Enter potassium. It has the ability to regulate the amount of sodium trying to move into your bloodstream.

Exactly how potassium does its job is still a mystery. It is known, however, that potassium is necessary for proper cellular function and salt balance, says George Bakris, M.D., assistant professor of medicine and pharmacology at the University of Texas Health Science Center in San Antonio.

STROKE PROTECTION

Potassium also appears to be part of the armor against stroke-associated death. At least that's the conclusion of a long-term study conducted jointly by the University of California, San Diego, School of Medicine and the University of Cambridge School of Medicine in England.

After following the diets of 859 Californians for more than a decade, researchers found that those who consumed the least amount of potassium had the highest incidence of

DON'T SWEAT OVER SPORTS DRINKS

It's mid-August, the second day of your hiking trip, and you're sweating like a racehorse near the finish line. Your hiking companions are swigging sports drinks like there's no tomorrow. Are you missing out on something?

Maybe so—if the drinks contain potassium.

When you perspire, you lose more than water. You also lose trace amounts of potassium and other electrolytes, important minerals that separate into electrically charged particles inside the body. Adequate potassium is needed to help muscles contract and relax. If your potassium level dips, your muscles may flex but not relax. The result: a cramp. What's more, a lack of potassium can impair your muscles' ability to use glycogen, the sugar that is their main source of energy.

In other words, a prolonged, sweaty workout could lead to weak, spasm-prone muscles. Worse, severe dehydration can lead to heatstroke.

Even so, many experts believe that, unless you are an endurance athlete competing in a hot environment, elec-

stroke-associated death. But not one stroke-associated death occurred among the people whose diets contained the highest levels of potassium.

Perhaps even more amazing is a study from India in which researchers found that potassium lowered both blood pressure and cholesterol (another stroke risk factor) in those with mild hypertension in just two months.

But such results are not surprising to Dr. Tobian. "I'm convinced that the best protection against aging arteries and modern diseases such as stroke and high blood pressure is to eat a primitive diet," he says. One with plenty of potassium.

trolyte sports beverages are probably unnecessary. That's because your body automatically rebalances its electrolyte levels through a regular diet of potassium-rich foods.

"For most exercisers, the important thing for preventing heatstroke and muscle cramps is getting fluid into your body," says Herman Johnson, Ph.D., of the United States Department of Agriculture's nutrition lab at the Presidio of San Francisco. "Plain water will do the trick."

But other experts argue that plain water is too "plain" for heavy exercise. "During a sweaty workout, more potassium may be depleted from the muscles than is measured by standard tests," says Robert Hackman, Ph.D., associate professor of nutrition at the University of Oregon in Eugene. When you're sweating heavily, he says, you need fluids containing potassium to prevent muscle cramps and fatigue.

These fluids need not be commercial sports drinks, however. "Sipping orange or grapefruit juice during and after a heavy workout is enough to make up for potential potassium losses," says Dr. Hackman. In between workouts, make sure you eat plenty of fruits and vegetables.

A ROLE AGAINST CANCER?

A number of population studies, supported by preliminary studies in animals, indicate that there might even be a connection between potassium and cancer prevention.

"The potassium/sodium balance appears to play an important role in regulating cellular growth," says Birger Jansson, Ph.D., professor of biomathematics at the M. D. Anderson Cancer Center in Houston, where the research is taking place. When the balance tips toward a surplus of sodium, he explains, cells can grow abnormally and the likelihood of cancer increases. Ample potassium, however, appears to retard abnormal cell growth and lower the risk of cancer.

"We and scientists at other labs found that laboratory animals fed high-potassium, low-sodium diets had fewer tumors and a longer lifespan than rats fed the opposite diets," says Dr. Jansson. "While the study results are preliminary, I believe it's safe to assume that eating more fruits and vegetables and reducing the intake of salt helps reduce not only your risk of cardiovascular disease but also cancer."

How Much to Aim For

Of course, getting plenty of potassium doesn't mean you should be getting it by eating banana splits. "To protect against heart disease and stroke, you need to follow other good eating habits for maintaining healthy arteries," says Dr. Tobian. That means a low-fat diet and plenty of fruits and vegetables—Grok's main menu.

"A good diet and a regular program of aerobic exercise is as important as increasing potassium," says Dr. Tobian. "The more they become a part of you, the more potassium will benefit you."

Studies show that roughly 3,000 milligrams a day are needed to protect against stroke. "That's not hard to achieve when you consider that a typical balanced diet offers between 2,000 and 2,500 milligrams of potassium a day," says Dr. Tobian.

Indeed, in the California study, people who added only about 400 to 450 milligrams of extra potassium a day—the amount in one banana—to their normal diets were able to reduce their risk of stroke death by 40 percent.

But, if you're a fast-food fan or you generally don't eat plenty of fruits and vegetables, you'll have to work a little harder to get 3,000 milligrams a day.

And if you are at risk for high blood pressure or stroke, you may need twice that, says Dr. Tobian. But be sure to check with your doctor before taking any potassium supplements.

POTASSIUM-BOOSTING TIPS

Getting more potassium is a snap if you learn to follow a few rules and make some simple substitutions, according to Dr. Tobian.

Take a juice break. "Instead of a coffee break, I drink grapefruit juice three times a day. At 400 milligrams of potassium per cup, that's 1,200 milligrams right there," he says.

Take your mother's advice. "Vegetables are loaded with potassium," says Dr. Tobian. "They're really the key to eating a healthy primitive diet." Consider, for example, that a cup of cooked asparagus has 558 milligrams of potassium; a cup of baked butternut squash has 580 milligrams.

Go natural. As a general rule, go for more fresh food and less packaged, canned or fast food, says George Webb, Ph.D., associate professor of physiology and biophysics at the University of Vermont College of Medicine in Burlington. "The canning process usually involves boiling the food, which leaches out the potassium," says Dr. Webb. "The tasteless result is then flavored with table salt."

Take peas, for instance. A half-cup of cooked fresh peas offers 217 milligrams of potassium and just 2 milligrams of sodium. But 1/2 cup canned peas delivers only 147 milligrams of potassium and 186 milligrams of sodium.

Go down to the farm. Although fruits and vegetables are the best sources of potassium, other sources are easy to find. Low-fat dairy products, fish, poultry and lean meat can also contribute to your daily intake.

Combine dishes to double your potassium. There are plenty of tasty ways you can bring potassium-rich foods together. Try a half cantaloupe with a scoop of ice milk, for example. Toss potassium-rich lentils in your spinach salad or bake fish with a layer of glazed apricots.

LESS PROCESSING—MORE POTASSIUM

The more a food has been processed, the more potassium it is likely to have lost. Compare the potassium content of the fresh or minimally processed foods below with their more processed versions.

FOOD (1 cup)	POTASSIUM (mg.)
BEETS	
Fresh	530
Canned	252
CAULIFLOWER	
Fresh	404
Canned	250
FLOUR	
Whole-wheat	444
White	109
MUSHROOMS	
Fresh	555
Canned	201
RICE	
Brown	137
White	57

Season lightly with salt substitutes. Salt substitutes containing potassium chloride can help limit your salt intake while boosting your potassium intake. But you shouldn't rely solely on these products to meet your quota of extra potassium, warns Dr. Webb. "For one thing, we're not sure of chloride's role in blood pressure," he says. For another, potassium in food is absorbed more slowly and probably more effectively than man-made chemicals.

A note of caution: If you have kidney problems or take a potassium-sparing diuretic, you should avoid potassium chloride salt substitutes. Otherwise, you could be getting too much potassium. Check with your doctor.

You needn't go bananas. This sweet tropical fruit gets most of the attention as a prime potassium source. But it really isn't the highest source. While a banana has about 450 milligrams of potassium, a slice of watermelon has 602 milligrams and a cup of prune juice has over 700 milligrams.

Searching for something out of the ordinary? Try green plantains. They look like unripe bananas but taste like potatoes and pack an awesome 716 milligrams per cup. Try baking them in their skins, or boiling and mashing them like potatoes.

Buy real juice. Some artificially flavored beverages are just chemical versions of juice. Others contain only about 10 percent real fruit juice. Look for juice labeled "100 percent fruit juice." Or squeeze your own freshly made juice complete with bits of healthy fiber.

Walk past the white bread. Choose whole-grain breads instead. A slice of white bread contains 26 milligrams of potassium; a slice of whole-wheat contains more than twice that amount. You can also buy whole-wheat flour for baking and whole-wheat bread crumbs for stuffing and mixing into meat loaf.

Stockpile potatoes. "People call milk the perfect food, but potatoes should really win that title," says Dr. Webb. For starters, they are great sources of potassium: one baked potato supplies more than 800 milligrams. They're also very low in calories, providing you avoid the fried kind and skip the butter topping.

For a treat, try potato pancakes. Simply shred one or two potatoes without peeling, add some minced onion, and brown in a nonstick pan. Serve with applesauce or a dollop of nonfat yogurt for even more potassium power.

Load up on legumes. Beans have a very high potassium content and make great additions to salads and stews. A cup of cooked pinto beans, for example, supplies 796 milligrams of potassium; the same amount of navy beans has 719 milligrams, and lima beans have 730 milligrams per cup.

Don't boil food. Boiling leaches out potassium. Researchers have found, for example, that boiled potatoes lose up to half of their potassium, while steamed potatoes lose only about 6 percent. Similar results were found with carrots, beans and peas. You're better off steaming, baking, microwaving or stir-frying.

Add a little blackstrap molasses. Two tablespoons of blackstrap molasses contain more than 435 milligrams of potassium. Try swirling it in hot cereal or using it instead of honey in recipes.

Toss in brewer's yeast. One tablespoon of this concentrated source of B vitamins also gives you 152 milligrams of potassium. And you can add it to everything from soups and stews to blender drinks.

Mix in tofu. One cup of tofu contains 596 milligrams of potassium and 244 milligrams of calcium, another mineral that may do good things for blood pressure. Dice tofu and add to chili or substitute it for half the hamburger in lasagna.

Have a date or two. Ounce per ounce, dried fruits have even more potassium than fresh fruits do. That's because the water has been removed so the potassium is concentrated, says Dr. Webb. Three fresh apricots, for example, give you a respectable 314 milligrams of potassium. A cup of dried apricots, however, supplies a mighty 1,204 milligrams of the mineral. Try dried dates, prunes, raisins or figs on your morning cereal or as stand-alone snacks. They also make great substitutes for fatty sauces to flavor oven-baked poultry and pork.

Dried fruits, however, should be eaten sparingly—they're very high in calories.

Serve some soup. Homemade soup is an ideal way to bring lots of potassium-rich vegetables to your table—minus the high levels of added sodium found in many canned soups. In addition to old standbys like chicken or tomato soup, try pumpkin soup. A cup of canned pumpkin has 503 milligrams of potassium.

EASY OPTIONS FOR EXTRA POTASSIUM

Here's some good news: High-potassium foods are great for your waistline. Here are some high-potassium substitutions for high-calorie fare.

• Instead of cream pie to satisfy your sweet tooth, have a pear for dessert. One juicy pear gives you 208 milligrams of potassium.

• Grill chicken or fish instead of frankfurters. A single chicken breast has less fat than a frank and gives you 220 milligrams of potassium compared to just 143 milligrams in the hot dog.

• Try fruit spreads in place of butter. Apple butter spread on your toast offers 38 milligrams of potassium per tablespoon and virtually no fat, versus 6 milligrams of potassium and 11 grams of fat per tablespoon of margarine.

• Instead of iced tea on a sweltering day, reach for frozen melon balls kept in the freezer. Substitute the frozen balls for ice cubes in fruit drinks. Or toss them in a blender for a refreshing slushy cooler. Honeydew melon, for example, contains 461 milligrams of potassium per cup; casaba has about 357 milligrams.

High-Nutrition Recipes

CUBAN-STYLE PLANTAINS

Plantains are cooking bananas often featured in Caribbean cuisine. They're super sources of potassium, but unlike bananas, they cannot be eaten raw. Cooking softens their starchy texture and develops their flavor. Buy plantains that are fully yellow, firm and heavy. Use this recipe in place of potatoes when serving spicy chicken, fish or pork dishes.

4 plantains	3 tablespoons shredded
¾ cup skim milk	low-fat Cheddar cheese
¼ cup fat-free egg	2 cups chunky salsa,
substitute	heated
¼ cup minced scallions	

Peel the plantains using a sharp paring knife. Cut the flesh into ½" slices. Steam for 15 minutes, or until very tender. Place in a large bowl and mash with a potato masher. Stir in the milk, egg and scallions.

Coat a 9" pie plate with no-stick spray. Add the plantain mixture and smooth the top with a spatula. Sprinkle with the Cheddar.

Bake at 400° for 10 minutes, or until the mixture is heated through and the cheese is lightly browned.

Cut into wedges and serve topped with the salsa.

Serves 6
Per serving: *208 calories, 3.6 g. fat (13% of calories), 3 g. dietary fiber, 4 mg. cholesterol, 347 mg. sodium, 887 mg. potassium*

ORANGE SHAKE

Here's another high-potassium beverage—this one thick and creamy like a milk shake. (But it contains none of the fat found in regular shakes.) For variety, replace the dates with banana slices or strawberries.

About 1 cup orange juice	1½ cups frozen nonfat
½ cup chopped dates	vanilla yogurt

In a blender, combine the orange juice and dates. Blend on high speed until the dates are very finely chopped. Add the yogurt and blend until just combined. If the mixture is too thick, thin with a little additional juice.

Serves 2
Per serving: *338 calories, 0.4 g. fat (1% of calories), 4.9 g. dietary fiber, 0 mg. cholesterol, 82 mg. sodium, 539 mg. potassium*

GERMAN POTATO SALAD

Potatoes are one of the best vegetable sources of potassium. But to help safeguard the nutrient, steam the potatoes rather than boiling them. Contrary to popular opinion, potatoes are not fattening. And neither is potato salad—as long as you stay away from fatty mayonnaise or oil-based dressing. This version has a tangy vinegar dressing and is served warm, in the German tradition.

2 pounds small potatoes	2 teaspoons honey
2 ounces turkey bacon, cut into ½" pieces	½ teaspoon ground black pepper
½ cup diced sweet red peppers	⅛ teaspoon celery seeds
½ cup diced red onions	1 tablespoon cornstarch
⅔ cup defatted beef stock	2 tablespoons water
⅓ cup apple-cider vinegar	2 tablespoons minced fresh parsley

Scrub the potatoes and cut into thin slices. Steam until tender but not mushy, about 10 minutes. Transfer to a large bowl.

Meanwhile, in a large no-stick frying pan over medium heat, cook the bacon, peppers and onions until the bacon is crisp, about 5 minutes. Add to the potatoes and toss lightly.

In a 1-quart saucepan, whisk together the stock, vinegar, honey, pepper and celery seeds. Bring to a boil over high heat. Reduce the heat to medium.

In a cup, dissolve the cornstarch in the water. Add to the pan and whisk constantly until the dressing thickens, about 2 minutes. Pour over the potatoes and toss gently. Sprinkle with the parsley. Serve warm.

Serves 6
Per serving: *174 calories, 3.5 g. fat (17% of calories), 3.2 g. dietary fiber, 9 mg. cholesterol, 231 mg. sodium, 870 mg. potassium*

GRAPEFRUIT COOLER

Fruit beverages are a tasty and easy way to get potassium into your diet. This citrus refresher combines potassium-rich grapefruit juice with orange or tangerine juice. You may serve the drink over regular ice cubes, but for an extra bonus of potassium, make cubes from additional grapefruit juice.

4 cups pink grapefruit juice	3 tablespoons lime juice
½ cup orange or tangerine juice concentrate, thawed	2 cups sparkling mineral water

In a large pitcher, mix the grapefruit juice, juice concentrate and lime juice. Stir in the mineral water. Serve over ice.

Serves 4
Per serving: *144 calories, 0.3 g. fat (2% of calories) 0.7 g. dietary fiber, 0 mg. cholesterol, 7 mg. sodium, 603 mg. potassium*

CHAPTER 14

Antioxidants

Dietary "Rustproofers"

Butter turns rancid. The iron gate rusts. Fire burns. Paint dries. Arteries harden. People grow old.

It's all the same, more and more scientists believe. The same chemical reaction—oxidation—that coats an unseasoned skillet with an orange film of rust is being implicated in such diseases as cancer, cataracts and atherosclerosis. Even aging may be caused by the same process.

If you slice an apple and leave it exposed to air, it will soon turn brown. But soak that sliced apple in a vitamin C solution first, and it will stay glistening white.

That's because vitamin C is one of a handful of nutrients with power to protect cells from the damage of oxidation. While the evidence still is inconclusive, it nonetheless strongly suggests that increasing dietary intake of nutrients known as antioxidants may help save the body from the ravages of certain diseases.

"It's only a hypothesis right now," says Balz B. Frei, Ph.D., an assistant professor of nutrition at the Harvard School of Public Health in Boston, "but there's a lot of good circumstantial evidence. While we still need to conduct more experiments, it's a good idea to have enough of the antioxidants around in your body."

AIRING THE ISSUE

Oxygen breathes life into our bodies; without it, every living thing would die. But the same process through which the body burns food with oxygen to generate energy also sparks a dangerous—albeit quite natural and common—side effect.

Eventually, the oxygen merges with hydrogen to form simple water molecules. But along the way, it also forms highly reactive molecularly unbalanced substances, called free radicals, that have the ability to attack and harm cells.

No, free radicals aren't some anachronistic throwback to the 1960s. A free radical is a wounded molecule that lacks an electron, and it lashes out violently at other molecules, stealing an electron to regain its balance. The victimized molecule itself becomes a free radical, initiating a chain reaction that can eventually destroy cells and organs.

"The problem is you have to get rid of that chain reaction," Dr. Frei says. "One or a few free radicals can oxidize a large amount of cells. The damage can spread very rapidly, especially in fats."

We can't totally escape from free radicals. They're everywhere—created in the body by ultraviolet light, radiation, pollution, car exhaust, cigarette smoke and alcohol—just to name the more common problems. The exposure is thought to be implicated in atherosclerosis, cancer, cataracts, degeneration of the retina in the eye and even aging.

"In each disease, the oxidation process is basically the same. It merely differs in what molecules are being attacked," says Denham Harman, M.D., Ph.D., professor emeritus of the University of Nebraska's College of Medicine in Omaha and executive director of the American Aging Association.

The body does have a defense system against the onslaught. Enzymes manufactured by cells, for example, interact and neutralize some free radicals, but we can do little to increase the amount of those enzymes in our bodies.

So attention has been focused on antioxidant nutrients, whose levels in the body *can* be increased by what we eat and by what supplements we ingest. The principal antioxidants—vitamin C, vitamin E and beta-carotene—do seem to offer protection. And scientists theorize that the higher their concentrations in body tissue and fluids, the better protected we may be against oxidative agents. If you put LDL—low-density lipoprotein, the "bad" cholesterol whose oxidation may initiate artery blockage—in a test tube and bubble air through it, "it won't oxidize appreciably until all the antioxidants are used up," says David Kritchevsky, Ph.D., a professor at the Wister Institute in Philadelphia. If it works in a test tube, does that mean it works in humans? "We don't know," says Dr. Kritchevsky.

SACRIFICED FOR A GOOD CAUSE

In the test tube and in many animal studies, at least, the antioxidants work by sacrificing themselves to the oxidizing molecules. They're sort of suicide bombers for health, either sapping the oxidizing molecules of energy or offering them electrons before body cells can be attacked. In either case, the reactive oxygen is rendered harmless, but, unlike victimized body cells, antioxidants do not initiate or continue any destructive chain reaction. Nor do they become malignant.

Vitamins C and E are called scavengers because they react with free radicals before those troublemakers can reach body cells, Dr. Frei says. They are doubly effective because each vitamin molecule can donate two electrons, neutralizing two free radical molecules.

A POSSIBLE ROLE AGAINST CATARACTS

Seeing is believing, according to the cliché, and more people may be able to see more clearly without the obstruction of cataracts if they increase antioxidant nutrients in their diets.

Ophthalmologists are studying how vitamins may prevent or slow the age-related clouding of the eye's lens, a prime cause of blindness. Other research is attempting to determine if the same nutrients can prevent degeneration of the retina.

"The lens of the eye, unlike any other tissue in the body, is subject to the concerted insult of oxidation and light," says Allen Taylor, Ph.D., director of the Laboratory for Nutrition and Vision Research in the United Stated Department of Agriculture's Human Nutrition Research Center on Aging at Tufts University in Boston. "Because it is exposed almost constantly to the air and to light, it is a prime target for oxidation."

At the onset of cataract formation, the lens starts to harden, says Shambhu D. Varma, Ph.D., director of ophthalmology research at the University of Maryland School of Medicine in Baltimore. The lens cannot flatten or thicken to focus, and people become farsighted. People who are still relatively young can squint to adjust the eye's focal range and compensate for the rigidity of the lens. But as they age and the eye continues to be exposed to oxidative harm, small chalky spots begin forming on the lens. Light doesn't pass through it so easily, Dr. Varma says, and images sent to the

Water-soluble vitamin C circulates through the bloodstream and is found in all body fluids. Fat-soluble vitamin E collects in fat tissue and blood fats.

Beta-carotene's antioxidant power is different from that of

retina are no longer clear and well defined. Eventually, a white film coats the lens, and vision becomes cloudy.

Exposure of eyes and lenses to higher doses of antioxidant vitamins "seems to delay the onset or progress of cataracts," Dr. Taylor says. And Dr. Varma notes, "Slower development means prevention. We might be able to prevent cataracts or maybe delay their formation."

People with more beta-carotene and vitamin C in their blood often have lower incidences of cataracts, Dr. Taylor says. Vitamin E also seems to play a role.

The antioxidant trio also may be useful against macular degeneration, a disease that harms the membranes of the retina, where images fall and are sent to the brain. "When the central part of the retina begins to deteriorate, it can't transmit to the brain," Dr. Varma says. But preliminary research in animals suggests that vitamin C, beta-carotene and vitamin E may retard the degeneration.

Delivering antioxidants to where they're needed could run into a snag, though. "There's a general failure with eyedrops," Dr. Taylor says. "They are not a good way to get vitamins into the lens. The nutrients are not that stable in drop form, and the solutions that contain them could themselves be irritants."

The easiest and perhaps most effective way could be overall good nutrition, he says. "Increasing dietary consumption of the antioxidants can increase levels in the eye tissue."

vitamin E and vitamin C, according to Dr. Frei. "It's not clear why it has protective antioxidant properties," he says, because it does not scavenge free radicals and offer up electrons. It "quenches" reactive oxygen but does not chemically alter it.

"It's an energy transfer," he says. "Beta-carotene takes up energy from the reactive oxygen molecules and dissipates it."

None of the antioxidant nutrients necessarily is a more potent protector than the others. In fact, in the case of vitamins C and E, they may even work in concert. "In different diseases or at different organ sites, one antioxidant may be more important than another, but they're all needed," says Gladys Block, Ph.D., a professor of public health nutrition at the University of California in Berkeley. While they probably act in unison, they usually are studied separately.

VITAMIN C: A KEY PROTECTOR

Heart disease. Vitamin C may be the body's most important guardian against atherosclerosis, according to Dr. Frei, who conducted laboratory tests on the subject. In the oxidative theory of hardening of the arteries, "if there's no oxidation, there's no atherosclerosis," he says. But if the arteries are left unprotected, oxidation eventually occurs. The "bad" LDL cholesterol in blood becomes trapped inside artery walls and slowly oxidizes. Once oxidized, it is taken up by cells in the artery walls at an extremely high rate and transforms into "foam cells," precursors of artery-narrowing plaque that Dr. Frei calls the hallmark of early atherosclerosis.

High-density lipoprotein (HDL) cholesterol, the "good" cholesterol, also is found in artery walls and may prevent LDL oxidation by removing it. But antioxidant vitamins seem to prevent oxidation even without removing the LDL, Dr. Frei says. In laboratory tests, vitamin C completely protected lipoproteins in human blood against a variety of oxidants, including smoke. Beta-carotene and vitamin E became activated only after all vitamin C in the plasma had been expended, and they only partially prevented oxidation.

Cancer. Scientists speculate that vitamin C's antioxidant properties may also play a role in cancer protection. Numerous studies show that people who have a low intake of vitamin C are almost twice as likely to develop cancer of the mouth, voice box or esophagus. In another study, people who consumed less than 90 milligrams of vitamin C a day were 1½ times more likely to develop lung cancer than those who ingested at least 140 milligrams of the nutrient.

And in a study of 55-year-old pack-a-day male smokers, those who consumed low amounts of vitamin C either through food or supplements had a 25 percent chance of dying from lung cancer. But those who ate a lot of foods high in vitamin C, particularly fruit, or who took supplements had only a 7 percent chance of dying from the disease.

High vitamin C intake also has been correlated with lower risks of stomach, pancreatic, cervical, and rectal cancer. And postmenopausal women can reduce their risk of breast cancer by 16 percent, one study suggests, if they increase their consumption of the nutrient.

Low levels of vitamin C in men, according to researchers at the University of California at Berkeley, may offer a gateway to free radicals to damage sperm, possibly increasing the risk of birth defects.

Older people seem more likely to have low levels of vitamin C in their bodies. And, for reasons still not known, elderly men need to ingest more C than elderly women to maintain high levels of the vitamin in their bloodstream.

Where to find it. Good dietary sources of vitamin C include citrus fruit and juices, strawberries, red and green peppers, broccoli, cantaloupe, mangoes, tomatoes and tomato juice, watermelon, honeydew melon, brussels sprouts and cauliflower.

VITAMIN E: FREE RADICAL FIGHTER

Ischemia. During surgery, it often is necessary to cut off blood flow to an organ or a part of the body. This process, which is called ischemia, can also occur spontaneously because of disease, and when it happens in the heart, chest pain and even a heart attack could occur. In either case, when oxygen-rich blood flow is restored to the oxygen-starved tissue, free radicals are generated, and fats start to oxidize. That eventually could destroy vital organs. But, Dr. Kritchevsky says, "If vitamin E's around, this doesn't happen."

In people who received vitamin E supplementation 12 hours before heart bypass operations, hydrogen peroxide levels in their bodies—an indicator of oxidation—did not increase during surgery. Levels of the chemical did increase, though, in people who did not receive the supplement.

Other experiments have shown that vitamin E supplements diminish fat peroxides in blood and, in women, reduce the increase in blood clotting associated with long-term use of hormonal contraceptives.

Cancer. As with vitamin C, there is evidence that vitamin E may lessen the risk of developing cancer, and not just because it scavenges free radicals. The nutrient may also bolster the body's immune system, enabling it to eliminate cells already damaged by oxidation. Vitamin E also seems to prevent the transformation of nitrite food additives into cancer-causing nitrosamines in the stomach.

Selenium, a nutrient that seems to work in conjunction with vitamin E, also possesses antioxidant properties. Experiments show that this mineral can reduce the size and growth of tumors in animals, perhaps by strengthening the immune system. But too much selenium in the body is toxic, and research shows that when vitamin E in the diet is adequate, selenium is of limited and perhaps no importance.

Where to find it. Good dietary doses of vitamin E include wheat germ, peanut butter, almonds, filbert nuts, sunflower seeds, shrimp, and vegetable oils. Green leafy vegetables also contain some vitamin E.

A STOP-GAP MEASURE FOR SMOKERS WHO CAN'T STOP?

Smoke gets in your eyes, according to the song, but it also gets in your lungs and bloodstream, causing oxidative damage to cells.

The best approach to preventing lung cancer, emphysema and hardening of the arteries is, of course, to quit smoking. But if you're currently curled up with a Camel or musing with a Marlboro, you may take some comfort from what scientists are learning about antioxidant nutrients.

Vitamin E may be utilized by smokers to stave off the oxidation of fats in cells. A group of researchers from the University of Toronto Department of Medicine in Ontario suggests that "for smokers who cannot refrain from smoking, a possible means of reducing their total body lipid peroxidation is to administer additional antioxidants—vitamin E."

The authors of the study chose vitamin E because it appears to be the only fat-soluble antioxidant in blood and because it is generally safe even in large doses. Normal blood levels of the nutrient in smokers did not adequately prevent oxidation, but "substantial doses" of 800 milligrams a day did minimize the damage, according to the report.

Antioxidant treatment also holds out some hope for people who chew tobacco. Beta-carotene and vitamin A supplements given to a group of Indian fishermen over a six-month period resulted in remission of precancerous white patches in their mouths and prevented any new lesions from forming. Once supplementation ceased, the lesions reappeared, according to members of the British Columbia Cancer Research Centre in Vancouver. The good results are all the more startling, the researchers note, because the fishermen in the study continued to chew tobacco during the six months of the trial.

HOW MUCH DO WE NEED?

Way back in the early 1940s when the Recommended Dietary Allowances (RDAs) were first established for optimal nutrition, we needed guidelines for how much vitamin D was necessary to prevent rickets, how much vitamin C was required to ward off scurvy and how much vitamin B_1 would eliminate the chance of beriberi.

In the developed world today, we don't have to worry about pellagra, rickets and scurvy; we're plagued by cancer, atherosclerosis and diseases associated with aging.

"The RDAs have outlived their usefulness," says John H. Weisburger, M.D., Ph.D., of the American Health Foundation in Valhalla, New York. "There are no more deficiency diseases. We have enough nutrients to meet the RDAs. We need optimal amounts to prevent other diseases like heart disease, cancer and stroke."

What are those new, higher amounts? No one really knows for sure. But the levels, especially for the antioxidant vitamins, certainly are higher than the current RDAs. And partly because Americans don't eat anywhere near the recommended serving of fruits and vegetables, some experts say supplementation is a necessity.

"It's very clear that hardly anybody eats a well-balanced diet," says Gladys Block, Ph.D., of the University of California in Berkeley. According to one survey, about 17 percent of people eat no vegetables, only half eat a vegetable other than potatoes or a salad, and some 40 percent have no fruit or fruit juice. On any given day, only about a quarter of the American people eat fruits and vegetables rich in the antioxidant vitamins.

BETA-CAROTENE: THE A-PLUS NUTRIENT

Cancer. It once was thought that beta-carotene's principal benefit was that the body could convert it to vitamin A on an as-needed basis. (Overdoses of vitamin A can be toxic to the

"When we see what we're eating, we realize there are not a lot of the antioxidants in our diets," Dr. Block says. People should "dramatically increase their eating of fruits and vegetables because they have the E, the C, the beta-carotene. Those are very important agents in the body. Nature packaged them together, and we evolved on them."

The amounts of vitamins believed to be needed to counter oxidants in the body far exceeds the RDAs and may even go beyond what we're capable of ingesting through food. "The amounts in food are too small to get the values we're talking about," says Denham Harman, M.D., Ph.D., of the University of Nebraska College of Medicine and the American Aging Association. "You'd have to eat an awful lot of oranges, for example."

Dr. Harman suggests that people concerned about counteracting oxidants in their bodies take between 100 and 200 I.U. of vitamin E a day and 500 milligrams of vitamin C two to four times a day. (Supplementing at levels in excess of the RDAs should only be done in consultation with a physician.)

No optimal dietary amount has been established for beta-carotene, a lack that Dr. Weisburger calls "a gap in food and nutrition thought." He recommends between 10 and 20 milligrams of beta-carotene three times a week. "That gives you a certain blood level that is distributed to all tissues." Beta-carotene is not toxic and its dosage is "self-limiting," he says, because it isn't absorbed very well. Dr. Harman recommends 15 milligrams of beta-carotene every other day.

system.) No longer. As an antioxidant, beta-carotene seems to work its magic without its transformation into vitamin A. Moreover, while few studies point to an association between cancer protection and high levels of vitamin A in the body, research consistently demonstrates a significant link between high levels of beta-carotene and lower rates of certain cancers, especially in the lungs.

Of 11 studies of diet and lung cancer reviewed by one researcher, all found a decreased risk of disease with higher consumption of carotene-containing foods.

One of the most extensive long-term examinations of antioxidants and cancer, the Basel study of 2,974 men in Switzerland, determined that people with low blood levels of beta-carotene have "a significantly higher risk of death from [lung] cancer." Little correlation was found for vitamin A and lung cancer, and vitamin C was lower in most incidences of the disease. But beta-carotene levels were considerably lower in the men who had lung and stomach cancer. That led the researchers to "strongly encourage a higher intake of dietary carotenoids and carotene-containing supplements as a preventive measure against cancer."

Where to find it. Beta-carotene can be found in such foods as carrots, winter squash, pumpkin, sweet potatoes, apricots, cantaloupe, mangoes, peaches and dark green leafy vegetables such as spinach, kale and broccoli.

BRAKING THE AGING PROCESS

From wrinkling of the skin to degeneration of muscles and organs, growing old may be the cumulative bodily response to constant oxidation, experts like Dr. Harman propose. "The aging process may be simply the sum of the deleterious free-radical reactions going on continuously through the cells and tissues," he says. The reactions produce progressively more severe harm the longer they remain unchecked and the longer a person lives.

Doctors can't see free radicals; they can only infer their impact on aging by the clues they leave, such as age spots, the accumulation of oxidized blood fats and damage to organs. Theoretically, slowing oxidation of the body—the onset of the process or the chain reaction it causes—should retard disease and extend life potential. And that might be achieved, Dr. Harman proposes, by increasing the amount of antioxidant chemicals in the body.

Maximum life span of the human species has not been extended so far, but aging could be slowed down and life extended by combating diseases that shorten life with antioxidants. That would permit humans to live closer to their maximum life potential, he predicts.

"Conquest of cancer and cardiovascular disease, the two main causes of death, would extend life expectancy by up to ten years," Dr. Harman says. "While most of the research suggesting that antioxidant nutrients could prevent those diseases involves animals, the human data we do have corroborate the animal studies."

WHEN TO TAKE ANTIOXIDANTS

Most people take their vitamins—if they do, in fact, take their vitamins—at breakfast. They're swallowed with a few gulps of coffee or juice, perhaps accompanied by a piece of toast or a muffin. That's probably the worst meal of the day with which to take them, especially if you're looking for maximum protective benefits from the antioxidants.

The best time to take your vitamins is with the main meal of the day, says John H. Weisburger, M.D., Ph.D., of the American Health Foundation in Valhalla, New York, and it's better to swallow them at the end of the meal.

Beta-carotene and vitamin E are fat soluble, he says. "They won't be absorbed well in a nonfat meal." The typical breakfast of coffee or juice and perhaps cereal contains very little fat, he says, so the fat-soluble vitamins are whisked through the digestive system without being retained in tissue. Thus, there's no antioxidant benefit.

High-Nutrition Recipes

DIJON PASTA SALAD

This main-course salad is brimming with antioxidant nutrients: The peppers and broccoli have nice amounts of vitamin C; the carrots and kale are great sources of beta-carotene; and the shrimp, wheat germ and almonds contribute valuable vitamin E.

4	ounces tricolor rotelle	⅓	cup wheat germ
1	cup bite-size broccoli florets, lightly steamed	3	tablespoons white-wine vinegar
1	cup cooked baby shrimp	1	tablespoon Dijon mustard
½	cup thinly sliced carrots		
½	cup diced sweet red peppers	½	teaspoon dried dill
		½	teaspoon ground black pepper
½	cup nonfat yogurt		Kale leaves
½	cup nonfat mayonnaise	3	tablespoons sliced almonds

Cook the pasta in a large pot of boiling water until just tender. Drain and rinse with cold water. Place in a large bowl.

Add the broccoli, shrimp, carrots and red peppers. Toss well.

In a small bowl, whisk together the yogurt, mayonnaise, wheat germ, vinegar, mustard, dill and black pepper. Pour over the salad. Toss well.

Line individual plates with the kale. Divide the salad among the plates. Sprinkle with the almonds.

Serves 4
Per serving: *286 calories, 5.4 g. fat (17% of calories), 3.8 g. dietary fiber, 56 mg. cholesterol, 574 mg. sodium*

FRUIT SALAD SUPREME

What makes this salad supreme is its high complement of antioxidant nutrients: C, E and beta-carotene. The citrus fruits have plenty of vitamin C, the cantaloupe and mango kick in beta-carotene, and the nuts and seeds supply vitamin E.

1 pink grapefruit, peeled and sectioned	2 tablespoons orange juice
	1 tablespoon lime juice
1 large navel orange, peeled and sectioned	1 teaspoon grated orange rind
1 mango, sliced	¼ teaspoon poppy seeds
1 cup cantaloupe chunks	Lettuce
1 cup honeydew chunks	3 tablespoons sunflower seeds
1 cup strawberry halves	
½ cup raspberries	3 tablespoons sliced almonds
½ cup nonfat vanilla yogurt	

In a large bowl, toss together the grapefruit, oranges, mango, cantaloupe, honeydew, strawberries and raspberries.

In a small bowl, whisk together the yogurt, orange juice, lime juice, orange rind and poppy seeds. Pour over the fruit and toss to combine.

Line individual plates with lettuce. Divide the fruit among the plates. Sprinkle with the sunflower seeds and nuts.

Serves 6
Per serving: *144 calories, 4.6 g. fat (26% of calories), 4.3 g. dietary fiber, <1 mg. cholesterol, 20 mg. sodium*

CHAPTER 15

The 101 Healthiest Foods

Eat More of These

Don't eat this. Don't eat that. Is this what most of today's nutrition advice sounds like to you—all negative?

Well, take heart. There are plenty of wonderful foods that are good for you and that also happen to taste divine. You would be doing yourself a favor if you ate them more often. That's why we came up with the 101 healthiest foods—our list of the foods that modern medical research smiles on for a whole lot of reasons.

What they have going for them (besides tastiness) are several nutritional factors that have been associated with lower risk of disease. Factors like dietary fiber, omega-3 fatty acids, beta-carotene, calcium and other health promoters that may help forestall the development of diseases such as cancer and heart disease. The evidence linking some of these factors to lower risk is strong; the evidence for others, though less conclusive, is promising.

In making our choices, we analyzed the nutritional content of more than 1,000 foods. In general, we tried to select foods that contain significant amounts of at least four essential nutrients that keep your body functioning at peak performance levels.

But we also chose some foods for what they *don't* have. To do that, we aimed for foods that have less than 200 calories and fewer than 100 milligrams of cholesterol and 200 milligrams of sodium per serving. In the meat category, our primary concern was selecting cuts that had less than 30 percent of calories from fat.

But of course, we're not suggesting that you should limit your diet to these 101 foods. "Variety and moderation are important factors in a well-rounded nutritional program," says George Seperich, Ph.D., a food scientist and associate professor of agribusiness at Arizona State University in Tempe. "It would be unwise to assume that these foods can provide absolute protection from health problems—no diet can do that. But eating meals based on this list may increase your odds of living a more energetic and healthy life."

FINFISH

You can't go wrong by including finfish in your diet. A terrific source of protein, fish is a good *lean* alternative to red meat. Flounder, for instance, has less than one-fourth the total fat of sirloin steak. Some species, like haddock, have hardly any fat at all. In any case, whatever fat the fish you select does have may actually be good for you.

Fish has something called omega-3 fatty acids, a type of polyunsaturated fat that may help prevent cardiovascular disease. In fact, some fatty fish might be dynamite secret weapons against high cholesterol and heart attack because they have extra large amounts of omega-3's. Population studies have linked high fish consumption with lower rates of heart disease and stroke among Greenland Eskimos and Japanese fishermen. But omega-3's are just one of many reasons why nutrition experts recommend that you eat at least two servings of fish a week.

Fish is a good source of iron, and that iron—which is in a form that is easier to absorb than iron from plants—helps fortify your blood and protect you against anemia. Most species also are high in magnesium and potassium, two minerals that help regulate blood pressure. Fish is also a good source of the B vitamins, particularly B_{12}, which is necessary for a healthy nervous system.

Flounder (1) with under 12 percent of calories from fat, and **haddock** (2) with under 8 percent, are among the trimmest fish in the ocean. But remember, fattier fish are not all bad, thanks to those heart-protecting omega-3 fatty acids. Although all fish have some omega-3's, among the smartest choices are **bluefish** (3), **mackerel** (4), **trout** (5) and **herring** (6). Two fish, **tuna** (7) and **salmon** (8), deserve special attention. The largest of the tunas, sometimes weighing in excess of 1,000 pounds, fresh bluefin tuna is an especially good heart protector and one of your best buys when available. Although they have somewhat less nutritional wallop, canned white and light tuna also are powerful dietary allies.

Another terrific source of omega-3's, canned salmon, if you eat it with the bones, provides ample amounts of bone-strengthening calcium and vitamin D.

High-Nutrition Recipe

HERRING AND POTATO GRATIN

This fish dish would make a perfect brunch entrée. It features herring, which is a good source of healthy omega-3

*fatty acids. Be aware that kippered herring contains a fair
amount of salt, but you can remove some of it by rinsing and
soaking the fish. You could also substitute poached or baked
fresh herring.*

2	cans (3¼ ounces each) kippered herring	2	tablespoons unbleached flour
2	large onions, thinly sliced	2	cups 1% low-fat milk
2	teaspoons olive oil	½	cup seasoned dry bread crumbs
½	teaspoon ground black pepper		
6	medium baking potatoes, thinly sliced	3	tablespoons minced fresh dill

Drain the herring and place in a strainer. Rinse under cold
water for 1 minute. Transfer to a medium bowl and cover
with cold water. Set aside.

In a large no-stick frying pan over medium-low heat,
sauté the onions in the oil for 15 minutes, or until limp and
lightly browned. Stir in the pepper. Set aside.

Coat 6 (8-ounce) gratin dishes or ramekins with no-stick
spray. Divide half of the potatoes among the dishes.

Drain the herring and flake with a fork. Divide among the
dishes. Top with the onions, then with the remaining potatoes.

Place the flour in a medium bowl. Slowly whisk in the
milk to make a smooth mixture. Pour into the dishes.

In a cup, mix the bread crumbs and dill. Sprinkle over the
dishes.

Bake at 350° for 25 to 30 minutes, or until the potatoes
are tender and have absorbed most of the milk.

Serves 6
Per serving: *300 calories, 9.4 g. fat (28% of calories), 3.9
g. dietary fiber, 6 mg. cholesterol, 274 mg. sodium*

SHELLFISH

Although shellfish contains lots of cholesterol, that is offset by the fact that it also is filled with the same type of omega-3 fatty acids found in finfish, which may actually help *lower* cholesterol levels in your body.

In addition, shellfish is extremely low in saturated fat. That's important because researchers now believe that eating saturated fat is a far greater risk factor for heart disease than consuming dietary cholesterol.

The importance of shellfish doesn't end there, though. Every time you crack into a crustacean or pry a mollusk apart, you're really opening a vault of hidden nutritional treasures. In fact, certain shellfish could vie for the title of "Nature's Mineral Depository" because of their abundance of calcium, zinc, magnesium and iron.

Clams (9), for example, are so high in iron, it's a wonder they don't rust. Twenty steamers provide over 160 percent of the women's RDA, 250 percent of the men's RDA. But more astounding, those 20 clams provide 45 times the daily recommendation for vitamin B_{12}.

Ounce for ounce, **oysters** (10) are among the best sources of zinc. Six medium oysters provide five times the RDA for men, more than six times the RDA for women. Oysters are iron-rich, too, but the Atlantic-bred variety is about 25 percent richer in iron than Pacific-grown types. **Mussels** (11) deserve recognition, in part because they are such an inexpensive source of good nutrition.

But as wonderful as shellfish is, "you should be cautious about eating it raw," says John Peters, a seafood processing specialist with the University of Washington Sea Grant Marine Advisory Service in Seattle. "Adequate cooking will kill any harmful bacteria that might be present." But whether you cook it or not, "be sure you buy only from a reputable source," he says.

POULTRY

Loaded with protein, poultry is lower in total fat and saturated fat than most red meat. That's important because saturated fat can raise blood cholesterol levels, and it plays a major role in the development of heart disease.

"If you remove the skin and trim the fat, poultry is great. It's probably one of the simplest and most versatile meats to prepare," Dr. Seperich says.

Poultry also is a good source of iron, zinc and niacin. In fact, some of the best sources of iron on earth can be found flying in the sky. Both **duck** (12) and **goose** (13) are high in the most absorbable type of iron.

For nearly as much absorbable iron, but much less fat, try **turkey** (14) and **chicken** (15). With turkey, dark meat's the most iron-rich part. But turkey breast is undeniably one of the leanest meat choices you can make. A three-ounce serving of skinless, roasted white turkey meat has 133 calories, 2.7 grams of total fat and less than a gram of saturated fat. Gobbling on turkey also provides nearly one-quarter of the daily recommendation for vitamin B_6. Chicken breast is a healthy choice, too. With only 19 percent of calories from fat, it also may help lower your risk of cancer. In a study of 88,751 women conducted over six years, researchers concluded that the women who consumed the most beef, pork and lamb had a higher risk of colon cancer than those who ate more skinless chicken and fish.

MEATS

Once considered America's all-star entrée, red meat is showing up on fewer plates these days because of concerns about saturated fat and cholesterol. It's true that many red meats are laden with those two heart disease-causing villains. In some cuts, more than 50 percent of the calories come from fat. But with proper selection and preparation, eating moderate three-ounce servings of lean red meat two to three times a week can be a good supplement to a low-fat, low-cholesterol diet.

It makes sense to include some red meat in your diet because it's one of the best sources of iron. Beef has $1\frac{1}{2}$ times more iron than an equivalent serving of chicken or fish. Pork and lamb also contain more of this blood-strengthening nutrient than an equal amount of chicken. And, unlike the iron in vegetables, fruits or grains, the iron in red meat is readily absorbed by the body. Red meat also contains significant amounts of copper, manganese and zinc. These three minerals work together with calcium to build strong bones.

When buying meat, look for "select" grade—it has the least amount of fat. Before cooking be sure to trim all the visible fat off even the best cuts.

Preparation also is an important consideration. Broiling, for instance, is much better than frying because it allows fat to drip away from the meat. "If you bread and fry it, you're really undoing all the good that you did by buying that lean meat in the first place," says Margy Woodburn, Ph.D., professor and head of the Department of Nutrition and Food Management at Oregon State University in Corvallis.

While it's often difficult to find a cut of red meat that has less than 30 percent calories from fat, it's not impossible. **Pork tenderloin** (16), for example, gets only 26 percent of its calories from fat and provides 53 percent of the RDA for thiamine. With only 25 percent calories from fat, **top round steak** (17) is another tremendous nutritional bargain. A three-ounce serving of **eye round roast** (18) supplies nearly half the RDA for protein, yet only has 143 calories and 4.2 grams of fat. **Lamb foreshank** (19) is the leanest cut of lamb—29 percent calories from fat—and is a marvelous source of protein and zinc. On the wild side, **venison** (20) is low in both fat and cholesterol, and has less than 135 calories per serving.

High-Nutrition Recipe

SPICY VENISON STEW

Venison is a very lean meat that makes a tasty substitute for beef. This stew contains an interesting blend of spices that gives it a Middle Eastern flavor.

2	tablespoons unbleached flour	¼	teaspoon ground cinnamon
1	pound boneless venison, cut into 1" cubes	¼	teaspoon red-pepper flakes
1	tablespoon olive oil	1	clove garlic, minced
2	cups diced onions	3	cups defatted beef stock
1	teaspoon ground cumin	8	ounces medium no-yolk egg noodles
1	teaspoon ground coriander		
½	teaspoon ground black pepper		

Place the flour in a plastic or paper bag. Add the venison and shake the bag to coat the pieces.

In a 4-quart pot over medium heat, brown the meat in the oil. Stir in the onions, cumin, coriander, black pepper, cinnamon, red-pepper flakes and garlic. Mix well.

Add the stock. Bring to a boil. Cover and simmer for 1½ hours, or until the meat is tender.

Cook the noodles in a large pot of boiling water for 8 minutes, or until just tender. Drain. Serve topped with the stew.

Serves 4
Per serving: *464 calories, 8.4 g. fat (16% of calories), 3.7 g. dietary fiber, 96 mg. cholesterol, 102 mg. sodium*

BEANS

When Jack swapped his mother's cow for a handful of beans, he may have made the wisest trade in fairy tale lore. After all, beans (or legumes) are crammed with nutritious goodies, including fiber, which can promote regularity and help lower cholesterol. *Prevention* magazine adviser James W. Anderson, M.D., professor of medicine and clinical nutrition at the University of Kentucky College of Medicine in Lexington, advocates a diet high in legumes for cholesterol control. In small studies, Dr. Anderson has seen cholesterol levels drop 60 points in three weeks after adding beans to the diets of men with high cholesterol. In other studies, results indicate that beans help normalize blood sugar, which makes them a great dietary choice for those with diabetes.

Beans also are high in complex carbohydrates and low in artery-clogging fat, and they have no cholesterol. Compared to other plant foods, beans are loaded with protein and iron. Beans also are rich sources of B vitamins. Beans are a good choice for pregnant women because they are rich in folate, a B vitamin needed for healthy babies.

"Beans certainly deliver the goods," Dr. Seperich says. "The nice thing about them is there are so many varieties that you'll probably find at least one that appeals to your taste buds."

On the downside, beans—particularly dried ones—can produce a lot of flatulence. But using antigas products such as Beano can help relieve that problem.

Among the most popular dried beans are **pinto beans** (21), **kidney beans** (22), **lima beans** (23) and **lentils** (24)—not to mention **navy beans** (25), which have helped keep sailors going full speed ahead since the early nineteenth century. Like all other legumes, **peas** (26), **chick-peas (garbanzo beans)** (27) and tiny **adzuki beans** (28) are high in iron and other minerals. **Anasazi beans** (29) have a special attraction: all the nutrition of regular beans but less than 25 percent of the flatulence-causing sugars.

High-Nutrition Recipe

WARM LENTIL SALAD

One way to enjoy fiber-rich lentils is mixed into an herb-scented salad, such as this.

8	ounces lentils, rinsed	2	tablespoons minced celery
3	cups water	2	tablespoons defatted chicken stock
¼	cup diced onions	2	tablespoons olive oil
1	clove garlic, minced	2	tablespoons red-wine vinegar
¼	teaspoon dried savory	½	teaspoon Dijon mustard
	Pinch of dried rosemary		Shredded romaine lettuce
1	bay leaf		
1	cup diced yellow peppers		
1	cup shredded carrots		

In a 2-quart saucepan, combine the lentils, water, onions, garlic, savory, rosemary and bay leaf. Bring to a boil. Partially cover the pan, reduce the heat to medium and simmer for 20 minutes, or until the lentils are tender but not mushy. Drain. Discard the bay leaf.

Transfer the lentils to a large bowl. Add the peppers, carrots and celery. Toss lightly.

In a small bowl, whisk together the stock, oil, vinegar and mustard. Pour over the salad and toss well. Serve warm over the lettuce.

Serves 4
Per serving: *281 calories, 7.6 g. fat (23% of calories), 8.4 g. dietary fiber, 0 mg. cholesterol, 46 mg. sodium*

DAIRY PRODUCTS

Rich in calcium and vitamin D, dairy foods are vital to growth and help us develop strong bones and teeth. In fact, there are no better natural sources of calcium than milk and other dairy products. Eating lots of dairy foods may prevent osteoporosis, the gradual loss of bone mass that can lead to fractures. In addition, studies indicate that low calcium consumption is a risk factor for high blood pressure. The problem with some dairy foods is that they tend to be loaded with fat and cholesterol as well as calcium. But there is a way around that problem—stick to low-fat varieties. After all, there are many to choose from.

Skim milk (30), with only about 6 percent of its calories from fat, is probably the best choice. "Like other dairy products, skim milk is packed with nutrients. Yet, unlike many other dairy products, it has virtually no fat and a minimum amount of calories, making it a super diet food," says George L. Blackburn, M.D., Ph.D., associate professor of surgery at Harvard Medical School and chief of the Nutrition/Metabolism Laboratory at the Cancer Research Institute at New England Deaconess Hospital in Boston.

One percent low-fat milk (solids added) (31), with 20 percent of its calories from fat, **1 percent low-fat cottage cheese** (32), any other **low-fat cheese** (33) (such as sapsago or part-skim mozzarella) and **nonfat yogurt** (34) are other good high-calcium selections.

VEGETABLES

Eating plenty of vegetables every day won't make you invincible, but many of these plant foods certainly can be classified as dietary superheroes. Vegetables are the backbone of any good diet because they provide lots of complex carbohydrates and vitamins A and C. Yet veggies have virtually no fat and few calories, so they're great for weight-conscious eaters.

"If I had to choose just one vegetable to take with me on a long space flight, I wouldn't go because the nutritional value of vegetables is truly in their variety. By mixing them in your diet, you get a little bit of everything," Dr. Seperich says.

Vegetables contain fiber, which may help prevent a number of diseases including heart disease and colon and breast cancers. And some vegetables pack a mighty supply of calcium for rock-solid bones.

If you feel overly tired, particularly after exercise, adding more vegetables to your diet might help boost your energy. That's because most vegetables are high in magnesium and potassium, two minerals that combat weakness and fatigue. Better yet, eating veggies that have lots of potassium and magnesium may help prevent high blood pressure.

ORANGE-YELLOW VEGETABLES

This group of vegetables is an important source of beta-carotene, a substance that your body converts into vitamin A. Carotenes (including beta-carotene) may decrease the risk of lung, laryngeal, ovarian and other cancers. Researchers in California and Arizona also have found evidence that beta-carotene may prevent oral leukoplakias (precancerous sores inside the mouth). Carotenoids also might play a role in preventing cataracts by retarding oxidation of the lens in the eye.

Carrots (35), ounce for ounce, are one of the best sources of beta-carotene. **Winter squash** (36) (such as acorn, butternut and hubbard), **pumpkins** (37) and **sweet potatoes** (38) are delicious alternatives.

GREEN LEAFY VEGETABLES

Like squashes, carrots and other yellow-orange vegetables, greens are good sources of the carotenes your body uses to make vitamin A. In general, the greener the vegetable, the more carotenoids (including beta-carotene) it contains. Green leafy vegetables also have fair amounts of magnesium and potassium, which, along with calcium, may reduce the risk of high blood pressure. They also have moderate levels of vitamin C, a nutrient that may lower the risk of breast cancer.

Iron and calcium lurk in some greens, but our bodies can't use the minerals in these vegetables as efficiently as those from meats and dairy foods.

For a real nutritional boost, try **romaine lettuce** (39). A one-cup serving has more vitamin C than sweet cherries and twice as much folate as other types of lettuce. **Swiss chard** (40), a spinach look-alike, is actually a relative of the beet. For variety, try **endive** (41), **watercress** (42), **spinach** (43), **kale** (44), **arugula** (45) or **turnip greens** (46).

CRUCIFEROUS VEGETABLES

For a real anti-cancer diet, be sure to eat lots of cruciferous vegetables. These vegetables contain high levels of indole glucosinolates, compounds that are believed to have a variety of cancer-fighting effects. In particular, indoles may inactivate tumor-causing estrogen that targets the breast. Many of these vegetables are also high in insoluble fiber, vitamin C and folate.

When you think of cruciferous, think **broccoli** (47). This mighty veggie has loads of cancer-combating nutrients. Just ½ cup provides 100 percent of the RDA for vitamin C. One cup of raw broccoli has more vitamin C than an equivalent amount of cantaloupe.

Other major members of this family include **cabbage** (48), **bok choy (Chinese cabbage)** (49) and **cauliflower** (50). Thanks to modern horticultural wizardry, the best of cauliflower and broccoli are available in one plant: **broccoflower** (51). A serving of this hybrid crucifer has more vitamin C than broccoli and more beta-carotene than broccoli or cauliflower. Broccoflower has a sweet and mild flavor, without the cabbage taste that turns some people off to cauliflower.

Like broccoli, **brussels sprouts** (52) have a lot of calcium and iron for a plant source. The minerals aren't quite as easily absorbed as from animal sources, but some gets through nonetheless.

High-Nutrition Recipe

SESAME BROCCOFLOWER

Broccoflower combines all the nutritional benefits of broccoli and cauliflower in one handsome-looking package. Here it's sautéed with sesame seeds for a quick side dish— or even a main meal served over rice.

1   teaspoon canola oil
1   head broccoflower, cut into florets
¼   cup defatted chicken stock
1   tablespoon low-sodium soy sauce
1   teaspoon grated fresh ginger
1½ teaspoons toasted sesame seeds

In a wok or large frying pan over medium-high heat, warm the oil for 30 seconds. Add the broccoflower and stir-fry for 5 minutes. Add the stock, soy sauce and ginger. Cover and cook for 3 minutes, or until the broccoflower is crisp-tender. Serve sprinkled with the sesame seeds.

Serves 4
Per serving: *108 calories, 2.3 g. fat (26% of calories), 3.3 g. dietary fiber, 0 mg. cholesterol, 166 mg. sodium*

PEPPERS

Cruciferous plants are not the only vegetables that may have superb cancer-protecting qualities. Capsaicin, the substance that makes **chili peppers** (53) taste hot, may block the formation of cancer-causing compounds in cured meats. In addition, dieters may want to eat lots of foods seasoned with chili peppers, since capsaicin may help increase metabolism and hasten weight loss.

Brought to Spain from the New World by Christopher Columbus, **sweet or bell peppers** (54) are a phenomenal source of vitamin C. But if you really want a healthy dose of vitamins, then be sure to eat your peppers red. The ripened red pepper has about nine times as much vitamin A and twice as much vitamin C as the unripened green pepper.

ALLIUM VEGETABLES

Vegetables that are members of the allium family contain substances that seem to inhibit the formation of blood clots (a principal trigger for heart attacks). Some research suggests that eating a pound of allium vegetables each week may significantly reduce the risk of stomach and colon cancers.

Onions (55) and **garlic** (56) are probably the most familiar members of the allium family. Onions may help lower blood cholesterol. Garlic is a natural blood thinner and may help prevent clogged arteries. A favorite of the Roman emperor Nero, **leeks** (57) share the cancer-protective traits of other allium vegetables. Like onions, they also supply a fair amount of fiber.

HIGH-CARBOHYDRATE VEGETABLES

Potatoes (58) are a nutritionist's dream: good sources of vitamins C and B_6, copper, magnesium, phosphorus, potassium, iron and fiber. This low-calorie delight will also help keep your waistline trim, if you avoid the fatty toppings.

Corn (59) is no empty husk, either. The bran in corn may help lower blood cholesterol. And one ear of corn will give you nearly a fifth of the RDA of folate.

FRUIT

Fruit contains a healthy mixture of complex carbohydrates, natural sugars, fiber, vitamins and minerals. Like vegetables, fruit is a good source of beta-carotene and vitamin C, two nutrients that have been linked to reduced risk of breast and other cancers. Carotenoids such as beta-carotene also may reduce your risk of developing cataracts. Fruit is a good source of soluble fiber that helps control blood sugar levels and relieve constipation. Some soluble fiber may also help prevent colon cancer.

But fruit also is important because of what it doesn't contain. Most fruits have little or no fat. Excessive fat consumption has been linked to heart disease and breast and colon cancer. In addition, most fruit contains only a trace of sodium. That's important because salt may contribute to high blood pressure, a major cause of heart attack, stroke and kidney disease.

Remember that fruit as well as vegetables are less nutritious the longer they are stored or cooked. So your best bet is to eat fresh fruit raw.

CITRUS FRUITS

Citrus fruits are outstanding sources of vitamin C, carotenoids and other compounds that some researchers suspect may have natural cancer-fighting qualities. Most of us don't realize that citrus also is loaded with fiber, particularly in the stringy sections and inner peel. A day without an **orange** (60) is like a day without 116 percent of the RDA of vitamin C. Incidentally, oranges are the leading fruit crop in the United States. **Pink grapefruit** (61) gets its color from its stores of beta-carotene. Pink grapefruits have somewhat more vitamin C than white, but both are good sources of that important nutrient. Both orange and grapefruit juice, by the way, are especially good sources of vitamin C, magnesium and potassium.

Tangerines (62) have more beta-carotene than other citrus fruits. Civil War general Stonewall Jackson considered **lemons** (63) an indispensable part of his diet. He sucked on them incessantly—even as he rode toward battle. The Confederate hero could afford to indulge, since a ¹⁄₂-cup serving only has eight calories. Of course, few people these days suck on lemons, in part, because the acid in the raw fruit can erode tooth enamel. A better way to enjoy this tart fruit is diluted in lemonade or fresh-squeezed in sparkling mineral water. In the nineteenth century, British sailors were known as limeys because they ate **limes** (64) to prevent scurvy. Limes are an excellent way to add a tangy taste to fish and seafood.

HIGH-C FRUITS

The prime advantage of these fruits is their high vitamin C content. Most are also good sources of potassium. Once considered an exotic oddity from New Zealand, **kiwifruit** (65) is now grown in the United States and is popular worldwide. This fuzzy-skinned fruit with emerald green flesh is available year-round. One kiwi packs 124 percent of the RDA of vitamin C, which is 60 milligrams. **Acerola** (66), a West Indian fruit, is still a stranger to most Americans. It looks something like a cherry and tastes very tart, and just one contains 134 percent of the U.S. RDA. And don't forget other high-C contenders like **pineapples** (67), **honeydews** (68) and **pomegranates** (69).

BERRIES

Bursting with vitamin C, berries also are a great source of fiber. But remember that heat destroys vitamin C, so for the most nutritional benefits, try to eat uncooked berries whenever possible.

As sweet as a first kiss and as elegant as a Cole Porter tune, the **strawberry** (70) is one of nature's classic beauties. Strawberries also contain a substance called ellagic acid that seems able to fight off certain cancer-causing agents. But **blackberries** (71) and **blueberries** (72) can be equally delightful. Both are wondrous snacks, but blackberries have more vitamin E. Another great natural snack, **raspberries** (73) only have 60 calories per one-cup serving.

HIGH-FIBER FRUITS

Although most fruits are rich in fiber, some are naturally more hefty sources of this important dietary component that may relieve constipation, lower cholesterol and prevent colon and other types of digestive cancer. Most of the fiber in these fruits is pectin, which helps control appetite by creating a feeling of fullness in the stomach. In addition to their pectin, **apples** (74) have significant amounts of boron, a mineral that may help strengthen bones and keep you alert. **Pears** (75) and **bananas** (76) are two other top fiber sources. Bananas also have lots of vitamin B_6. Ten **cherries** (77) provide one gram of fiber, much of it soluble. Sour cherries have significantly more vitamin A and more vitamin C than sweet ones.

ORANGE-YELLOW FRUITS

These fruits, which include **cantaloupe** (78) and **apricots** (79), are good sources of beta-carotene, which may help prevent certain types of cancers. **Papaya** (80) has more vitamin C than oranges. **Mangoes** (81) are a great addition to yogurt, salads and vegetable dishes.

High-Nutrition Recipe

ISLAND PARADISE SALAD

This delicious salad combines tropical fruit with lettuce, peppers and a citrus-based vinaigrette. Serve it as a light lunch on languid summer days. Here's a surprise: Papaya seeds are edible—they have a peppery flavor similar to radishes.

2	pink grapefruit	2	tablespoons honey
1	papaya	1	teaspoon olive oil
1	mango	¼	teaspoon ground black pepper
1	sweet red pepper, diced		
2	scallions, thinly sliced		Pinch of celery seeds
2	tablespoons minced fresh coriander or parsley		Pinch of ground red pepper
3	tablespoons lime juice	2	cups torn red-leaf lettuce
3	tablespoons nonfat yogurt	1	bunch watercress

Peel the grapefruit, removing the outer white pith. Working over a bowl to catch the juices, remove each segment from its surrounding membrane. Squeeze the membranes to extract extra juice. Measure out ¼ cup of juice and set aside.

Peel the papaya, halve and scoop out the seeds; reserve about 1 tablespoon of the seeds. Cut the flesh into cubes.

Peel the mango and carefully slice the flesh from the inner pit. Cut the flesh into cubes.

In a large bowl, toss together the grapefruit, papaya, mango, peppers, scallions and coriander or parsley.

In a small bowl, whisk together the reserved grapefruit juice, lime juice, yogurt, honey, oil, black pepper, celery seeds and red pepper. Pour over the salad and toss to combine.

Divide the lettuce and watercress among individual plates. Top with the salad. Sprinkle with the reserved papaya seeds.

Serves 4
Per serving: *148 calories, 1.7 g. fat (9% of calories), 4 g. dietary fiber, 0 mg. cholesterol, 18 mg. sodium*

DRIED FRUITS

Because the water has been taken out, dried fruits often have more calories than fresh fruits. But they also become concentrated storehouses for fiber and a variety of minerals, including copper, iron, magnesium, potassium and zinc. No sour grapes, please, when you speak of **raisins** (82). They have a combination of minerals that may help lower high blood pressure. Golden raisins have a bit more vitamin B_6 and riboflavin than darker varieties. Other outstanding dried fruits include **dried peaches** (83), **prunes** (84) and **figs** (85).

GRAINS

Any way you slice them, grind them or bake them, grains in some form should be an essential part of your diet. Whole grains are important sources of thiamine, iron, riboflavin, magnesium and vitamin B_6. Better yet, they're great low-fat, high-fiber foods loaded with complex carbohydrates. Even refined, processed grains such as the flour used in white bread are fairly nutritious when enriched with thiamine, riboflavin, iron and niacin.

Grains also can be one of a dieter's best friends. "Grains help satisfy your appetite. They make you feel like you've had a good meal. That's important because if you don't feel like you're full, you're more likely to snack on foods that have a lot of empty calories," Dr. Woodburn says.

Dietitians say we should be eating at least six servings of grains, cereals or breads daily. But remember that one serving is only a single slice of bread or $1/2$ cup cooked cereal, rice or pasta. However, choosing the best grain foods could be a daunting task. Here's a sampling of some of our favorites.

Most grains aren't very high in calcium. But **amaranth** (86), a little-known, highly nutritious grain, is an exception. (It can be boiled and eaten like rice, popped like popcorn or ground into flour and used in hundreds of recipes.) Once an integral part of Aztec religion and culture, amaranth has more protein than most other grains. **High-fiber cereal** (87) and **whole-grain bread** (88) are usually fortified with calcium, iron and a variety of vitamins. The sprouting part of the wheat seed, **wheat germ** (89) really does deserve its reputation as a health food. Packed with vitamins and minerals, it can be added to many foods including breads, cookies, cereals and milk shakes. **Brown rice** (90) is more nutritious than white rice. Only the inedible outer husk has been removed. **Whole-wheat pasta** (91), **buckwheat** (92), and **barley** (93) are other superb grain foods. **Oatmeal** (94) and related foods have been shown to lower cholesterol. In South America, the Incas believed a steady diet of **quinoa** (95) ensured a long, fruitful life. It's one of the best plant sources of protein.

OILS

Cooking oils have one unfortunate thing in common—they're 100 percent fat. They also are incredibly calorie-rich (just one tablespoon of oil has at least 119 calories). But despite that, oils can remain a part of your diet if they're selected wisely and used sparingly. All oils are combinations of three types of fatty acids—saturated, monounsaturated and polyunsaturated. Saturated fats have been linked to higher cholesterol levels and increased risk of heart attack. Fortunately, liquid cooking oils are mostly polyunsaturated and monounsaturated fats.

Kudos for **olive oil** (96), which is high in monounsaturated fat and is excellent in salad dressings. It is also frequently used for cooking pastas and vegetables. And finally, three cheers for **canola oil** (97), also known as rape-seed oil. It is one of the few plant sources of heart-disease-fighting omega-3 fatty acids.

NUTS AND SEEDS

Yes, nuts and seeds are loaded with fat—up to 95 percent fat. But in most cases, much of that fat is either polyunsaturated or monounsaturated. But within their tiny shells, nuts and seeds have more than fat. A few nuts, such as **walnuts** (98) are also high in omega-3 fatty acids, the same heart-protecting substance found in fish. In addition, nuts and seeds are good sources of minerals, especially iron, potassium and magnesium. However, nuts should be eaten in moderation because of their high fat and calorie content. Barely a handful can contain more than 160 calories.

Chestnuts (99) are the exception to the high-fat, high-calorie tendency of nuts. With about 70 calories per serving, this lean nut derives less than 8 percent of its calories from fat. Fresh chestnuts usually are available from September to February. You can roast them in the oven, but be sure to pierce the husk first to prevent the nut from exploding when it's heated. **Dried sunflower seeds** (100) get 78 percent of their calories from fat, but more than half of that fat is polyunsaturated. Sunflower seeds also are good sources of calcium, copper, iron, magnesium, potassium and zinc. **Dried pumpkin seeds** (101) are comparable to sunflower seeds but have slightly more zinc.

High-Nutrition Recipe

SAVORY GLAZED CHESTNUTS

Chestnuts are one nut you can eat with abandon. That's because they contain only a trace of fat, unlike almonds, pecans and other common nuts. Although they're delicious as a snack when simply roasted, you can serve them as a vegetable.

12	ounces unshelled chestnuts	1	tablespoon maple syrup
8	ounces pearl onions, peeled	1	tablespoon balsamic vinegar
1	cup defatted chicken stock	1	teaspoon Dijon mustard Pinch of dried marjoram

Cut an X in the flat side of each chestnut. Place in a 3-quart saucepan and cover with cold water. Bring to a boil. Cook for 1 minute. Remove from the heat.

Using a slotted spoon, remove 1 chestnut at a time. Remove the peel and inner skin. Set aside.

In a large no-stick frying pan, combine the onions, stock, syrup, vinegar, mustard and marjoram. Bring to a boil over medium-high heat. Cover, reduce the heat to medium-low and simmer for 5 minutes.

Add the chestnuts. Cover and simmer for 8 minutes, or until the chestnuts and onions are tender. Using a slotted spoon, transfer to a bowl.

Cook the remaining liquid over medium-high heat until it

is reduced to about ¼ cup. Return the chestnuts and onions to the pan. Cook for another minute, until the liquid is reduced to a glaze and the chestnuts and onions are well coated.

Serves 4
Per serving: *183 calories, 2 g. fat (10% of calories), 3.4 g. dietary fiber, 0 mg. cholesterol, 57 mg. sodium*

CHAPTER 16

Water

The Best Toast to Your Health

The gray-haired honeymooners joked about their stamina as they raced each other through lush Hawaiian undergrowth. Finally, the waterfall appeared before them, plummeting hundreds of feet from the top of a green-shrouded cliff and crashing into a deep, shimmering pool. The pristine-looking, crystal-clear liquid invited the breathless couple to quench their thirst, but a small sign at the base of the fall stopped them. "Warning: Water not safe to drink."

The couple's desire to drink was thwarted, they later learned, by feral pigs running loose in the mountains. Like all living things, pigs need water. But by drinking from streams and excreting wastes in and near the water, the animals spread bacteria, like *Leptospira*, that can cause serious illness in humans. The lovers left, still thirsty but ready to swear off water for the rest of their trip.

It turned out to be a vow impossible to keep. No one on this "Water Planet" can live without that precious liquid for more than a few days. After all, we're made mostly of water. Sixty percent of most adult bodies are pure water. Infants are true "water babies," weighing in at 80 percent water. By retirement age, the ratio drops to around 50 percent. There is water in every cell of the body and in every type of body tissue, although, as you must suspect, teeth and bones harbor much less fluid than muscle, while blood is fully four-fifths water. Virtually every biological process going on inside us takes place in a watery medium as well.

WATER POWER

To help sort out its many functions, consider water's three major roles.

1. Transporter. Water in the body helps digest the salad you had for lunch and loads the blood with the dissolved nutrients, which it carries to each living cell. In the process, water helps carry toxins and waste products away from cells, to the lungs, skin or kidneys to be excreted. Water also helps solid wastes move through the intestines. Without water we would be poisoned by the by-products of life.

2. Temperature regulator. A healthy body's temperature hovers at 98.6°F—regardless of the weather outside or the great amount of heat generated inside us—thanks to self-adjusting blood vessel thermostats and the cooling effects of perspiration evaporating from the skin.

3. Lubricator. Without water to lubricate them, our joints would stop moving and we would stiffen up like statues. Our lungs would not be able to inflate or deflate.

TAKING IT ALL IN

Ironically, there is no "official" recommended daily allowance or requirement for water, yet all the other nutrients we require in a day could take a bath in the amount of water we need.

Experts say we need *at least* two quarts, or eight 8-ounce glasses, of water every day.

PERCHANCE TO DRINK, PER DAY, HOW MUCH?

"I see people carrying bottles of water everywhere today. It wasn't like that a few years ago," says Howard Flaks, M.D., a Beverly Hills weight-loss specialist and proponent of H_2O. People are catching on to the wonders of water, but there is still some confusion about just how much they should drink.

To clarify things, specialists at the International Sportsmedicine Institute in Los Angeles worked out a "recipe" for refreshment and rehydration that anyone, from professional athlete to sedentary fan, can follow.

According to Leroy Perry, D.C., president of the Institute, a non-active, healthy adult, should be drinking ½ ounce water per day for each pound of body weight. A 160-pound person, therefore, should sip ten 8-ounce glasses of water throughout the day.

An active or athletic person will do well to drink ⅔ ounce for each pound of weight. In that case, a 160-pound person on the go should down 12 or 13 glasses of water throughout the day.

"Generally, a large percentage of the water we need comes from what we drink," says Howard Flaks, M.D., a Beverly Hills, California, weight-loss expert.

"Some of our fluid intake comes from solids in the diet," says Dr. Flaks. Yes, and he's not talking about ice cubes, either. It's no surprise that watermelon is 92 percent water, but lettuce swims in at 96 percent. Baked fish is still 76 percent H_2O. A potato? Seventy-five percent water. Surprisingly, that seems only a little drier than milk, at 88 percent.

"A small amount of fluids the body uses originate as products of metabolism released in the body," says Dr.

Flaks. That is, when the body burns its carbohydrate, fat and protein fuels, energy and carbon dioxide are released, and water is produced. In a sense the water of metabolism is like ashes left after a fire, except the body uses this liquid by-product as a liquid asset.

So what's the best source of this liquid gold?

Make it pure and simple. Plain water may not be the best-tasting beverage around but it's the one experts recommend most. "I recommend drinking fluids in the form of pure water," says Dr. Flaks. "Eight glasses a day for a healthy person."

"Unfortunately, most of our fluid needs are met by flavored fluids with lots of calories without many nutrients," says George L. Blackburn, M.D., Ph.D., associate professor of surgery at Harvard Medical School and chief of the Nutrition/Metabolism Laboratory at the Cancer Research Institute of New England Deaconess Hospital in Boston. "We need to break that habit by consuming a cup of water before we drink the other," he suggests.

Fruit juices are not recommended because of their high sugar content. And forget coffee and cocktails as substitutes for filling your daily quota. Besides their obvious negatives (caffeine and alcohol), they also serve as diuretics, sometimes increasing your body's need for fluids.

Make it a habit. Most people do not tank up enough. Although the body *can* extract part of the water it needs from solid foods, many physicians prescribe eight to ten glasses of fluid *in addition to* the amount drawn from other sources. That may seem like a great deal, but the benefits from getting plenty of "hydro-power" can be great as well.

The full benefits may be best reaped, though, by spreading out your intake of water throughout the day. Drinking is not like showering. The inner body needs a steady supply of water, not a once- or twice-a-day dunking.

LETTING IT ALL WASH OUT

What exactly does the body do with all the water it craves? "Just as we wash the outside of the body, we need to cleanse the inside of the body as well," explains Dr. Flaks. "We remove the stagnant, dirty water in the body by replacing it with fresh, clean water." It's like a circulating fountain. Water flows in, through and out. But instead of spouting from the tops of our heads, water leaves the body via four major routes: The kidneys and urinary tract, the intestinal tract, the skin and the lungs. Tear ducts and the nasal passages are a fifth, small-volume exit route.

Our average daily wastewater output is one to two quarts, and we eliminate most of it as urine. The water in urine spends much of its prior "internal" existence in the bloodstream, doling out nutrients to cells and collecting wastes in turn. Next, the blood races through the hard-working kidneys at a rate of about $1/2$ cup per minute—that's up to 180 quarts per day—where waste products and extra water are filtered out. The kidneys pass the contaminated water to the bladder, where it collects until you urinate. If there is not enough water to handle the body's waste products, the kidneys may not be able to work efficiently, and wastes can contaminate the blood and tissues.

Although as much as eight to ten quarts of water pass in and out of the stomach and intestines every day, very little of it is excreted with the solid wastes it helps to form. In a healthy person only about 2 to 4 percent of the water output leaves the body through the intestinal tract.

Much more water than that exits through the skin in the form of perspiration. "Sweat is absolutely essential. It's a primary way your body regulates its internal temperature," says Norman Levine, M.D., professor and chief of dermatology at the University of Arizona Health Sciences Center in Tucson. When all systems are go, the body burns up nutrients and pumps out a lot of excess heat in the process. The body keeps itself cool by sending water through millions of sweat glands at the skin surface, where it evaporates, carrying heat away from the body.

Some of the body's water output also leaves through the lungs. Breathe in and the fluid between the outer and inner layers of the lung helps you collect air. Breathe out and away go carbon dioxide and water. You can see evaporated water leaving your body when you exhale in chilly air.

ABOVE AND BEYOND

Given the need to closely match water input with output, just how much should we really be drinking? As we've already noted, eight glasses a day is only a rule of thumb. There are actually almost as many exceptions to this rule as there are people.

Add such dehydrating factors as exercise, illness, hot or dry weather, stress, dieting and even air travel to the equation, and water needs chance. You may need more water when you're menstruating or pregnant, if you're overweight or aged. Check with your doctor. In many cases, consuming extra water is absolutely vital to good health.

If you fit any of the following profiles, it is essential to keep a watch on your water consumption.

The aging. "Elderly people do not get enough water because they do not recognize thirst as well as they did when they were young," says Susan Schiffman, Ph.D., a professor of psychology and psychiatry at Duke University located in Durham, North Carolina, who is an expert on the senses and how they change with age. And although increasing age brings a decreasing need for fluid, water and all its attendant functions are still prime concerns for the aged and people who care for them. Watch your loved ones for signs of water retention or dehydration, such as dry lips and skin, dwindling urination, confusion and high body temperature.

"I find that, for the elderly, offering flavored drinks is a better way to get them to drink water," says Dr. Schiffman, "because with their loss of the sense of smell—more so than the loss of their sense of taste—flavored drinks are more appealing. Water does not have a flavor, so there's less motivation to drink."

Exercisers. The old ticker starts humming, the limbs start swinging, and before long, the sweat starts flowing. A heavy-duty workout in hot weather could drain as much as six or seven quarts of water out of your body. A loss of—or failure to replace—just 3 or 4 percent of your vital fluid can definitely slow down all the action in your deprived cells.

There's no need to allow dehydration worries to dampen your fun. Just think—and drink—ahead. The experts typically recommend a hydrating routine like this: Before your workout, sip at least a cup of water. Every 15 to 20 minutes during your exercise, make it a point to chug ½ to ¾ cup, and soon after your routine is finished, enjoy another cupful.

The overweight. "Certainly, overweight people tend not to drink enough water," says Dr. Flaks. And that can actually make them look even heavier. "When people are not drinking enough, a lot of what appears to be fat is often retained water," he explains.

WATER WORRIES

It's easy enough to say we need to drink more water. But we're also aware that what looks cool, clear and inviting can also be downright dangerous—as the couple in Hawaii found out. In fact, pollution in drinking water is such a concern that the Environmental Protection Agency (EPA) has set safe-level standards for contaminants that may be health-threatening.

In fact, say the experts, some levels of contamination—

though considered harmless—are hard to avoid. That's because there are so many water sources—surface waters such as rivers and reservoirs, ground water, municipal water companies and private wells and springs—and so many possible sources of contamination—industrial and mining by-products, agricultural chemicals, natural and man-made radiation, leaking underground fuel tanks, air pollutants washed down with rain, unlawfully dumped wastes, sewage and corroded plumbing.

"Any public water supply system that does not meet the requirements set by the EPA must inform the public and take remedial action," says Daniel Henry, information specialist with Geo/Resource Consultants working at the EPA Office of Ground Water and Drinking Water. If there is a problem, the water company will suggest temporary solutions to your drinking water supply problem until it is able to solve the problem. This may range from boiling the water to drinking bottled water at their expense.

Some forms of contamination, however, are much more likely to occur between the water plant and your spigot. The possibility of lead leaching from old water pipes is a prime example. Private wells or springs are also especially prone to contamination by bacteria. If it's been a while (a year or more) since you had your tap water tested or treated, now's a good time to call your state health office or department of environmental regulation for a list of EPA- or state-certified testing labs.

If your water proves to be tainted, or if it is safe but smells, tastes or looks unacceptable to you, you may be a good candidate for an in-home water treatment system, especially if you have a private well. There are four basic types of units to choose from: activated carbon, reverse osmosis, distillation and water softeners. The type and brand of system you choose will depend on exactly which contaminants you want to get rid of.

BETTER WATER FOUR WAYS

Choosing a water treatment system for your home can be mind-boggling. Here's how the four types of systems work to reduce undesirables in drinking water, according to Nancy Culotta, manager of the Drinking Water Treatment Program at NSF International, a nonprofit product testing foundation in Ann Arbor, Michigan.

Activated carbon. These filters work by passing water through a carbon bed that absorbs contaminants, including chlorine, volatile organic chemicals, and in some cases, lead, color, herbicides, hydrogen sulfide, pesticides and turbidity (fine, suspended particles). Carbon filters that attach directly to your faucet may cost around $100, while large units range upward in price to $300.

Reverse osmosis. These systems force water through a membrane that rejects contaminants and stores the processed water in a tank. They help reduce arsenic, cadmium, chlorine, chromium, color, giardia cysts, iron, lead, nitrate, radium, sulfate and turbidity. Countertop and under-sink models range from about $200 to $500.

Distillation. By boiling off and then recondensing water, these systems remove contaminants such as arsenic, cadmium, chromium, giardia cysts, iron, lead, nitrate, sulfate and turbidity. Prices range from $400 for countertop models to around $2,500 for the largest models.

Water softeners. They replace the calcium and magnesium that make water hard with sodium to soften water. (If you are concerned about sodium intake, you may want to leave one cold-water tap unconnected to the system for drinking water.) They also may reduce the levels of cadmium, iron, and radium. Whole-house water-softening systems cost from $575 to $1,750.

NSF International, 3475 Plymouth Road, Ann Arbor, MI 48105, offers a free book listing certified treatment units to help you choose one that will suit your particular needs.

Is Bottled Water a Good Buy?

You may instead opt to get your water from the multibillion-dollar bottled-water industry. Whether you buy it in a supermarket or have it delivered to your home, you should know that bottled water is produced under rigorous quality control. Most bottled water sold in the United States is derived from natural springs and wells. About one-fourth of the bottled water sold comes from municipal water sources. In order to be sold as bottled water, however, water from these municipal sources must undergo additional treatment and quality control procedures.

Bottled spring, mineral and carbonated waters are all subject to the same EPA standards as any other publicly consumed water. Bottlers are not allowed to make health claims, and the products are sold primarily to people who like the way they taste . . . or *don't* taste, as the case may be.

If you purchase individual bottles of water at the market, you should take a few simple precautions to keep it wholesome.

"Bottled water is a food and should be handled as any other food product," says Lisa Prats, vice president of the International Bottled Water Association. Store bottled water in a cool, dry place, away from direct sunlight and household chemicals. After the bottle is opened, if all of the product is not consumed, be sure to recap the bottle and store it in a cool, dry location or in the refrigerator.

CHAPTER 17

Food Additives

A Mixed Blessing

Peter Gross, M.D., didn't believe in allergic reactions to food additives until he was doubled over with severe abdominal cramps.

Hospitalized four times in two years, the Hackensack, New Jersey, internist underwent nearly every conceivable test to determine the source of his agony. "All of them showed allergic reaction. The question was what was causing it," he says.

His wife, a health writer, suggested he keep a food and medicine diary. Sure enough, when Dr. Gross listed the ingredients of the items in the diary on a spreadsheet along with his symptom flare-ups, one common element stood out like a thug in a police lineup: Yellow Dye No. 6, an artificial coloring often used in drugs and processed foods.

Further testing confirmed the culprit. And since eliminating the foods and drugs containing the dye from his diet, Dr. Gross has been pain-free. "I just learned to read labels," he says.

Fortunately, most of us don't have to scrutinize lengthy ingredient listings *that* closely. If you're like most healthy Americans, those sometimes-ominous-sounding three-syllable food additives are harder to pronounce than to digest.

Normally, research shows, our bodies have little trouble tolerating the smorgasbord of strange-sounding ingredients designed to keep TV dinners oven-fresh, turn green citrus fruit sunshiny orange or tantalize our palates with ersatz flavors.

THEY'RE EVERYWHERE

In fact, chemical additives are so common in processed foods that more than 2,500 are approved for use by the Food and Drug Administration (FDA). And let's not forget that more familiar-sounding substances can be additives as well. Sugar, salt and corn syrup are the most common, found in everything from peanut butter to breakfast bars. And adding vitamins and minerals during processing sometimes takes nutrients where nutrients have never gone before.

Calorie-cutters like Simplesse, the revolutionary fat replacer, and Nutra-Sweet are the food additives of the future. Fat and sugar substitutes already top the list of some two dozen new additives heading for store shelves each year, says Manfred Kroger, Ph.D., professor of food science at Pennsylvania State University in University Park. "There's money to be made," says Dr. Kroger. "The public is buying diet products like wild."

Other additives—like MSG (monosodium glutamate), sulfites and certain colorings—are less popular, having been fingered for causing headaches, rashes and other reactions in an unfortunate, sensitive few.

In fact, the late Benjamin Feingold, M.D., an allergy specialist, made headlines during the 1970s by claiming there was a connection between hyperactivity in children and food additives. By following an additive-free diet, Dr. Feingold claimed, 50 percent of hyperactive and learning-disabled children would undergo a dramatic improvement in behavior.

Although Dr. Feingold's assertions have been questioned and disproven by his scientific brethren, for many people, concerns about the broader health risks of some food additives linger. Sodium nitrite, a common lunch meat preservative, for example, has long been suspected as a possible contributor to some cancers.

Of course, food manufacturers point out that any minute health threat created by additives pales in comparison to deadly diseases like botulism caused by spoiled (albeit preservative-free) food. Many health food purists, on the other hand, advocate avoiding additives at all costs, forcing you, perhaps, to forsake some of your favorite foods.

Perhaps the best approach, says Dr. Kroger, is "Know thyself." "If you have an individual sensitivity, once you know the effect a certain ingredient or food has on your health, you can try to steer clear of it. For example, if you're sensitive to alcohol, you should even check the label before buying a chocolate confection. The same with MSG, sulfites, caffeine, whatever." If you prefer to avoid as many additives as possible, stick to a healthy diet rich in fresh fruit, vegetables, whole grains, low-fat meats and dairy products. These are less likely to contain additives.

TAMING THE TINKERING

Additive use is a bit more sophisticated today, but there's nothing new about tinkering with food. The ancient Egyptians used sulfites to stop bacterial growth and fermentation in wine. They also used extracts from beetles for food coloring. Vegetable dyes from juniper fruits or beech-root juice were popular colorings in the Middle Ages, although wary kings began to employ "garglers" to test their meals—perhaps for additives that did not originate in the kitchen. Saltpeter became the meat coloring and preservative of choice for aspiring chefs in Germany and Austria, according to seventeenth-century cookbooks.

But as time marched on, less scrupulous elements began their assault on the food supply. As early as 1887, muckraking journalists at *New York World* published a list of the additives that at the time appalled even the staid *Journal of the American Medical Association*. Observed *JAMA:* "On reading the list one is amazed at the ingenuity and dishonesty of civilized, Christian man." Among the ingredients found in milk by the *World*: "Water principally, flour or starch, boiled white carrots, milk of almonds, sheep's brains, gum tragacanth, carbonate of soda, chrome yellow for coloring."

On the heels of similar revelations, Congress passed the Pure Food and Drug Act in 1906 and the Federal Food, Drug, and Cosmetic Act in 1938. While the laws were among the first attempts to regulate additives, they didn't pack much clout: In fact it was up to the FDA, not the manufacturer, to prove an additive's "harmfulness."

The Food Additives Amendment of 1958 and Color Additive Amendments of 1960, however, solved this dilemma by requiring manufacturers to establish that their products were safe. The 1958 legislation led to the creation of a list of ingredients that were deemed free from the need for further investigation. These ingredients are called GRAS, or Generally Regarded As Safe. Another much-debated amendment, introduced by Representative Delaney in 1972 and passed by Congress, banned for human consumption any additive that caused cancer in lab animals.

But the cyclamate scare of 1969 raised questions about the coveted GRAS status. After research indicated that this artificial sweetener, already on the GRAS list, appeared to cause cancer in rats, cyclamates were taken off the GRAS list and disappeared from the U.S. marketplace. A White House Conference in 1969 led President Richard M. Nixon to order the FDA to review the entire GRAS list for potentially toxic substances.

Experts chosen by the Federation of American Societies for Experimental Biology reaffirmed the safety of 70 percent of the additives, while painting the rest varying shades of gray.

BETTER LIVING THROUGH FORTIFICATION

Among the most beneficial additives are vitamins and minerals blended into food. Not only do they enhance the nutritional value of many foods, in some cases added vitamins are also used to improve appearance and taste, according to the Institute of Food Technologists' Expert Panel on Food Safety and Nutrition.

Vitamin C, also called ascorbic acid, is perhaps the most versatile, improving bread, making wine and beer clear and enhancing the pink color of cured meat while inhibiting the formation of harmful substances. Because ascorbic acid is good at stopping oxygen's detrimental effects on foods, it's often added to sodas and fruit drinks. Vitamin E or tocopherols are antioxidants used in bacon, baked goods, butter, lard, margarine, rapeseed oil, safflower oil and sunflower seed oil.

Beta-carotene, a source of vitamin A, is used to add color to some margarines, shortening, butter, cheese, confections, baked goods, ice cream, egg nog, macaroni products, soups and juices.

Even though the last of their reports was issued in 1982, over 150 substances have yet to be reaffirmed as GRAS.

When animal tests showed that saccharin, an artificial sweetener, caused cancer, the FDA sought to remove it from the marketplace. But Congress chose, despite the Delaney Clause, to allow saccharin sales to continue, as long as the products included a warning label.

But for the most part, the only thing standing between you and these often helpful but sometimes harmful ingredients is still the FDA. The FDA alone is charged with the awesome task of policing our food supply.

The most common use of vitamins is to fortify, restore or enrich a food's nutritional value. In fact, the addition of vitamin D to milk and iodine to salt are credited with preventing major nutritional deficiencies like rickets and goiter in the United States.

The most frequently fortified foods: breakfast cereals. Even the most sugary breakfast concoctions are commonly fortified to provide at least 25 percent of the Recommended Dietary Allowance for ten vitamins and six minerals. Also on the list of fortified foods are bread, margarine, nonfat dry milk, evaporated milk, infant formulas, breakfast bars and liquid and solid meal replacements, according to the institute.

A surge of interest in fiber by consumers has led food manufacturers to add cellulose, pectin, starch, and other naturally derived fibers to foods. Although it may seem like a good idea, the FDA does not encourage indiscriminate food fortification. In fact, adding nutrients to fresh produce, meat, poultry or fish products, sugar, or snack foods is discouraged. However, fortifying is recognized as often necessary to restore nutrients lost in processing.

So where does that leave the consumer? While the FDA attempts to police the industry, for your own peace of mind, it pays to have a bit of background on some of the most discussed additives.

ASPARTAME: A SWEET INNOVATION

Also known as NutraSweet brand sweetener, this additive appears in over 5,000 foods and beverages, from frozen desserts to diet soft drinks. There's little doubt about the reason for its popularity: Aspartame is 200 times as sweet as sugar with 95 percent fewer calories. And according to The

CHEMICALS WITH A MISSION

You've seen them in everything from cereal to salad dressings. But have you ever wondered just what those additives are doing in your food? Here's a short list with some of their job responsibilities.

Acetone peroxide. Used as a dough conditioner and bleaching and conditioning agent in many baked goods.

BHA. Used alone or with BHT as an antioxidant to help stabilize fat in dehydrated potato shreds, dry beverage and dessert mixes, shortenings and potato flakes.

Calcium disodium EDTA. Used as a color or texture protector in canned soft drinks, canned white potatoes, dressings, beer, mayonnaise, processed dry pinto beans, cooked and canned crabmeat, clams and shrimp and lemon- or orange-flavored spreads.

Polydextrose. Used as a bulking agent, partial sugar replacer, formulation aid, humectant (helps maintain moisture) and texturizer in custards, pudding-filled pies, cakes, cookies, salad dressings and hard and soft candy.

Polysorbate 60. Used as an emulsifier (to ensure consistency) in whipped toppings, cake mixes, icings, dressings and milk and cream substitutes.

Sodium lauryl sulfate. Used as a whipping aid in marshmallows and angel food cake mix.

Sodium nitrate. Used as an antimicrobial agent and color fixative, with or without sodium nitrite, in smoked, cured meats, fish and poultry.

Sodium stearoyl lactylate. Used as a dough strengthener in pancakes and waffles, a formulation aid in dehydrated potatoes and an emulsifier in snack dips, cheese substitutes and gravies.

NutraSweet Company, the additive—which is made from
two naturally occurring amino acids, aspartic acid and
phenylalanine—has been found safe in nearly 200 animal
and human studies, making it "the most tested food ingredient
ever approved by the FDA."

But the substance is not without some drawbacks. Products
containing aspartame must carry a warning label "Phenylke-
tonurics: Contains Phenylalanine" on the label. The notice is
a red flag for about 1 in 15,000 Americans who has phenylke-
tonuria, a disease that makes it nearly impossible for the individual to metabolize the amino acid phenylalanine.
Diagnosed at birth, the disorder has been linked to mental retardation, epilepsy and other neurological problems.

The tip-off on the label is required by the FDA because
many of the foods using aspartame would not normally contain phenylalanine. Other concerns have been raised about
the safety of aspartame. Over 5,000 people have contacted
the FDA in the 11 years since aspartame was approved for
tabletop use, claiming that the product had caused a variety
of symptoms. The FDA analyzed these complaints carefully
and found no cause-and-effect relationship. In addition,
clinical studies to investigate these complaints, conducted in
U.S. and foreign medical schools, have confirmed the safety
of aspartame.

MSG: THE INVISIBLE ADDITIVE

Sometimes even reading food labels isn't enough. Consider the case of the 32-year-old woman who suffered six
moderate to severe migraines a month. The pain was so bad
she missed at least one day of work a month for a year.

On the advice of her doctor, the woman avoided foods
that had monosodium glutamate listed on the label, but her
headaches continued. That is, until she learned that hydrolyzed vegetable protein and some natural flavors contain

MSG naturally. Soon after switching to brands of mayonnaise and mustard without those mysterious ingredients and adopting other MSG-avoidance tactics, the woman's migraines decreased to one a month.

While some studies show that roughly 30 percent of people who eat Chinese food suffer from headache, tightness of the face, dizziness, diarrhea, nausea and abdominal cramps, this case shows that MSG reactions are no longer a problem strictly in Chinese restaurants. Purveyors of Oriental fare actually only account for a fraction of the 85 million pounds of MSG used in the United States each year—enough for five ounces per person.

Food manufacturers love the additive because it enhances flavor in processed products like frozen dinners, potato chips, soups, sauces, canned meats, lunch meats and broths.

And yet, ingredient labels that list pure MSG are rare. Manufacturers are aware that MSG occurs in hydrolyzed vegetable protein, hydrolyzed plant protein and some flavorings, so they are getting the flavor boost with these additives instead.

But a migraine is still a migraine. And researchers have demonstrated that three to five grams of MSG for those unable to tolerate the additive is enough to trigger severe headaches.

NITRITES: A NECESSARY EVIL?

Scientists studying historical cookbooks and medical records discovered what may have been more than an interesting coincidence: The first detailed descriptions of large bowel cancer and multiple sclerosis in Germany and Austria did not appear until the early nineteenth century, a short time after the use of nitrates to color and preserve meat began.

There's little debate in the scientific community over the cancer-causing ability of nitrosamines, substances formed during the breakdown of nitrates and nitrites. Nitrites are the most commonly used preservative in meats. They are added to bacon, bologna, corned beef, frankfurters, sausages, ham and some fish and poultry products. The problem is that today there are no better alternatives. Nitrates are found naturally in vegetables like spinach, beets, celery and rhubarb.

The good news is that the way to prevent cancer-causing nitrosamines from forming from the nitrites in your morning bacon may be as close as your glass of orange juice. Further research is needed, but scientists have discovered that when nitrites are bathed in a solution containing vitamin C, the additive's ability to convert to nitrosamines is effectively blocked, says Leonard Cohen, Ph.D., head of the Section of Nutritional Endocrinology at the American Health Foundation in Valhalla, New York.

SIMPLESSE: THE FAT REPLACER

The introduction of Simplesse, the fat substitute developed by researchers at the NutraSweet Company, heralds a new era in food additives. Food manufacturers have replicated lots of flavors over the years—artificial flavors account for more than one-third of the taste in the marketplace today—but never that of fat.

"Nobody looking into their crystal ball can say whether this is good or this is bad. This is progress, and we ought to make the best of that," says Dr. Kroger.

Among the benefits: If used in the maximum number of applications, Simplesse could reduce the fat content in the U.S. diet by 14 percent, research shows. Among potential drawbacks: use of Simplesse could increase U.S. protein consumption, already higher than desired. Also, there have been no published long-term health investigations of human subjects who have eaten Simplesse.

Developed in 1982, Simplesse is the trade name for microparticulated protein, made by a patented process that shrinks the size of the protein in egg white or skim milk—

PESTICIDE RESIDUES LINGER ALONG
WITH WORRIES

Pesticides aren't actually considered food additives. But judging from the results of the Food and Drug Administration's (FDA) own Market Basket Survey, they probably should be. According to the FDA, pesticide residue lurks beneath the bountiful exterior of roughly one-third of our produce.

The Environmental Protection Agency (EPA), however, contends that no more than 1 to 2 percent of all produce contains pesticide in amounts considered poisonous. Deaths from eating poisoned produce are almost nonexistent. But no one is sure about the long-term risks of cancer. While risks are generally considered very low, the cancer/pesticide connection is hard to establish.

But since the Alar apple scare of 1989 (sparked by claims by the Natural Resources Defense Council that the chemical, which was commonly used to make apples crisper, could cause cancer), consumers are more willing than ever to buy fruit and vegetables grown without the use of chemicals. In fact, 75 percent of consumers cited in a Rand Corporation study said they considered the use of pesticides, herbicides, additives and preservatives "a serious hazard." Those consumers who were most concerned indicated that they were willing to pay a "substantial premium to avoid these residues."

The EPA approves the use of pesticides and establishes residue tolerance levels for food. Residue tolerances are

without changing its chemistry, according to researchers. A similar but less advanced process is used to turn soybeans into simulated meat products.

If the transformation is less than spectacular, the results have drawn raves. In coffee ice cream taste tests, a product

between 100 and 1,000 times lower than the level that caused "no effect" in test animals. The EPA admits, however, that it's nearly impossible to determine how much residue might be harmful to humans.

Companies trying to get EPA approval for a pesticide's use must submit toxicology studies and pesticide residue reports that show how much pesticide is expected to remain in a crop.

To make sure that pesticide residue levels meet safety requirements, the FDA each year tests 15,000 to 18,000 shipments of food, including produce, seafood, milk and processed goods. Under another program, four times a year the agency buys more than 200 different supermarket food items from across the country that are representative of the diet of U.S. consumers. The foods are then prepared and analyzed for pesticide residues and other chemicals.

According to a 1991 FDA report, domestically grown items with the highest percentage of samples found containing residues include cranberries, grapefruit, lemons, oranges, peaches, nectarines, tangerines, pumpkins, strawberries, pears, fruit juices and barley.

The FDA says that the analytic methods used are capable of detecting only about half of the pesticides with established EPA tolerances, but the results are believed to be representative of residue levels.

Consumers can limit the amount of pesticide residues in foods by thoroughly washing fresh fruit and vegetables, removing the outer leaves of leafy vegetables and sometimes trimming the skin.

using Simplesse was rated nearly as high as fat-laden super premium ice cream. In fact, the participants rated the Simplesse product above super premium in aftertaste, color and "overall liking." Manufacturers credit the taste to Simplesse's "mouth-feel"—the closest thing to fat ever made in the lab.

And research shows that the fat content of foods with Simplesse drops dramatically. One tablespoon of traditional mayonnaise-based salad dressing contains 12 grams of fat, while one tablespoon with Simplesse has less than 1 gram. A four-ounce serving of super premium ice cream that normally contains 15 grams of fat also has less than 1 gram of fat when made with Simplesse.

There are at least two groups of people who will never enjoy the benefits of this fat substitute: those allergic to eggs or milk. Studies show they'll also react to the Simplesse.

But that probably won't prevent the introduction of Simplesse into dozens of foods like cheeses, yogurts and salad dressings.

Already, several other companies are developing their own fat substitutes. Procter and Gamble, the consumer products giant, is attracting attention with Olestra, a nondigestible cooking oil additive. Hercules, a multinational chemical and aerospace company, has launched Slendid, a fat replacement made from citrus peels for use in baked goods, frozen desserts, soups, cheeses, sauces and yogurts, among other products.

SULFITES: ASTHMATICS BEWARE

The reaction was sudden and alarming: Just two minutes after he was fed a mixture of sulfites and applesauce, the two-year-old asthmatic began to cough and wheeze. His pulse, blood pressure and respiratory rate all shot up. Because the boy was being closely monitored by a doctor, he was not in danger. But his reaction confirmed the diagnosis: sulfite sensitivity.

A common preservative primarily used to keep medicines potent and food looking fresh, sulfites are known by several names, including potassium or sodium sulfite, bisulfite, metabisulfite and sulfur dioxide.

Unfortunately, there was little government concern over

the use of sulfites on fresh fruit and vegetables until after 17 unrelated deaths in 1985, most of which were connected to the use of sulfites at salad bars.

These deaths led the FDA to ban the preservative, which formerly had GRAS status, from nearly all raw or fresh fruits and vegetables in 1986.

"That's where most asthmatics were getting their exposure and having their reactions," says Ronald A. Simon, M.D., head of the Division of Allergy and Immunology at the Scripps Clinic and Research Foundation in La Jolla, California. "Then, because people became so aware of sulfites, the manufacturers began to pull them out of many other foods. Even in the foods they continue to be in, they are there in lower amounts."

But while sulfites do a remarkable job keeping food looking fresh, studies show that between two and five percent of asthmatics in the United States are extremely sensitive to sulfites.

Although it's unclear what actually triggers the reaction among asthmatics (one theory is individuals sometimes inhale the sulfur dioxide gas generated by the sulfites added to the food), there's no doubt about the consequences. Most reactions are characterized by severe bronchial spasms, which can occur within minutes after eating foods containing sulfites. During a reaction, sulfite-sensitive patients with asthma should immediately use their metered-dose inhalers and have epinephrine ready.

Although banned from nearly all fresh foods, the use of sulfites by food and beverage manufacturers continues. Foods that most commonly contain sulfites include shrimp, dried fruit, cider and vinegar. A single five-ounce glass of sweet white wine may contain up to 50 milligrams of sulfites. The only fresh vegetable that may still be sprayed with sulfites is potatoes.

To protect consumers, the FDA requires that packaged foods containing ten or more parts per million (ppm) of sulfites must say on the ingredient label that they contain sulfites. Foods with less than ten ppm should not be a problem even for the most sensitive patients.

Sulfites can be added during food manufacturing, processing or delivery and are used as sanitizing agents for food containers and fermentation equipment.

However, most people do not have to be concerned about sulfites, says Dr. Simon. "There are these rare reported cases of hives or a more systemic allergic reaction we call anaphylaxis but they are so few and far between that I don't think the average person has to worry about it."

Anaphylaxis, the worst possible allergic reaction, often includes hives, throat swelling, low blood pressure, shock and perhaps even death. "In our opinion, those people who have that kind of anaphylactic reaction to sulfites probably are truly allergic to sulfites—not simply sensitive to sulfur dioxide gas," says Dr. Simon.

A simple skin test performed by any allergist can determine if you're sensitive to sulfites.

TARTRAZINE: COLOR IT POPULAR

Remember Dr. Gross, the internist from Hackensack? He's not the only one who's had trouble with food colorings.

Dr. Gross reacted to Yellow No. 6, the third most commonly used coloring. Red No. 40, commonly found in maraschino cherries, is the most popular coloring used by food manufacturers. Close behind, in second place, is tartrazine, or as it's known in the industry, Yellow No. 5.

By 1975, the number of reported cases of tartrazine reactions became large enough to make this dye "a major health concern," according to Joseph R. DiPalma, M.D., professor emeritus of pharmacology and medicine at the Hahnemann School of Medicine in Philadelphia. In 1980, the FDA, while still maintaining approval of tartrazine, issued new

---

AVOIDING SULFITES? THEN START HERE

The following products often contain sulfites.
• Alcoholic beverages—beer, cocktail mix, red wine, white wine, wine coolers
• Condiments—olives, relishes, pickles, salad dressing mixes, wine vinegar, sauerkraut, pickled pearl onions
• Fresh fish and fish products—clams, crabs, lobsters, scallops, shrimp
• Processed fruit—dietetic fruit or juices, dried fruit, fruit juices and drinks, fruit pie fillings
• Processed foods—avocado mix; dried vegetables, including green vegetables and potatoes; pickled vegetables; vegetable juice; hominy; dry soup mixes
• Snack foods—apple bits, dried fruit, fruit-filled crackers, trail mix containing dried fruit bits

---

regulations that required listing of the dye on the labels of all drugs and food packages. The FDA estimates at least 50,000 Americans are sensitive to tartrazine.

The amount required to provoke tartrazine sensitivity varies from 25 milligrams down to as little as 0.00085 milligrams each day. Most people consume an average of 13 milligrams daily.

Products that may contain tartrazine include orange and lime drinks, ice cream and sherbets, gelatins and puddings, salad dressings, cheese dishes, cake mixes and icings, seasoned salts and confections.

Tartrazine has also caused its share of problems as a coloring in drugs. When a 50-year-old Milwaukee woman suffering from skin rash did not respond to treatment for six weeks, her physician recommended that she replace her estrogen tablets with others not colored with tartrazine. Soon after, the rash went away—until the woman was inadvertently served a relish containing tartrazine.

CHAPTER 18

Ethnic Foods

Healthy Eating from Around the Globe

In the days when Fords and Chevys ruled American roads and meat and potatoes ruled American menus, the closest many of us came to ethnic foods was chop suey from a can.

Today, Americans are as likely to drive a Honda as a Ford and as eager to feast on grilled Indonesian chicken saté or Spanish seafood paella as pot roast.

Yes, American food has gone global. And that's an international trade imbalance that can only result in a surplus—a surplus of health.

Unlike the Anglo-Germanic food that shaped the typical meat-and-milk American diet, this Asian-Mediterranean-Latin-influenced fare tends to be light and healthy. It's also infused with out-of-this-world flavor from tongue-tingling curries and chilies to sweetly sublime cinnamon and papaya.

You don't have to venture far to see evidence of the ethnic food boom. You can, for example, buy whole-grain Arabian pita bread at the local sandwich shop or dip into Lebanese hummus spread (pureed chick-peas) at the church buffet. Red-hot Mexican salsas outsell catsup in some parts of the country. In other areas, instant cup-of-Indian-style-lentils is giving chicken noodle soup a run for its money.

A stroll through almost any supermarket is a crash course in world gastronomy. Oriental bok choy, tofu and "tree ear" mushrooms are nestled next to the carrots and broccoli. Jade-tinged olive oil from Sicily and amber-colored sesame oil from China share shelf space with Crisco. Oodles of noodles stretch down the aisle with pastas ranging from whole wheat to buckwheat; there's skinny pasta for thick, Italian sauces and squiggly pasta for thin Japanese soups.

Open the newspaper and you'll see such tasty recipe alternatives to Tuesday's meat loaf as Moroccan orange pistachio couscous (cracked wheat) to Thai peanut-and-pepper grilled shrimp.

The Timing Is Right

The explosion of ethnic food in America is a direct result of the influx of immigrants arriving from the Pacific Rim and Latin countries. And it couldn't be better timing, according to Aliza Minear, Ph.D., director of health and nutrition education at the Scripps Clinic in La Jolla, California. "People are seeking ways to cut back on calories, fat, salt and sugar and still have a satisfying, tasty meal. Eating ethnic foods fills the bill nicely."

Many ethnic diets are built around complex carbohydrates—grains, greens and other plant foods, says Dr. Minear. They provide a lot less artery-clogging fat and a lot more cholesterol-busting fiber than you'd get from the traditional meat-and-dairy-based American diet. They also provide more disease-fighting nutrients. Among them: potassium to control blood pressure, nondairy calcium to stave off osteoporosis and beta-carotene to combat cancer.

Indeed, many nutrition experts believe that adopting ethnic food choices may be the ideal solution for combating obesity, heart disease, cancer and other chronic diseases linked to the usual American, high-fat, low-fiber diet.

Trying to "fix" our usual foods by engineering leaner hamburgers or fat-free cakes is not the best way to promote healthful eating, according to Marion Nestle, Ph.D., professor and chairperson of the Department of Nutrition, Food and Hotel Management at New York University in New York City. "People feel they are giving up something and may feel deprived."

But shifting to a plant-based cuisine that is highly flavorful makes eating light a whole new satisfying way of eating, not a sacrifice.

SPICING IT UP: THE HEAT IS OPTIONAL

Spices can make low-fat, low-sodium dining a blast instead of a bore. A little salsa on a baked potato, for example, and you'll never miss the butter or salt.

Not all ethnic foods are fiery hot, though. For instance, while many Mexican dishes include palate-paralyzing chilies, others use subdued spices such as cinnamon and nutmeg along with a squeeze of tangy lime juice. A good cookbook with a spice chart can help you select flavor combinations to suit your palate.

On the other hand, if you can stand the heat, you may want to include a chili or two in your diet.

Capsaicin, the "hot stuff" in hot peppers, appears to lower cholesterol in lab animals in a way similar to some cholesterol-reducing drugs. After rats were fed capsaicin and other spices, it more than doubled the rate at which cholesterol was bound to bile acids, a process that helps whisk this troublemaker out of the body.

More hot food news for thought: It turns out that capsaicin not only burns your mouth but burns calories by increasing metabolism.

THE MEDITERRANEAN MODEL

You'd think that the country with the highest standard of living would produce the world's best diet. In fact, from a health standpoint, the standard American diet ranks among the world's worst.

Studies show that the healthy eating award goes to more "primitive" lands. As it turns out, countries in the Mediterranean Basin—the birthplace of civilization—have perfected one of the healthiest diets in the world.

Here, in the sun-drenched countries of Greece and Italy, for example, people still toil long hours in fields and dine on foods of their forefathers: fresh-picked green vegetables seasoned with garlic and olive oil, hearty minestrone soup laced with robust red beans, hunks of whole-grain bread, a plate of chewy pasta. It's also in this region that heart disease—America's number one killer—is as rare as marbled steaks and creamy milk shakes.

In a long-term landmark study begun some 40 years ago, Ancel Keys, Ph.D., of the University of Minnesota School of Public Health in Minneapolis, compared the mortality of men from Italy, Yugoslavia, Greece, Finland, the Netherlands, the United States and Japan. Dr. Keys found that the men living in countries with the highest fat intake—America and Finland—also had the highest death rate from heart disease. Among Greeks and Italians and other people in the Mediterranean Basin, however, the rate was only half that of Americans and Europeans.

And while the American/European meat-and-dairy diet is filled with saturated fat, the Mediterranean diet relies on olive oil, a monounsaturated fat that may actually lower cholesterol levels. Dr. Keys observed that these folks drizzled the "nectar of the olive" on tomatoes and pasta, sautéed zucchini in it and made marinara sauces with it.

Subsequent research has underscored olive oil's amazing health benefits. In one study involving 8,000 Italian men and women, for example, the regular olive oil users had significantly lower blood pressures as well as blood sugar levels, than those who used butter or polyunsaturated oil.

"Olive oil isn't a medicine," says Maurizio Trevisan, M.D., of the State University of New York at Buffalo School of Medicine and Biomedical Sciences who conducted the Italian study. You can't, for example, eat a greasy double cheeseburger and expect a salad drenched in olive oil to shield your heart.

Rather than adding olive oil to your usual diet, says Dr. Trevisan, you should use it sparingly as a *substitute* for saturated fat. "Your primary goal should be to reduce fat overall, eat a variety of vegetables and increase your intake of grains and fresh fruit," he says. Do this, and you'll truly be reaping the rewards of the Mediterranean diet.

THE LOW-FAT ASIAN WAY

Studies show that you'd also do well to take a few dietary tips from the Orient. Although Japan's high-tech industry has soared to heights matching Mount Fuji's, many of her people eat the same simple, ultra-low fat diet consumed by the Japanese for centuries. This may be a big reason why Japan's people live longer than any other people on the planet and suffer fewer diet-related chronic diseases than people who regularly indulge in fatty foods.

In the Honolulu Heart Program study conducted by the National Heart, Lung and Blood Institute, researchers looked at 8,000 men of Japanese descent who lived in Japan or America. They found that the Japanese-American men had three to four times more heart disease than the men living in Japan.

The higher incidence of heart disease in Japanese-American men can be explained because they strayed from their low-fat diet of their ancestors, according to Grant N. Stemmermann, M.D., director of the Japan-Hawaii Cancer Study in Honolulu.

"In Japan, a person typically starts the day with rice and miso soup made from soybeans," says Dr. Stemmermann.

A BUYER'S GUIDE TO OLIVE OIL

Heart-healthy olive oil may be used in place of other cooking oils. But *which* olive oil do you choose? Like fine wine, olive oil varies in bouquet, color and taste. Generally, the more full-bodied, the better the grade of olive oil. Mediterranean cooks prefer different grades to prepare different dishes. Here's a guide to the standard grades, set by international agreement.

Virgin olive oil. Oil that is pressed (never chemically extracted) from the fruit only, not the pit. In U.S.-produced oils, which account for less than 3 percent of the olive oil sold in this country, "virgin" means the oil is from the first pressing. Not to be used in high-temperature cooking (high heat breaks down flavor) but excellent for light sautéing and adding to cooked sauces and dressings.

Extra-virgin olive oil. Top quality, and most costly, oil from the first pressing. Acid levels are under 1 percent, and the oil has a greener color and richer flavor. Best used in cold pasta salads or drizzled over crisp greens, veggies or poached fish or chicken.

Pure olive oil. (Called refined oil in the United States.) Oil that's been refined and filtered to reduce acidity. Lighter in color and aroma, with less of an olive taste. Can be used in stir-frying.

Extra-light olive oil. An American invention, it's extra-refined and pale in color with a mild flavor, but it contains the same amount of fat (13 grams per tablespoon) and calories (120). Use it as you would any highly refined oil such as sunflower.

"In contrast, a typical Japanese-American breakfast is ham and eggs." The saturated fat score? Japanese: one gram. Americans: six.

In similar studies from Stanford University School of

Medicine comparing Chinese men in China with Chinese men in North America, the latter group had four to seven times more colorectal cancer than the former group. They also had more saturated fat in their diets.

MORE VEGETABLES, LESS MEAT

The most striking difference between the world's healthier diets and the standard American diets is this: Meat is not the centerpiece of meals.

Even meat-laden Italian dishes such as lasagna that Americans adore are reserved for celebratory feasts in the homeland. And in Third World locations, meat may be an even rarer treat. "Meat is expensive and hard to come by in many non-Westernized countries," says New York nutritionist Denise Webb, Ph.D., author of *The International Calorie Counter.*

An everyday Italian dish is more likely to be a plate of fiber-rich white beans and fresh-picked greens, for example. Or tomato and mushroom polenta (cornmeal mush). Unfortunately, many traditional dishes get "beefed up" once they cross U.S. borders.

A typical meal in China, for example, is a mound of steamed rice, lots of vegetables and a few bits of pork or beef. The Americanized version, however, serves the reverse: lots of meat, a little rice, with deep-fried egg rolls and enough soy sauce to send your sodium levels over the pagoda.

Likewise, a typical Americanized version of Mexican food is beef-stuffed burritos smothered in sour cream and Cheddar cheese. Authentic Mexican food is less artery-clogging. A common meal consists of cholesterol-fighting beans (like chick-peas or pinto beans), cabbage and corn or squash, for instance.

The bottom line: Most traditional ethnic cuisines could be classified as vegetarian or nearly so—and that may be their major health advantage, studies show.

Results from the Nurses Health Study from Harvard Medical School, involving 89,000 nurses, showed that the women who ate red meat infrequently had less than half the risk of colon cancer of their omnivorous colleagues.

Consuming certain vegetables may boost the health advantage even more. Take broccoli, for example. The people of Asia and Italy are fond of this bright emerald veggie and include it in countless stir-fried and pasta dishes. And they may be healthier for it.

The reason? Broccoli is higher in nutrients including vitamin C, iron and B vitamins than most other plant foods. What's more, broccoli, a member of the cabbage family, is a great source of beta-carotene. Studies show that regular consumption of beta-carotene-rich vegetables helps ward off heart attacks, strokes and cancers.

It's more than possible that Japan's lower incidence of lung cancer is because of their higher intake of beta-carotene-rich vegetables, from broccoli to seaweed, according to Dr. Stemmermann.

CALCIUM? PROTEIN? NO PROBLEM!

Except for some Indian dishes such as chicken masala that contain yogurt and butter, the world's healthiest cuisines are generally devoid of dairy products. You won't find the buttery sauces, creamy salad dressings, and mounds of cheese that typically blanket American food.

Yet, even with few milk-based foods, the people in many ethnic cultures manage to get enough calcium to keep their bones strong.

How? The answer, once again, is vegetables. Lots of them. In a study conducted at Creighton University in Omaha researchers found that the calcium in the Chinese vegetable bok choy, and also kale and spinach, is as readily absorbed as the calcium in milk. The bonus: There's very little fat. "Bok choy has the highest calcium-per-calorie ratio of any food," says the study's director, Robert Heaney, M.D., professor of medicine at Creighton. There's about 79 milligrams of calcium in a ½-cup serving, and only ten calories.

How do these cultures obtain protein without red meat? Often the answer lies in the deep blue sea. Fish favorites among the Japanese and Mediterranean peoples include mackerel and sardines, to name a few. Like all fish, these varieties are loaded with protein, but they also contain omega-3 fatty acids, a type of fat that has been found to keep cholesterol in check.

BEYOND BARBECUE SAUCE

Grilling using flavors from around the world is a mouth-watering way to prepare low-fat foods, according to Linda Burum, California ethnic food expert.

The soy sauces of the Orient, the balsamic vinegars of Italy, the limes of Latin America and yogurt dressings of the Middle East all naturally tenderize lean cuts of meat, chicken and fish. This means you don't need to add fat or rich sauces, says Burum.

Using these natural tenderizers as a base, you can add zip with almost any spice. To add a Latin-style flavor to shrimp, for example, soak in lime juice laced with cayenne pepper. Or grill chicken Thai-style, using rice vinegar, garlic and peanut-chili sauce. Flavorless, protein-rich tofu (soybean curd) takes on a delightful, meaty taste when marinated in Chinese hoisin sauce, (spicy brown paste from ground soybeans, garlic, sugar, vinegar and sesame sauce). Grill it, chop it and toss it in salads.

Fiber Has a Starring Role

Unfortunately, most Americans get only half the protective amount of fiber they need. In contrast, high-fiber foods make up the bulk of the fare on most world menus.

Take Indian food, for example. You may associate this highly flavored food with the richly sauced lamb dishes typically served in Indian restaurants in this country. In India, however, rich meat dishes are reserved for royalty, according to Neela Paniz, owner of the Bombay Cafe in Los Angeles. A common everyday dish is dahl—a thick, split lentil stew served in dozens of ways and seasoned with a dazzling array of spices to suit every palate. Moong dahl, for example, is yellow split peas with fenugreek and cumin.

Lentils have virtually no fat and provide lots of protein and iron, and like other legumes they're super sources of soluble fiber. It's believed this type fiber may help flush out cholesterol before it builds up on artery walls. Studies conducted by James W. Anderson, M.D., professor of medicine and clinical nutrition at the University of Kentucky College of Medicine in Lexington found that adding 1½ cups of legumes a day to the diet lowered cholesterol 26 points in 30 days.

Grains are another potent fiber source in ethnic cuisines. Greeks eat chunks of crusty whole-grain bread at every meal. Mexicans eat cornmeal tortillas. In India, chapati, the flat whole-grain griddle-bread, is used in place of forks and knives to sop up every morsel of lentil stew. And in North Africa, couscous makes a complete high-fiber salad when combined with fresh oranges and dried figs.

Rice is the main ingredient in meals eaten by half the world's population. Rice types range from the chewy arborio in Italian risotti and the fluffy basmati in Middle Eastern pilafs to the sticky Asian rice, custom-made for chopsticks and dipping into fish sauces.

NOODLE KNOW-HOW

People from Italy to Asia have long known what Americans are now discovering: that pasta can be a nutritious, quickly fixed, low-calorie meal. (One cup is only 120 calories if you don't add creamy sauces.) Pasta is also the perfect companion for tossing with vegetables and bits of grilled seafood and for soaking up tomato-based marinaras or other savory sauces. There's a dizzying number of noodles on the market. Here's a bit of background to help you sort through them.

Italian pastas. Most are made with wheat flour, usually durum wheat, which is high in gluten, making the strands hard and firm. Semolina flour is durum wheat that is more coarsely ground than other wheat flours. It makes an even firmer, less elastic noodle, ideal for the curved "elbow" macaroni, for example. Semolina pasta also holds up to a thicker sauce. Pasta may also be made with flour from spinach, beets, corn, even Jerusalem artichokes. These flours add color but do not add much in the way of nutrition and may only impart a faint flavor.

Stir pasta while cooking to prevent sticking. It's done when it's *al dente* . . . chewy . . . not mushy. Rinsing is not necessary unless you're using the pasta in a cold salad.

From Italy to Asia, there's literally pasta in every pot. Noodles come in all shapes and colors of the rainbow. In Japan, for example, noodles may be made from buckwheat or mung bean flour, and are served for breakfast, dinner and late-night snacks.

When mild-tasting grains and pastas are married with the melange of spices, spectacular dishes are born. Pesto, made with fresh-picked basil and pungent garlic, for example, can transform a simple plate of linguine into an unforgettable Italian feast.

Asian pastas. Rice vermicelli, also known as rice sticks, are delicate in flavor and complement most Oriental meat, fish and vegetable dishes. Wheat noodles are made with or without eggs, and include ramen, somen and udon—each with a different shape for a different purpose. Ramen, for example is squiggly, and is often sold with packets of instant miso soup. Bean thread pasta, made from mung beans, is slippery, transparent noodles. They have little flavor but soak up tastes of everything they are cooked with, making them great in soups and stews. Buckwheat noodles, called soba, taste slightly nutty and can be eaten hot in broth or chilled and dipped in ginger-spiked soy-based sauces.

Try soba sprinkled with bits of broccoli, red pepper, carrots and other fresh vegetables. Just toss with light soy sauce, rice vinegar, sesame oil and ginger for a filling, low-fat meal.

"Don't overcook," says Linda Burum, California ethnic food expert and author of *Asian Pasta.* "Overcooking is the cardinal sin in noodle preparation." Place cooked noodles in a colander, drain, then refresh under running water, swirling in a colander. Place in a bowl and sprinkle with sesame oil.

Many of these seasonings have a health bonus of their own. Studies show that garlic, once believed to ward off evil spirits, may ward off heart attacks by reducing cholesterol and keeping blood clots from forming.

A Sweet Ending

Gooey Greek baklava aside, the healthiest cuisines generally feature Mother Nature's own dessert: raw fruit.

Melon and mangoes, popular meal-enders in Mexico and

SHOPPING FOR REAL ETHNIC FLAVOR

You're dying to try the recipe for Mexican spicy-chocolate chicken mole sauce, but where do you find ancho chilies in the middle of Maine? In your mailbox, of course.

Dozens of mail-order firms offer global ingredients that haven't yet made their way to your local supermarket, health food store or deli. We can't list them all here, but the sampling below will give you an idea of what's available.

Latin American. *G. B. Ratto and Company, 821 Washington Street, Oakland, CA 94607.* This one-stop "food hall" has been in the ethnic food business since 1897 and offers an impressive array of Mexican and Latin ingredients including quinoa, black beans, blue corn tortillas and Mexican chilies from mild to four-alarm hot.

Asian. *The Oriental Food Market, 2801 West Howard Street, Chicago, IL 60645.* If you can't find wasabi (Japanese horseradish), for example, or other ingredients for your Asian recipes, these folks will send it to you. Among their hundreds of mail-order offerings are more than two dozen types of teas, a multitude of noodles and

the Caribbean, for example, are chock-full of potassium. One study has found that adding about 400 milligrams of potassium to your daily diet—an amount easily supplied by a cup of cubed honeydew melon, for example—cuts your risk of fatal stroke almost in half.

Dessert or main course, we're not suggesting that all ethnic food is healthy, fat-free or low calorie. Thai mangoes and sticky rice made with coconut and cream, for example, packs a whopping 16 grams of fat. Miso and pickled vegetables, so popular in the Far East, can send your sodium levels into the ozone.

canned, preserved and dried items from dried lotus root to boiled ginkgo nuts.

Italian. *Balducci's Mail Order Division, 11-02 Queen's Plaza South, Long Island City, NY 11101-1908,* is the Tiffany's of Italian food. They stock everything for your Mediterranean meal from polenta with sun-dried tomatoes to rare, aged balsamic vinegars.

Middle Eastern. *Sultan's Delight, P.O. Box 140253, 25 Croton Avenue, Staten Island, NY 10314.* Here you'll find everything from falafel, lentils, tabbouleh and tahini to ready-to-serve stuffed grape leaves and sweet-flower water. They can even send you belly dancing music and finger cymbals for dining entertainment (you provide the dancer).

Indian. *Cinnabar Specialty Foods, 214 Frontier Drive, Prescott, AZ 86303.* Their Barbados Honey Pepper Sauce can transform fish fillets or fresh vegetables into a meal to remember. Other homemade chutneys are made from mangoes, pears and peaches. And their Tandoori paste mixes with yogurt to infuse ordinary chicken with extra-ordinary flavor. A sampler pack offers you a choice of four products to try.

"The idea is to pick and choose the best foods from the world's banquet to create a healthy diet," says Dr. Minear.

Ten Ways to Eat Global Foods at Home

By adopting and adapting ethnic foods, you can trim fat, boost fiber and other nutrients and improve your health. Here are some tips.

1. Add new ingredients in small amounts. "Adapting your palate to new foods is like adapting to fine wine," says Sandy Kapoor, R.D., associate professor in the School of Hotel and Restaurant Management at the California Polytechnic Institute in Pomona. Introduce unfamiliar foods in small doses, says Dr. Kapoor. Instead of serving a lentil dahl dish as the main meal, try it as a side dish first. Toss some Asian noodles in your usual chicken noodle recipe. Throw in bok choy while steaming spinach.

2. Substitute high-fiber, low-fat ingredients. Substitute whole-wheat tortillas for white flour varieties in Latin American dishes, for example. You can lighten up an Alfredo sauce by using Parmesan and nonfat yogurt instead of cream. Use polyunsaturated or olive oil instead of ghee (clarified butter) in Indian dishes and in place of lard when making Mexican refried beans.

3. Save meat for feasts. Three times a week, serve a hearty fish dish. A good one is Spanish paella, made with mussels and shrimp, crimson peppers and sunshine-yellow rice. Mussels provide about the same amount of protein as hamburger and are a better source of iron than sirloin. Their succulent flavor can satisfy without buttery sauces.

4. Go with the grain. Try tabbouleh salad made from bulgur, scallions, tomatoes, cucumbers, radishes, mint and a dash of lemon juice. One serving has less than 100 calories and less than a gram of fat, but it's packed with fiber as well as B vitamins, iron and calcium.

5. Invite a legume for lunch. Try a Greek salad made with white fava beans. Or puree chick-peas, to make a high-fiber dip for carrot sticks that's lighter and livelier than sour cream. Just blend with garlic and a squeeze of lemon.

6. Have butterless bread every day. To add a little zip, rub the surface with olive oil and lemongrass. Or try tahini, a peanut-butter-like spread made from ground sesame seeds. It's high in protein as well as vitamin E.

7. Phase in more fruit. Instead of coffee for breakfast, try a *licuado*, the Mexican nondairy version of a smoothie. Blend together potassium-rich cantaloupe with vitamin C–rich papaya, for example. (If the mixture is too thick for your liking, add a bit of juice.) Other great combos: strawberries and guava for double vitamin C punch. If you blend with a bit of watercress as they do in Mexico, it boosts the iron content.

8. Don't save the pumpkin for pie. This beta-carotene-rich vegetable is too good to reserve for just dessert. Try it in a dish like African pumpkin soup or Moroccan pumpkin-yogurt stuffing. For recipes, consult some ethnic cookbooks.

9. Go ahead, experiment. Ordinary vegetables come alive with a little creative cookery using exotic seasoning combinations. Transform steamed cauliflower into an Indian delight with cumin and cinnamon, for example.

10. Don't be afraid to mix and match. "Some of the best chefs now cross-pollinate cuisines," says California food expert and author Linda Burum, whose books include *Guide to Ethnic Restaurants in Los Angeles*. One popular restaurant combines Middle Eastern and Mexican food, for example. They grill Middle Eastern-style chicken with lemon, olive oil and rosemary, slice it and stuff it in a Mexican fajita (a thin, whole-grain tortilla). Topped with roasted chilies and a Middle Eastern yogurt-tahini sauce, it's fabulous!

High-Nutrition Recipes

FETTUCCINE WITH PESTO SAUCE

Pesto is a much-loved Italian sauce made from fresh basil, garlic, olive oil, cheese and pine nuts. It's a wonderful change of pace from tomato sauce when on most any type of pasta. This recipe cuts back on the fat found in traditional recipes by substituting chicken stock for part of the oil.

1	cup tightly packed fresh basil	1	tablespoon pine nuts
1/2	cup chopped fresh parsley	2	cloves garlic, minced
2	tablespoons grated Parmesan cheese	1 1/2	tablespoons olive oil
		1/4	cup defatted chicken stock
		8	ounces fettuccine

Place the basil, parsley, Parmesan, pine nuts and garlic in the bowl of a food processor. Process with on/off turns until finely chopped. With the machine running, pour in the oil. Scrape down the sides of the container. With the machine running, slowly pour in the stock. Continue to process with on/off turns until a thick paste is formed.

Cook the fettuccine in a large pot of boiling water for 8 minutes, or until just tender. Drain and return to the pot. Off heat, add the pesto and toss to coat the pasta.

Serves 4
Per serving: *295 calories, 8.4 g. fat (25% of calories), 1.5 g. dietary fiber, 2 mg. cholesterol, 72 mg. sodium*

PORTUGUESE CHICK-PEAS

This hors d'oeuvre was enjoyed by one of our editors when she visited Lagos, Portugal. It also makes a great salad for two—serve it on a bed of mixed greens.

1	can (19 ounces) chick-peas, rinsed and drained	2	tablespoons minced fresh coriander
2	tablespoons diced onions	1	tablespoon olive oil
1-2	cloves garlic, thinly sliced	1	tablespoon water-packed tuna, mashed into a paste
2	tablespoons red-wine vinegar	4	thick slices crusty bread

In a large bowl, toss together the chick-peas, onions, garlic, vinegar, coriander, oil and tuna. Chill well. Serve accompanied by the bread.

Serves 4
Per serving: *151 calories, 5.4 g. fat (31% of calories), 4.2 g. dietary fiber, <1 mg. cholesterol, 395 mg. sodium*

PAELLA

This Spanish classic pairs modest amounts of poultry and seafood with rice and vegetables. Feel free to use other seafood, such as clams or small lobster tails.

2 teaspoons olive oil	½ teaspoon saffron threads
3 skinless chicken thighs, cut in half (see tip below)	12 large shrimp, peeled and deveined
1 teaspoon fresh rosemary leaves	12 mussels, scrubbed
2 cups medium-grain white rice	1 cup peas
4 cups defatted chicken stock	2 canned pimientos, thinly sliced
1 can (28 ounces) plum tomatoes, drained	2 cloves garlic, minced

In a very large ovenproof frying pan or paella pan, warm the oil over medium heat. Add the chicken and sauté for about 15 minutes, or until golden and almost entirely cooked through. Use tongs to transfer the pieces to a plate; sprinkle with the rosemary.

Add the rice to the frying pan and sauté over medium heat for 2 minutes. Add the stock, tomatoes and saffron. Stir with a wooden spoon to loosen browned bits from the bottom and also to break up the tomatoes. Bring to a boil.

Add the chicken (with any accumulated juices), shrimp, mussels, peas, pimientos and garlic. Bring to a boil and stir to mix the ingredients. Remove from the heat and cover the pan with a lid or foil.

Bake at 350° for 20 minutes. Remove from the oven and let stand, covered, for 20 minutes. Lift the chicken and shellfish to the surface of the dish to show them off.

Serves 6
Tip: *Cut the chicken thighs in half crosswise through the bone. Either use a sharp, heavy cleaver or ask the butcher at your supermarket to cut the thighs when you purchase them.*
Per serving: *390 calories, 5.2 g. fat (12% of calories), 2.5 g. dietary fiber, 58 mg. cholesterol, 166 mg. sodium*

COUSCOUS SALAD WITH ORANGES AND FIGS

Couscous is a staple of North African cuisine. This tiny pasta cooks up quickly and makes an ideal base for interesting salads. In the Moroccan tradition, we've combined the couscous with fresh oranges and dried figs. When fresh figs are in season, use them for a real taste treat.

1½ cups defatted chicken stock
¼ cup currants
1 teaspoon ground cumin
½ teaspoon turmeric
⅛ teaspoon ground red pepper
1 cup couscous
1 cup cooked peas
1 cup chopped orange sections

4 dried brown figs, quartered
2 tablespoons minced fresh parsley
1 tablespoon minced fresh mint
3 tablespoons lemon juice
2 tablespoons olive oil

In a 1-quart saucepan, combine 1¼ cups of the stock with the currants, cumin, turmeric and red pepper. Bring to a boil. Stir in the couscous. Remove from the heat, cover the pan and let stand for 10 minutes, or until all the liquid has been absorbed.

Fluff the conscuous with a fork and transfer to a large bowl. Lightly toss with the peas, oranges, figs, parsley and mint.

In a cup, mix the lemon juice, oil and the remaining ¼ cup stock. Pour over the couscous mixture and toss to combine.

Serves 4
Per serving: *381 calories, 8.1 g. fat (19% of calories), 11.2 g. dietary fiber, 0 mg. cholesterol, 40 mg. sodium*

PART 3

ALL SYSTEMS ARE GO WITH GOOD NUTRITION

CHAPTER 19

The Brain

Food for Thought

When your boss breathes down your neck and steams up your collar, are you sometimes more capable of coping with the pressure and performing at your best? It could be because you first fed your head with breakfast. Do you feel mellow-minded or sleepy after eating spaghetti for lunch? It's probably because you've effectively injected your brain with a dose of a tranquilizing drug. Are your kids not performing as well as you'd like in school? It could be because they haven't taken their multivitamins.

You probably don't think about your brain the way you do about your heart or lungs or stomach or intestines. It is the essence of what you are. It defines your sense of self, what you think, what you believe, what you feel. But ultimately, it is an organ, just like any other in the body, and it needs to be adequately nourished to best do what it does.

What does it do? Technically, it coordinates the transmission of nerve impulses from one cell to another through the secretion of brain chemicals called neurotransmitters. The billions of nerve cells, called neurons, aren't wired together directly to interact; if they were, they'd be able to perform only one function. Instead, they're separated by imperceptibly thin gaps called synapses. Messages from one neuron to another travel across synapses through any of a number of neurotransmitters that are released from the nerve endings like a message in a bottle. How we feel, how we behave, and how well we do at our tasks depends on what neurotransmitters traverse the synaptic ocean to the neural shore on the other side, setting off a wave of reactions that triggers different responses in different parts of the brain.

To maintain the smooth firing of those neurotransmitters, the brain needs the whole array of vitamins and minerals. For energy, the brain requires glucose, sugar ingested from simple and complex carbohydrates. And for the production of some neurotransmitters as well as for repair and replacement of tissue, nerve cells and certain chemicals, the brain needs amino acids, which are obtained from protein.

From the digestive tract, glucose, protein, vitamins and minerals enter the blood, where they circulate to nourish the entire body. "But the brain gets them first," says John Fernstrom, Ph.D., professor of psychiatry and pharmacology at the University of Pittsburgh's School of Medicine. "The brain gets first choice of the nutrients available in the body."

Although it has the right of first use, the brain discriminates when it comes to what and how much of a certain element is allowed in. A buffering layer of cells, the blood/brain barrier, stands guard over the chemicals and nutrients in blood vessels like a bouncer at a nightclub, checking I.D.'s, rejecting riffraff that could cause problems and regulating the number so the room doesn't get too crowded.

The existence of that filtering system and the first-use concept traditionally led neuroscientists and psychologists to assert that the brain always is amply nourished and that individual meals and snacks never could influence mood or behavior by altering brain chemistry. But researchers are increasingly discovering that the quantity and quality of food can, in fact, tip the mental scale and—sometimes subtly, sometimes more obviously—affect behavior and mental performance.

LEAN BODY, FAT HEAD

You'd be smart to eat a low-fat diet, but you'd be stupid on a *no*-fat diet.

Fats and fatty acids are "absolutely essential" to the brain during development, according to Carol E. Greenwood, Ph.D., at the University of Toronto Faculty of Medicine in Ontario. And they're probably just as integral during the course of your lifetime.

The brain and nervous tissue have high concentrations of fatty acids, Dr. Greenwood says, but neuroscientists differ over how important fatty acids are once you're fully grown. Some say fat plays no role once the body is developed. But she argues that it does, citing the regeneration of all tissues (including the brain) over a person's life. "While the brain doesn't have any new cells developing once we have our full complement, these membranes still have to turn over and renew themselves," Dr. Greenwood says. "So we need fat for that. Damaged nerve cells also can repair themselves or sprout new terminals. All of these processes, while they won't require as much fat as we would developmentally, show that the brain will still have a degree of sensitivity to fat intake," she says.

All fats aren't born equal, of course, and new research suggests that nonanimal fats are better for the brain, Dr. Greenwood says. In tests she has conducted, she has found that rats fed soybean oil performed better at cognitive skills than those animals fed lard. She stops short of saying that lard-fed rats performed worse, though. The rats fed soy oil performed more like rats on the typical laboratory chow diet, whose fat content comes from nonanimal sources.

MIND BEFORE MATTER

There's no deficiency of irony in the fact that while Recommended Dietary Allowances (RDAs) for nutrients are based on avoiding physical impairment, the brain often shows signs of undernutrition long before the rest of the body. "What's enough to prevent physical symptoms of vitamin deficiencies may not be adequate to prevent impaired mental function," says Stephen Schoenthaler, Ph.D., who has studied the relationship between nutrition and behavior as a professor of sociology and criminal justice at California State University, Stainislaus in Turlock. "You can't assume subclinical malnutrition isn't there in the absence of physical problems."

The mental dysfunctions associated with vitamin malnutrition have been known, Dr. Schoenthaler says, since World War II, when the armed services experimented with conscientious objectors, systematically feeding them diets lacking in one specific nutrient to gauge the consequences. During the experiments, "impairment of mental function always occurred first," he says.

Today, under more stringent research standards, it's more difficult to quantify, analyze and verify the frequently subtle shifts in mood and behavior. Physical symptoms are easier to study, Dr. Schoenthaler says, which is one of the reasons why RDAs remain based on them.

BREAKFAST: FOR CHAMPIONS

The connection between good nutrition and mental performance can be seen as early as the first meal of the day. Both children and adults perform better at school or at work if they've broken their night-long fast with a filling, nutritious meal. Generally, children who are reasonably well fed don't show any noticeable decline in school achievement if they miss an occasional breakfast, according to Bonnie Spring, Ph.D., a professor of psychology at the University of Health Sciences/Chicago Medical School, who's extensively studied the effects of food on behavior. "If the kids are basically well nourished," she says, "you see very minimal consequences. They can probably get away with skipping breakfast for the day, pull together and function okay. They have enough reserves."

But if the children are at all undernourished, missing breakfast "is not advisable," Dr. Spring says. If these kids miss the first meal of the day, by late in the morning, "they don't concentrate as well, and their problem-solving ability deteriorates." For them, "you do see improvements in school, which suggests there are long-term benefits of eating breakfast."

The mechanism behind the enhanced learning associated with breakfast is difficult to pinpoint, Dr. Spring says. "Who knows to what extent the benefit is due to nutrition or other factors that come along for the ride," such as better attendance because of less illness or better motivation because of a boost in mood and outlook. Whatever the reason, "there's enough evidence that something positive is happening when they eat breakfast."

A SMART PILL TO SWALLOW

If your children can't always eat that breakfast, it may be wise for them—and you, too—at least to swallow a good multivitamin containing a full 100 percent of the RDAs for all essential nutrients. In a 12-week test of 615 children, Dr. Schoenthaler found that students who took a supplement offering a full day's supply of vitamins and minerals did significantly better on intelligence tests than those taking pills providing half that amount, twice that amount or nothing at all. The kids displayed improvement in "fluid" intelligence, the ability to reason and make analogies, but not in pure rote learning or memory, the ability, say, to recall dates or facts.

The improvement—45 percent of the kids taking 100 percent of the RDAs gained at least 15 points on intelligence

THE THINKING PERSON'S VITAMIN GUIDE

Every vitamin worth its alphabetic assignation is required by the brain for some mental function. Here are some of the most significant.

B_{12} before all. All of the B vitamins are especially important for optimal brain development and function, but B_{12} seems to be the most crucial. A dearth of the nutrient, also called cobalamin, has been linked to everything from paranoia, restlessness, irritability and manic depression to confusion, chronic fatigue syndrome, memory loss, phobias and insomnia. Mental problems often can develop long before the more physical sign—pernicious anemia—shows up in a blood test. The anemia itself can cause some of the same symptoms as well as listlessness, lower IQ, learning disorders and short attention span.

Why should a deficiency of B_{12} cause mental impairment? Researchers think it's because, along with dietary fat, B_{12} is vital to the growth and maintenance of the tissue that encases and protects the brain's nerve fibers, the myelin sheath. Without enough B_{12}, the myelin sheath degenerates, exposing the nerves and causing the mental disorders.

Few people, except some strict vegetarians, develop B_{12} deficiencies for dietary reasons; most people eat enough animal-derived foods, the only sources of the nutrient. Most deficiencies are caused by an inability of the body to absorb the vitamin, according to John Lindenbaum, M.D., a professor of medicine at Columbia University in New York City. People with atrophic gastritis, in which the stomach doesn't secrete a protein necessary for B_{12} absorption, and those who have had part of their colons removed are especially susceptible, Dr. Lindenbaum says.

Feeling better with folate. You're more likely to develop a deficiency of folate, or folic acid, than of B_{12}, although both these B vitamins interact in the body and a lack of either can bring on a case of the blues. Many psychiatric patients "show a high instance of folate deficiency," according to Simon Young, Ph.D., a professor in the Department of Psychiatry at McGill University in Montreal. Some association has been found between low folate in the body and depression-like symptoms. When people with such symptoms were treated with folate, Dr. Young says, their symptoms improved.

There also is a correlation with the neurotransmitter serotonin, whose presence in the brain seems to soothe and relax.

Those with low serotonin levels in their brains have not only lower moods but lower amounts of folate in their bodies, according to Dr. Young. When supplemented with folate, these people lift both their serotonin counts and their spirits.

B_6 and the blahs. Many women who complain of premenstrual tension are deficient in vitamin B_6, says John Dommisse, M.D., a psychiatrist in private practice in nutritional and metabolic psychiatry in Portsmouth, Virginia. And the estrogen in some oral contraceptives and in the estrogen replacement therapy for postmenopausal difficulties and osteoporosis can cause a deficiency of this nutrient. Depression often is the result of a deficiency because, Dr. Dommisse explains, B_6 is needed to produce serotonin. Other mental signs of a B_6 deficiency include anemia-like symptoms, irritability and fatigue.

A need for niacin. This B vitamin also needed for a healthy myelin sheath, was used back in the 1950s and 1960s to treat schizophrenia, Dr. Dommisse says, but the connection today between niacin and the mental condition is regarded as unproven. Nonetheless, a chronic shortage causes the hallucinations, confusion and nervous disorders associated with the classic deficiency disease pellagra. Less severe niacin deficiencies can cause anxiety, fatigue, loss of short-term memory and depression.

Riboflavin for a better start. Riboflavin (vitamin B_2) deficiency can retard brain growth in children, leading to abnormalities in behavior as adults. Hypochondria, depression and lethargy could result from a marginal deficiency of riboflavin before other physical symptoms manifest themselves, according to some experts.

Thiamine versus the bottle. Heavy drinkers run the risk of developing a chronic deficiency of thiamine (vitamin B_1). People who frequently use aspirin or antacids also are especially susceptible to thiamine deficiency. That could be particularly dangerous because some researchers suggest that a thiamine deficiency causes brain damage even before overt signs of harm exist. Symptoms include fatigue, confusion, depression and loss of memory. Thiamine supplementation reverses the symptoms in very early stages, but once more advanced, the damage becomes irreversible.

Adrift without C. Scurvy, the classic vitamin C–deficiency disease, can result in depression, hypochondria and hysteria, Dr. Dommisse says, and less severe deficiencies have been shown to trigger edgy feelings of anxiety and overexcitement as well as depression and fatigue.

tests, as opposed to 20 percent of the children taking pills without nutrients—was seen even in pupils who otherwise would be considered well fed, Dr. Schoenthaler says.

The results raise intriguing questions, he says. Because the kids receiving 50 percent of the RDAs didn't perform as well as those receiving 100 percent, are the RDAs really adequate for optimal mental function? And if providing twice the RDA doesn't improve intelligence scores, is an excess of one vitamin interfering with the absorption of others, toppling the nutrient balance? "Getting more than is needed is not necessarily better," Dr. Schoenthaler says.

Students in another, much smaller study also scored gains in intelligence tests after taking additional vitamins and minerals. The authors of this British study theorize that pupils who increased their scores with supplementation may have had nutrient deficiencies because, while not malnourished, they may have been ingesting too many calories from junk food.

ADULTS ARISE AND SHINE

While the impact of eating or missing breakfast has been examined extensively in children, comparatively few studies have assessed the intelligence and performance effects on adults. Nonetheless, there are several known consequences of not eating a morning meal. "As a general rule, when people eat breakfast, they are more alert by midday than they were when they first woke up in the morning," Dr. Spring says. "When they skip breakfast, they're about equal. In other words, they don't fully wake up." Alertness and reaction time suffers markedly on an empty stomach. "Breakfast skippers aren't sleepier than when they woke up," she says, "but they are no better than when they first rolled out of bed."

Don't depend on coffee. The traditional wake-up call, coffee, may produce results similar to breakfast's effect, but with no nutritional benefit and actually at some nutritive cost. People profess to be more alert after drinking coffee, and it does help to keep you awake and to some extent sharpen reaction time. But controlled performance tests often don't confirm the stimulant effect. Chronic coffee and caffeine consumption can, of course, lead to coffee jitters, along with insomnia, anxiety and perhaps even paranoia or depression. There's evidence that heavy users may perform less well than light or moderate users or nonusers. And caffeine interferes with the body's absorption of iron, enough so that chronic intake could cause a potentially energy-robbing deficiency.

Although researchers don't know for certain, caffeine seems to work by blocking the brain chemical adenosine, a natural tranquilizer. It also stimulates production of the neurotransmitters epinephrine and norepinephrine, which stimulate the mind.

Even though you may be sleepier without breakfast in your belly, comprehension and problem-solving skills late in the morning remain relatively unaffected—unless you're under emotional stress or the demands of deadline pressures. "When you're in a casual pace and not under any stress, you work fine" and there's no effect on intellect from not eating breakfast, according to Dr. Spring. "But if you add emotional stress or a deadline, you see an impairment in such things as math skills and reasoning skills." People also become more anxious and irritable, she says.

Aim for a balanced breakfast. The kind of breakfast you eat makes little difference, unless, again, you're under some form of duress or deadline demand. "There's some evidence that a balanced breakfast is better," Dr. Spring says. If working under stress, a meal comprised equally of carbohydrates and protein—for example, oatmeal or cereal for carbohydrates and a slice of lean ham or a large glass of skim milk for protein—offers a "significant advantage" in mental performance compared to the high-carbohydrate load of a bagel or two.

THE ELEMENTS OF BRAIN POWER

Minerals, too, are important for proper brain development and functioning. Research indicates that maternal mineral and trace element deficiencies before birth may cause irreversible brain damage in infants, while behavioral problems caused by malnutrition after birth can be reversed by supplementation.

Pump iron into the brain. Even without the low red blood cell counts found in anemia, a less-than-adequate amount of iron in the diet can cause mental problems, according to Harold H. Sandstead, M.D., of the Department of Preventive Medicine and Community Health at University of Texas Medical Branch in Galveston. Children have been examined more extensively in this regard than adults, he says, and most studies show that those who have problems in learning and comprehension are low in iron, which carries oxygen to the brain as well as to all other organs in the body.

"Iron is essential," Dr. Sandstead says. "Iron deficiency may be rather subtle—affecting attention, learning, concentration and other functions. But with iron repletion, things improve."

The possibility of iron deficiency should be considered if your children are hyperactive, have short attention spans and are irritable. Adults with an iron deficiency are often irritable and suffer from headaches.

Zinc to think. Researchers link zinc shortage to a variety of mood changes. A severe lack induces depression, lethargy and irritability, but supplementation reverses

SEROTONIN: THE MOOD MAKER

By the time the lunch hour rolls around, meal composition assumes a much greater importance to the brain, determining how you feel for the remainder of the day. While carbohydrates supply glucose necessary for the brain's energy, they

those problems, according to Dr. Sandstead. Less drastic deficiencies impair memory, but "it's improved in certain areas with repletion." Low levels of zinc in the bloodstream also have been associated with more aggressive behavior, less curiosity, hyperactivity, mental retardation and dyslexia, says John Dommisse, M.D., a psychiatrist in private practice in nutritional and metabolic psychiatry in Portsmouth, Virginia.

More magnesium might be needed. Magnesium deficiency might be more common than most experts believe, Dr. Dommisse says, because processing removes much of this mineral from food. When the brain is low in magnesium, people could become depressed, agitated, confused and irritable. They also may experience tremors and twitches.

Low calcium and confusion. While calcium commonly is associated with strong bones, it also may bolster the brain, Dr. Sandstead suggests. Even short-term deficiencies of either calcium or magnesium can cause tremors in some people. When those two minerals are not in intravenous feeding solutions, he says, "hospital patients become confused."

Chromium puts a shine on stress. Because the brain gets its energy from glucose, this trace mineral plays an important role, for it is involved in the body's release of insulin for sugar metabolism. More related to behavior, though, chromium seems to help the body manage stress, Dr. Dommisse says.

also trigger the production of serotonin, a widely studied neurotransmitter associated with a variety of emotional states. It calms and relaxes, perhaps even inducing sleep under the right circumstances. It also tends to counteract feelings of stress and anxiety and enhances your ability to concentrate. Low brain serotonin, on the other hand, is associated with insomnia, de-

A SLAVE TO THE CRAVE?

Ever had a yen for orange juice or broccoli? Is it because you just like the taste, or is it because your brain is detecting a deficiency of vitamin C in your bloodstream? Is your mouth watering for a steak or seafood dinner? It may not be the atavistic carnivore in you at all. It simply may be the high-carbohydrate, low-protein lunch you had.

What you eat or don't eat not only sometimes determines your mood; it often determines what you'll ingest for your next meal. And the mood itself also plays a role in what you eat.

"You have to consider both," says Michael D. Chafetz, Ph.D., a clinical neuropsychologist and author of the book *Nutrition and Neurotransmitters.* "What you eat can determine your mood, and what your mood is directs what foods you eat. There's a change in eating pattern to feed the mood."

The precise mechanism is unknown, but the effect is seen all the time. When rats are given premeal snacks to judge later eating behavior, "we find that if it's a carbohydrate snack, the animals prefer a main meal of protein, and vice versa," says Carol E. Greenwood, Ph.D., at the University of Toronto Faculty of Medicine in Ontario.

pression, aggression, and hypersensitivity to sound, touch, heat and pain, according to Dr. Fernstrom.

No other neurotransmitter is as easily manipulated by food as serotonin, which the brain manufactures from the amino acid tryptophan. In a blatant bypass of the blood/brain barrier, the more tryptophan that reaches the brain, the more serotonin is produced. But you cannot raise brain tryptophan by eating high-protein food, because it has to vie against higher concentrations of all the other amino acids in

"The signal," Dr. Greenwood says, "is serotonin," a neurotransmitter whose level in the brain is increased by eating carbohydrates and decreased by eating protein.

Anxious or depressed people often have lower brain levels of serotonin, and they seem to intuitively learn that eating high-carbohydrate foods as disparate as rice pilaf or chocolate cake improves their outlooks, eases the depression and soothes their nerves by increasing the production of the neurotransmitter. Similarly, people who receive medication to increase serotonin in their brains "tend to decrease carbohydrate intake," Dr. Chafetz says. They tend to want protein.

While serotonin plays a role, "it doesn't explain all of the phenomenon," Dr. Greenwood says. "We don't know yet what it is, but it's a whole-body issue dealing with the overall balance of the right foods for health."

That's obvious when you consider studies showing an innate desire for salt when the body is low in sodium, or for vitamin C when levels of that nutrient have dipped, Dr. Chafetz says. "We can't specify a mechanism like we can with carbohydrates, but it's suggestive." Perhaps, he theorizes, when your body is low or high in a nutrient, certain brain receptors aren't seeing enough of it in the blood or are gauging too much, and they send appetite-influencing signals accordingly.

the bloodstream rushing to the brain. Amid the competition, tryptophan is barely noticed and has little effect.

But it gets a virtual free ride up to the brain when you eat carbohydrates, which also contain small amounts of amino acids, including tryptophan. The reason is that sugars in carbohydrates stimulate the release of insulin, which draws most of the other amino acids into muscle cells. Tryptophan is unaffected by insulin's attraction, and so it freely cruises up to the brain, which then uses it to make more serotonin.

WHEN A RICE CAKE IS A SHOT IN THE ARM

If you're like most people, when you eat a high-carbohydrate, low-protein lunch or dinner, you calm down, relax a bit, get sleepy and sluggish.

But what if you don't? What if you find yourself invigorated after a heavy dish of spaghetti or a bowl of rice? Not to worry; you're just a carbo craver.

Some folks—often those suffering from premenstrual tension or seasonal affective disorder (wintertime depression), for example, "selectively overeat carbohydrates," says Bonnie Spring, Ph.D., at the University of Health Sciences/Chicago Medical School. "With unbalanced, high-carbohydrate meals, they get activated."

The reason, as with other triggers of food/mood reactions, is serotonin, a chemical in the brain that is responsible for feelings of serenity and placidness. The amount of serotonin in the brain can be increased by eating a high-carbohydrate meal.

People who crave carbohydrates "act as if they have a long-term deficiency in serotonin," Dr. Spring says. People who have a normal amount of serotonin get sleepy after eating a high-carbohydrate meal. "They trip the sleep mechanism because they're getting a rise in serotonin," she says. But those with a deficiency of the neurotransmitter feel better after a high-carbohydrate food because they're edging their serotonin level up to a normal level.

"They're giving themselves a high-carbohydrate load that is acting like a shot in the arm," Dr. Spring says. "It's correcting the deficiency in brain serotonin and improving their mood, almost as if they were self-medicating."

During midafternoon snacktime, if you find yourself habitually reaching for a carbohydrate food to make you feel better and get you through the rest of the workday, don't let your conscience bother you, Dr. Spring says. "You're probably one of those people who will get activated by carbohydrates." Your only concern should be to "keep the fat down. Eat ginger snaps or rice cakes or angel food cake," she says, "not potato chips."

Until the Food and Drug Administration (FDA) took tryptophan supplements off the shelves of health food stores, there was a more direct way to deliver this amino acid to the brain. But a problem arose in the manufacturing of synthetic tryptophan by a certain company, according to Dr. Spring. "It's inaccurate to describe it as an impurity," she says, "but something unusual was done to it so that it caused a white blood cell disease in people who consumed it." The FDA pulled all brands of tryptophan from the market for its investigation merely as a precaution, but "there's little doubt it was the particular manufacturer." Increasing brain levels of the amino acid through eating should be no cause for concern because tryptophan is a common, natural substance in foods.

When most people eat a high-carbohydrate lunch, they become sleepy and sluggish by the middle of the afternoon. Eating some protein along with the carbohydrates, though, counteracts the serotonin slump, because the brain uses the amino acid tyrosine found in protein to produce norepinephrine and dopamine, two neurotransmitters associated with invigoration, motivation, mental acuity and quick thinking.

Early food/mood research suggested that a pure-protein meal would spike the neurotransmitter punch to give you vim and vigor for the rest of the day or evening, Dr. Spring says. Newer studies have found, though, that brain levels of tyrosine are not so readily affected, although enough reaches the brain to counteract tryptophan's production of serotonin.

What does this mental menu mean? Basically, you do have some options available to you.

Vary the protein/carbohydrate mix. If you want to fall asleep or feel lethargic after lunch or dinner, go for the high-carbohydrate, no-protein option. If not, "add meat sauce to the pasta or cream cheese to the bagel," Dr. Spring says. "You'll feel more invigorated and alert than if you ate a meal without protein."

Consider your timing. "On a day-to-day basis, with the kind of meal patterns most people have with protein and carbohydrates, it's unlikely we'd see a mood effect," notes Carol

DOES ALZHEIMER'S START IN THE WOMB?

If scientists ever find a nutritional way to avert Alzheimer's disease, the preventive path may start before birth.

Rats born to mothers fed extremely high doses of choline, a natural substance found in almost all foods, display better memory retention, and their brains seem to age much more slowly than rats not fed the nutrient.

"These are particularly exciting findings," says Christina Williams, Ph.D., an associate professor of psychiatry at Barnard College of Columbia University in New York City and part of a team of researchers studying, under a grant from the National Institute of Aging, how to prevent the brain deterioration of Alzheimer's. She says she hopes a variation of choline treatment one day could serve as an inoculation against memory loss in old age.

Choline's role in memory has long been examined because it is the precursor of the neurotransmitter acetylcholine, which courses through the cholinergic system, the memory and recall portion of the brain that appears to degenerate under Alzheimer's. Under certain circumstances, such as when the cholinergic neurons are being used actively to store memory, intake of exceedingly high doses of choline results in production of more brain acetylcholine.

Because of that, scientists initially thought that supplemental choline would help stave off or reduce the effects of the disease. A number of tests were conducted, many of them using lecithin, a choline-rich fatty substance found in soybeans and egg yolks, but "it's a relatively ineffective treatment," Dr. Williams says. "You can get a transient increase in memory, but you have to keep eating a huge amount of choline. And it doesn't work all the time in all people."

But because there are certain sensitive developmental periods during which memory-related parts of the brain form, it could be a question of *when* choline supplementation is started. And the answer to that may be found in mother's milk.

"In mother's milk, choline is remarkably high—more than in blood plasma," Dr. Williams says. And during the first week after birth, choline levels in mother's milk are exceptionally high. "Mothers are already supplementing choline to their kids," she says.

That at least says something about comparing labels on commercial infant formulas, which "differ quite dramatically in choline content," Dr. Williams says. (Soy-based formulas usually are highest in the nutrient.)

Instead of trying to treat aging adults already afflicted with a brain-degenerating disease or even trying to prevent it in adulthood, Dr. Williams and her colleagues decided to study choline supplements in unborn rats, giving them doses through the diets of their mothers, then testing their memories as they aged.

The rats fed choline prenatally performed 10 to 20 percent better on memory tests than their unsupplemented counterparts, Dr. Williams says. And as they aged, "they still behaved like a young adult," with memory retention between 20 and 30 percent better than their untreated peers.

"We're somehow strengthening the cholinergic system to withstand age-related changes," Dr. Williams says.

These experiments have been conducted exclusively on rats, and Dr. Williams foresees no human tests for quite some time. Dosages have been 10 to 20 times the amount of choline normally thought required by the body. "They're very high amounts, super amounts," she says, "but then choline is not lethal or toxic at all." But it's more than you can get from food alone.

Rather than rushing for the choline capsules just yet—the most common supplemental form is lecithin, which Dr. Williams says is "not good" because it primarily is fat—perhaps you should obtain more of the nutrient through diet. Almost all foods contain choline, according to Dr. Williams, but particularly good sources include spinach and other green vegetables, seaweed and eggs.

E. Greenwood, Ph.D., an associate professor in the Department of Nutritional Sciences at the University of Toronto Faculty of Medicine in Ontario. "But that doesn't mean we can't use the observations and play with them," altering performance by changing what we eat and when we eat it.

"Maybe that tells us that if we have dessert," she suggests, "it's better not to eat it with dinner but about half an hour before bed," when a carbohydrate punch will help us more easily greet the Sandman. "You're not changing the number of calories you eat in a day, but you're waiting for when you're most likely to get the positive benefit of carbohydrates."

Don't go overboard on calories. Just be aware of how much of everything you eat. High-calorie cramming will make you browse the drowse section of your mental folds regardless of your meal composition. "When you're eating a very high calorie lunch, all bets are off about protein or carbohydrates," Dr. Spring says. "We don't understand what the mechanism is, but you get about a 10 percent decline in performance after a high-calorie meal. No matter what you eat in that kind of meal, you're going to get sleepy."

CHAPTER 20

The Immune System

Defensive Dining

Imagine this urgent supply order from your body's front lines of defense: "Hey, what's the story? You forget we're here? We're just about out of zinc, our B_6 supply is going fast and we haven't had any vitamin E since you ate that avocado *last year*! Listen, we like pretzels and diet soda as well as you do, but we need some *real food*! Eat some bloody vegetables, will ya? And throw down a few oysters while you're at it."

Having a supply officer for your immune system's legions of infection-fighting white blood cells would certainly be a help. He would let you know in no uncertain terms just what you need to bounce back from a cold, the flu or other viral infections. You'd know what to pile on your plate to prevent infections after burns or surgery, perhaps even to avoid cell changes that can lead to cancer.

Just as real soldiers suffer serious morale problems when their C-rations are cut back, the cells of your immune system could go AWOL if they're not getting the high-quality nutrition they need to fight off infections and disease.

Researchers have known for many years that any nutritional deficit bad enough to produce classic deficiency diseases, such as kwashiorkor (caused by protein shortage) or scurvy (caused by lack of vitamin C), can also lead to life-threatening drops in immune function.

And researchers are now finding that compromised immunity can also occur with borderline nutritional deficiencies and may even occur in people whose diets meet the current Recommended Dietary Allowances (RDAs).

"Some nutritionists get upset hearing this, but the fact is that the RDAs may not be the optimum amount to prevent certain diseases like cancer," says Ronald Watson, Ph.D., research professor at the University of Arizona College of Medicine in Tucson. Dr. Watson is studying the immunity-enhancing effects of beta-carotene, a compound in fruits and vegetables that is thought to help protect against cancer.

The list of nutritional deficiencies associated with poor immune function is long. It includes protein, vitamins A, E, C, B_6 and B_{12}, folate, beta-carotene, iron, and magnesium, plus the trace minerals selenium, copper, manganese and zinc.

Before detailing how some of these nutrients may enhance your immune system, though, we need to know how your body's defense works.

MEMBERS OF A MIGHTY ARMY

Researchers—and writers—often find themselves using military terms to describe the immune system. They talk about invaders, attacks, counterattacks and defense systems. "In fact, the comparison is an accurate one," says Terry M. Phillips, D. Sc., Ph.D., director of the immunogenetics and immunochemistry lab at George Washington University's Medical Center and coauthor of *Winning the War Within.* "It seems the more we learn about the immune system, the more amazingly appropriate the army analogies become," Dr. Phillips says.

That system is a complex, total body system of cells that kills off bacteria, viruses, parasites and fungi and also detects and destroys virus-infested or damaged cells that may be or may become cancerous.

A FORMULA FOR PEAK IMMUNITY

The limp lettuce and quivering gelatin on hospital dinner trays may not be what the immune system craves. But if you're sick enough to require a nasogastric feeding tube, you might be getting exactly the nourishment you need—or as close to it as researchers can now determine. This kind of nutritional support drips nutrients directly into your stomach through a tube inserted through your nose.

A few of the more than 300 feeding formulas now available contain "a veritable kitchen soup of everything that's known to enhance immune function," as one researcher puts it. Marketed as "immuno-stimulating" formulas, these liquids contain varying proportions of key ingredients.

Most contain fish oils and other omega-3 fatty acids that are thought to enhance immune response and dampen inflammatory response; arginine, an amino acid associated with enhanced immune function and preservation of body protein; nucleotides (bits of genetic material) whose restriction is thought to result in depressed immune function; and more than the Recommended Dietary Allowance of vitamins E, A, C, B_6 and other B-complex vitamins, zinc and copper, along with beta-carotene, selenium and a host of other essential nutrients.

How well do these formulas work? In a study at University Hospital in Philadelphia, surgical cancer patients receiving one such formula had less than a third as many infections and were released from the hospital five days sooner than patients receiving a standard liquid formula.

At Shriner's Burn Institute in Cincinnati, severely burned patients get feeding formulas made up just for them. "We give astonishing amounts of vitamin A, for example," says Michele A. Gottschlich, R.D., Ph.D., director of nutritional services. "A healthy person would develop a toxicity to such large doses, but we don't see toxicity in our patients because the need is so great. In fact, it boosts the immune system."

Because the nutritional needs of critically ill patients can vary, not everyone will do best on the same formula, Dr. Gottschlich says. "So ask your doctor about the formula he has chosen for you, and why."

Cells of the immune system patrol the bloodstream, line our bronchial passages and lurk in our lymph nodes, just waiting for security to be breached. When it is, they spring into action. Some move into the area of infection, then call for reinforcements. Some multiply rapidly, producing several hundred thousand of their own kind in a single day. Some send out orders with a series of biochemicals (cytokines) that tell other cells what to do, where to go, even when to back off, Dr. Phillips says.

DIGEST AND CONQUER

Some cells are for general defense. They'll go after anything that isn't you, and they don't need to wait for orders from headquarters to do so.

General defense cells include all the "feeding" cells, called phagocytes. Two of the most common of these cells are neutrophils and macrophages.

"Neutrophils might be considered the foot soldiers of the immune system," Dr. Phillips says. They move quickly, swimming through your blood and oozing amoeba-like through the cells of your blood vessels to attack. A neutrophil flows around its prey, envelops it inside its body and then secretes digestive enzymes on it.

Macrophages are big eating cells, slow but tough. Each one can eat an infinite number of bacteria, as long as they don't eat them too fast. When a chemical signal brings an invasion to their attention, macrophages will ooze on over to see what the trouble is. Once they get into the fray, they liven up.

"Macrophages also do garbage detail. They devour the remains of invading microorganisms as well as the cellular casualties from your own immune system," Dr. Phillips explains.

After it digests a virus or bacteria, a macrophage burps out pieces of the offending substances (antigens) and puts them on its surface. It then presents the antigens to a different class of immune cells, known as lymphocytes, described below. When the lymphocytes get a look at the antigens, a whole different component of the immune system kicks in—one primed to go after specific targets, like that virus that's been percolating in your gut all day.

NATURAL KILLERS

The target-specific portion of the immune system includes two general types of lymphocytes: B-cells, formed in the bone marrow, and T-cells, formed in the thymus, a lymph gland behind the breastbone.

"B-cells are the admirals of your body's defense system," Dr. Phillips says. "They deploy antibodies into your bloodstream and other body fluids." (These Y-shaped protectors help to neutralize some invaders themselves, or work with a "chemical warfare" cohort, called complement, to subdue other foes.) B-cells also keep the war records of previous battles so that any repeat invasion by a former foe is immediately countered.

T-cells come in three types. Killer T-cells do the dirty work of killing any cells in your body that have been invaded by viruses. T-helper cells and suppressor T-cells regulate the magnitude of the immune response and help bring things back to normal when the infection is conquered.

Natural killer cells are closely related to killer T-cells but aren't as picky about what they'll go after. They can recognize cells infected by viruses, and some tumor cells, and kill them.

THE NUTRIENTS THAT MATTER MOST

All these specialized cells depend on what you eat to do their jobs: They need good nutrition to develop in the bone marrow or thymus, to multiply rapidly in response to an infection, to protect themselves during the heat of battle and to generate the biochemicals that orchestrate an effective immune response. Let's see why some of these nutrients are so important.

CAN YOU FIGHT THIS INFECTION WITH FOOD?

You're feeling miserable with a head-pounding cold, or is it really a touch of the flu you're battling? In any case, your nagging conscience is chiding: "No wonder you're sick. The way you eat."

So, since you're already laid up, does it matter what you eat *now*? You don't have much appetite anyway, so why not tickle your taste buds with that quart of Rocky Road in the freezer? Or would you feel better faster if you started drinking plenty of vitamin C–rich orange juice and scheduled some zinc-packed foods like oysters for supper?

"You *should* eat better, but realize that eating better over that short period of time is not going to cure your cold or flu," says Ananda Prasad, M.D., Ph.D., of Wayne State University in Detroit.

It's possible that eating well may provide some immediate immune system benefits, like maintaining fighting levels of vitamin C and zinc. (These nutrients tend to be used up fast during an infection.) But it's long-term good nutrition that improves immune function most, researchers say.

"If you have optimal nutrition status, you will be able to fight any infection better," Dr. Prasad says. "And optimal status takes at least several weeks to establish, and can take months, depending on your nutritional needs."

If a cold or the flu does rev up your resolve to eat better, make sure you continue to eat well even after you start to feel better, says Thomas Petro, Ph.D., associate professor of microbiology and immunology at the University of Nebraska Medical Center in Omaha. "That's because your body needs time to rebuild damaged tissue and restore a possibly battered army of immune cells, and unless it has the nourishment to do so, you're at risk for another infection soon down the road," Dr. Petro says.

Vitamin B₆: The Booster

Remember wheat germ, blackstrap molasses and brown rice? These perennial health food staples are chock-full of vitamin B_6. Your immune system may like them no better than you do, but eating them or other B_6-rich foods may do you both a lot of good.

Vitamin B_6 may help your immune system produce antibodies and your thymus to churn out the hormones that allow T-cells to mature into deadly, target-specific killers. B_6 and other B-complex vitamins are also needed for cells to replicate (make more of themselves). Low levels of some B vitamins means your body will be unable to produce the large numbers of immune cells it may need for a major attack, says Simin Meydani, Ph.D., of the U.S. Department of Agriculture's (USDA) Human Nutrition Research Center on Aging at Tufts University School of Nutrition in Boston.

Even though B_6 and other B-complex vitamins are found in whole-grain and fortified baked goods and cereals, some people don't get enough of these nutrients or may need more than the RDA for optimum immune function, Dr. Meydani says.

She and researcher Robert M. Russell, M.D., professor of medicine and nutrition at Tufts, discovered that when healthy elderly people had vitamin B_6 taken almost completely out of their diets, their immune response went down, as expected. What wasn't anticipated was the finding that the amount of vitamin B_6 needed to restore immune function was much higher than the current RDA of about two milligrams.

Vitamin E: The Shield

Researchers know that vitamin E protects immune cells from what could be called stray bullets, harmful free radicals generated during immune system battles and the process of destroying bacteria and viruses. These battles involve chemical reactions that use oxygen—so they're called oxidative reactions. These oxidative reactions generate free radicals.

"As long as they have plenty of vitamin E incorporated into their outer membrane, immune cells are shielded from these reactions," explains Jeffrey Blumberg, Ph.D., chief of the Antioxidants Research Laboratory, also at the research center on aging at Tufts. "If immune cells lack sufficient antioxidant protection, however, their own reactions can injure or even kill them."

Vitamin E also affects the immune system by reducing the formation of a biochemical called prostaglandin E2 (PGE2), says Dr. Blumberg. PGE2 inhibits immune function. "So by giving vitamin E, we are turning one of the immune's system's 'off' switches back on," he explains. "We've also shown we get increases in interleukin-2, which is a T-cell growth factor, by giving vitamin E."

In one study, Dr. Blumberg found that older people given supplemental vitamin E had marked improvement in certain tests of immune response. One of the tests, a skin-patch test exposing the skin to certain toxins, measures the body's ability to fight antigens. (A poor response on this test is associated with increased death rates.) "However, after giving older people vitamin E supplements, their response to the skin-patch test was more like that of younger people," Dr. Blumberg says.

His subsequent research shows that vitamin E enhances immune response in older men after exercising. "That's important because this immune response helps repair tissue damaged during exercise; it may even be important in building new muscle," he explains.

VITAMIN C: THE PROTECTOR

Do you naturally crave orange juice when you're feeling out of sorts? Maybe that supply officer's message is getting through. "Pour me a tall, cool one."

Like vitamin E, vitamin C is an antioxidant. So it helps to control the potentially damaging reactions that occur when immune cell meets bacteria, and the shooting starts. But because vitamin C is water soluble, not fat soluble, it provides protection not in the cell membrane, but in the watery fluid within cells, and surrounding cells.

"Vitamin C deficiency has been shown to weaken a number of immune system functions," says Adrianne Bendich, Ph.D., senior clinical research coordinator in the Human Nutrition Research Division of Hoffmann-La Roche in Nutley, New Jersey. "Cells just don't multiply, communicate or mature into target-specific fighters as well when vitamin C levels are low."

Studies show that when adequate vitamin C is present, the number of frontline infection fighters—T-cells and B-cells—increases. Studies with higher-than-normal intakes of vitamin C have had mixed results, Dr. Bendich says. "Some studies show improved immune response; others do not."

Research seems to show that vitamin C helps smokers and people with asthma retain immunity in the lungs, Dr. Bendich says. "Both cigarette smoke and the inflammatory response of asthma generate lots of free radicals that can damage lymphocytes in the lungs," she says. "Vitamin C seems to offer these cells some protection."

Studies show that certain immune cells, especially neutrophils, have concentrations of vitamin C up to 150 times the amount typically found in cells, and that vitamin C is quickly used up during infection fighting. So you may really need those extra glasses of orange juice when you're sick, researchers say.

BETA-CAROTENE: TUMOR DOOMER?

Do natural killer cells like a hearty lunch of carrots and sweet potatoes before resuming their day's work? Some research seems to indicate they do.

Those foods, along with other red, yellow, orange and dark green fruits and vegetables, are packed full of beta-carotene,

SAVING LIVES WITH VITAMIN A

In some parts of the world, people die for lack of what we take for granted. That's because nutrition in some countries is so bad and the chances for all kinds of infections so good that a person's immune system never has a fighting chance.

Even in the face of across-the-board malnourishment, though, it appears that vitamin A can save lives.

In southern India, where vitamin A deficiency is rampant, the distribution to 15,000 preschool children of supplements that provided the Recommended Dietary Allowance of this nutrient reduced death rates by more than half in just one year. And in Napal vitamin A cut children's deaths by a third.

"These children were dying mostly of pneumonia and fevers, or diarrhea and dysentery," says Keith West, Jr., Dr.P.H., director of the Vitamin A Project at Johns Hopkins Hospital in Baltimore. (The Vitamin A Project is aimed at solving health problems related to vitamin deficiencies in developing countries.) "We don't know all the details of how the vitamin A works, but we do know that it plays a role in a large number of activities within the body that involve defense against infection."

Vitamin A reduced death rates most dramatically in children who were the most poorly fed. "It seemed to work even in children whose growth was stunted, which would indicate chronic malnourishment," Dr. West says.

a nutrient associated with reduced risk for several kinds of cancer. Some researchers believe beta-carotene may even reverse early cell changes that could lead to cancer.

In one study, Harinder S. Garewal M.D., Ph.D., assistant director for cancer prevention and control at the University of Arizona Cancer Center in Tucson, gave high doses of beta-carotene (30 milligrams a day) for six months to a group of 24 people with precancerous growths in their mouths. Seventeen responded to the treatment; their lesions decreased in size by at least 50 percent, and in several patients they disappeared altogether.

University of Arizona researcher Dr. Watson homed in on immune system changes in these same 24 people. "We found that 30 milligrams a day or more of beta-carotene caused significant increases in the number of natural killer cells and T-helper cells," he says. Both are important parts of the body's tumor surveillance and disposal system. "Levels of cells with interleukin-2 and transferrin receptors, both indicators of lymphocyte activation, also rose," he says.

"Theoretically, all those things should be good for cancer resistance," Dr. Watson says.

A typical American consumes about 5 milligrams of beta-carotene a day, about a carrot's worth.

Getting plenty of beta-carotene is also a safe, low-fat way to get enough vitamin A, a nutrient that has a profound impact on many immunological functions. Your body converts beta-carotene to vitamin A, but only as needed—thereby eliminating any potential for vitamin A overdose.

ZINC: THE VITAL LINK

Abraham Lincoln's army dined on Chesapeake Bay oysters and won the war. Your own internal army might thrive on an occasional serving of these tasty mollusks, too. Why? Because oysters are a great source of zinc, a mineral involved with many aspects of immune function.

"Our research shows that zinc is very important, especially for thymic-dependent lymphocyte functions," says Ananda Prasad, M.D., Ph.D., professor of medicine at Wayne State University in Detroit and a pioneer researcher in the role of zinc in immune function. "The thymus gland helps T-cells to mature and become target specific," Dr. Prasad says. These cells also hold the body's memory of an invader, which allows it to respond more quickly should an infection recur.

Zinc is also necessary for the frenzy of immune cell reproduction that takes place during infection, and for the production of cytokines, those biochemicals that whip immune cells into action, Dr. Prasad says.

Studies show that people deficient in zinc have a variety of immune system weaknesses and are much more prone to infection. "Adding adequate zinc to the diet has been valuable in improving immune response," Dr. Prasad says.

In the United States, some people get only 8 to 10 milligrams of zinc a day, well below the RDA of 12 to 15 milligrams, Dr. Prasad says. "Older people, dieters and people who eat little or no meat and lots of fiber are most likely to develop zinc deficiency-related immune problems," he says.

AN EATING PLAN FOR IMMUNE POWER

How can you possibly eat everything you need for optimum immunity without overeating?

The goal is to choose a wide array of nutrition-packed foods that are low in fat and calories, says Susanna Cunningham-Rundles, Ph.D., associate professor of immunology at New York Hospital-Cornell University Medical Center in New York City. "That doesn't happen by chance. You need to plan meals, and know what to pick up at the grocery store or when dining out."

The single most important thing that most people can do to improve their nutrition? "Eat more fruits and vegetables," Dr. Cunningham-Rundles says. Aim for two servings of fruits and three servings of vegetables a day, she suggests. "You *can* expand your tastes by exposing yourself to foods you've never had before, in a cheerful way, not like it's medicine."

WHEN IMMUNITY GOES ASTRAY

What do rheumatoid arthritis, multiple sclerosis and lupus have in common? All three are *autoimmune* diseases. Their symptoms are caused by misguided immune cells attacking the body's own tissue. In the case of arthritis, it's the joints that come under attack, for multiple sclerosis it's the central nervous system, for lupus it's the kidneys, skin, heart and joints.

"Little research has been done on nutrition and autoimmune diseases compared to nutrition and immunity in general, and most studies so far have been done in animals," says Carl Keen, Ph.D., professor of nutrition and internal medicine at the University of California at Davis. So researchers are extremely wary about making any kinds of dietary recommendations. Still, research suggests that in the future, dietary manipulation, along with other treatments, may help some of these diseases.

Among the findings so far: omega-3 fatty acids, found in fatty fish like mackerel and salmon, apparently help suppress the inflammatory reaction in autoimmune diseases and perhaps provide other, still-unknown benefits. "There are many different hypotheses about how these oils work in immune function, but the details have yet to be worked out," Dr. Keen says. "The few preliminary studies done so far in humans show some potential for benefit."

Antioxidants like vitamins A, E and C might also play a role in slowing organ damage from autoimmune disease, but research is needed to confirm that possible role, Dr. Keen says. "On the other hand, it's also possible that these nutrients could speed up damage in some cases by boosting immune function in a system out of control."

Animal studies also show that deliberately inducing deficiencies of nutrients needed for immune function, such as zinc or specific amino acids, sometimes prolong the lives of animals with autoimmune diseases. "But doing that sort of thing just wouldn't be at all advisable in people," says Dr. Keen, "since the nutritional deficiencies create all sorts of other problems."

Once you've started to widen your dining horizons, here are some specific ways to zero in on what you need.

Snack on vitamin C–rich fruits and vegetables. These include grapefruit, oranges, strawberries, cantaloupe, honeydew melons, mangoes, watermelon, fortified fruit juices, red and green peppers, broccoli, potatoes (white or sweet), tomatoes, brussels sprouts and cauliflower.

Chow down on foods high in beta-carotene. Sweet potatoes top the list, along with carrots, spinach, winter squash, kale, cantaloupe, apricots, broccoli and other colorful fruits and vegetables.

Zero in on zinc. Add shellfish (oysters are your best source); beef; wheat germ; fortified, ready-to-eat breakfast cereals; chicken; turkey and pumpkin seeds.

Seek out vitamin E. Eat wheat germ, peanut butter, almonds, filbert nuts, sunflower seeds, shrimp and vegetable oils. Green leafy vegetables also supply some vitamin E.

Get your fair share of vitamin B$_6$. It's easy with chicken; fortified, ready-to-eat cereals; sweet green or red peppers; turkey; brown rice; soybeans; oats; whole-wheat products; peanuts; bananas; plantains and walnuts.

Add vitamin A. Eat the same foods that provide beta-carotene (in the body, beta-carotene is converted into vitamin A as needed) or with a low-fat source of preformed vitamin A such as fortified skim milk.

Fill up on folate. The list of foods that supply folate includes broccoli; green peas; fortified, ready-to-eat cereals; beans; baked potatoes and orange juice. Folate is needed to make all new cells, including the white blood cells of your immune system.

Add omega-3 fatty acids. Mackerel, salmon, bluefish, herring, trout and tuna are good sources. Fish oils rich in omega-3's help stop inflammation, and unlike some other fats, do not impair immune function. Indeed, they may enhance it.

Pump up iron intake. Lean red meats; fortified, ready-to-eat cereals; dark-meat chicken or turkey; fish; shellfish; beans;

nuts and seeds are good sources. Iron plays a major role in the chemical reactions that allow immune cells to zap invaders.

Concentrate on copper. Shellfish, nuts, sesame seeds, mushrooms and whole-grain cereals are good sources. Copper, like zinc, plays an important role in making sure your T-cells and antibodies are working optimally.

For more help in formulating an immune-boosting diet and selecting appropriate supplements, if necessary, see a doctor knowledgeable in nutrition, or a registered dietitian. Especially if you're cutting calories or have frequent or chronic illness, professional help can be invaluable, experts say.

High-Nutrition Recipes

SHRIMP CREOLE WITH BROWN RICE

This favorite Louisiana dish contains lots of immunity-bolstering nutrients, including vitamins C, B_6 and E, beta-carotene and copper.

3 cups defatted chicken stock	½ cup tomato sauce
1 cup diced sweet red peppers	½ teaspoon dried thyme
½ cup diced onions	⅛ teaspoon ground red pepper
½ cup diced celery	1 tablespoon sherry extract (optional)
1 clove garlic, minced	1 pound small to medium shrimp, peeled and deveined
1 tablespoon olive oil	
1 tomato, seeded and diced	
3 tablespoons unbleached flour	3 cups hot cooked brown rice

In a 1-quart saucepan over high heat, bring the stock to a boil. Keep warm over low heat.

In a 3-quart saucepan over medium heat, sauté the diced peppers, onions, celery and garlic in the oil for 5 minutes, or until the vegetables are wilted. Add the tomatoes and cook for 3 minutes.

Sprinkle with the flour and mix well. Stir in the stock, a little at a time, until it is well mixed with the flour, creating a smooth sauce. Stir in the tomato sauce, thyme, ground pepper and sherry extract, if desired. Cover and simmer over medium-low heat, stirring occasionally, for 25 minutes.

Add the shrimp. Cook for 5 minutes, or until the shrimp are pink and curled. Serve over the rice.

Serves 4
Per serving: *381 calories, 7.8 g. fat (19% of calories), 4.4 g. dietary fiber, 153 mg. cholesterol, 242 mg. sodium*

SWEET POTATO SALAD

Here's a nice change of pace from standard potato salads. The sweet potatoes add plenty of beta-carotene, which is not present in regular white spuds.

3	medium sweet potatoes (about 1 pound)	2	tablespoons minced scallions
1	tart green apple, diced	½	cup nonfat mayonnaise
½	cup chopped pineapple	¼	cup nonfat yogurt
¼	cup diced celery	2	tablespoons lime juice
2	tablespoons toasted slivered almonds		

Scrub the potatoes and cook in boiling water to cover for 25 minutes, or until easily pierced with a knife but not mushy. Drain and set aside until cool enough to handle. Peel and cut into ¾" chunks. Place in a large bowl.

Add the apples, pineapple, celery, almonds and scallions. Toss lightly.

In a small bowl, whisk together the mayonnaise, yogurt and lime juice. Pour over the salad. Toss well. Chill before serving.

Serves 4
Per serving: *197 calories, 2.4 g. fat (11% of calories), 4.4 g. dietary fiber, <1 mg. cholesterol, 422 mg. sodium*

BREADED OYSTERS

Oysters are an awesome source of zinc, an indispensable mineral in the war against infections. Baking eliminates all the fat traditionally used in deep-frying.

24 large frying oysters	1 tablespoon water
2 tablespoons unbleached flour	¼ teaspoon hot-pepper sauce
¼ cup fat-free egg substitute	1 cup dry bread crumbs

Drain the oysters and pat them dry on paper towels. Dredge each oyster in the flour to lightly coat it.

In a shallow bowl, lightly combine the egg, water and hot-pepper sauce with a fork. Dip each oyster in the mixture to coat it lightly. Then dip it into the bread crumbs to coat it completely.

Coat a large baking sheet with no-stick spray. Place the oysters on the sheet with a little space between them. Mist lightly with no-stick spray.

Bake at 450° for 10 to 15 minutes, or until the coating becomes crisp.

Serves 4
Per serving: *175 calories, 3.4 g. fat (18% of calories), 1 g. dietary fiber, 46 mg. cholesterol, 299 mg. sodium*

PORK WITH APRICOTS

Vitamin B$_6$ is a major player on the immunity team. And lean pork—such as tenderloin—is a good source of the nutrient. Combining the meat with apricots adds other vital nutrients, such as beta-carotene and vitamin C. If fresh apricots are out of season, substitute drained canned halves.

1 **pound pork tenderloin, trimmed of all visible fat and cut into 1" slices**	1 **tablespoon lemon juice**
2 **teaspoons olive oil**	½ **teaspoon Dijon mustard**
½ **cup defatted chicken stock**	8 **apricots, halved and pitted**
2 **tablespoons all-fruit apricot preserves**	8 **ounces medium no-yolk egg noodles**

In a large no-stick frying pan over medium-high heat, brown the pork in the oil for about 2 minutes per side. Remove to a plate.

Reduce the heat to medium. To the pan, add the stock, preserves, lemon juice and mustard. Stir to mix thoroughly. Add the apricots. Cover and cook for 3 minutes, or until the apricots are soft but not mushy. Add the pork and keep warm over low heat.

Cook the noodles in a large pot of boiling water for 8 minutes, or until just tender. Drain. Serve the pork and apricots over the noodles.

Serves 4
Per serving: *401 calories, 6.6 g. fat (15% of calories), 3.7 g. dietary fiber, 74 mg. cholesterol, 116 mg. sodium*

CHAPTER 21

The Heart and Arteries

Rolling Back the Risks

Even though you know it probably isn't the healthiest lunch, you're in a hurry, so you decide to eat just one slice of gooey pizza covered with pepperoni and extra cheese. But it tastes so good that you appease your growling stomach with another piece.

You figure you're merely eating a quick meal packed with carbohydrates to keep yourself energetic throughout the busy afternoon. Of course, you know—or at least should know—that this pizza is loaded with cholesterol and saturated fat, two of your heart's worst enemies. But two slices of pizza aren't going to kill you. Or are they?

Well, it depends. "No, a slice or two of pizza now and then *isn't* going to hurt you," says Gregory Kay, M.D., a cardiothoracic and vascular surgeon at the Hospital of the Good Samaritan in Los Angeles. "But if it's part of a daily pattern of eggs, hamburgers and other fatty foods, then you're looking at trouble."

Heart disease isn't caused by one food, one meal or one

day's menu. Heart disease often is the result of years of poor eating habits that include thousands of french fries, hundreds of eggs, hordes of hamburgers and yes, gobs of pizza.

Certainly there are other risk factors such as smoking, diabetes, lack of exercise and your family history that increase the risk of heart disease. But there's little doubt that over a lifetime what you eat does play a major role in determining your likelihood of suffering a fatal heart attack.

"In terms of the development of heart disease, 70 to 80 percent of your risk comes from what you eat," says Daniel Eisenberg, M.D., a Los Angeles cardiologist and assistant clinical professor at the University of Southern California School of Medicine.

CHOLESTEROL ISN'T COOL

Why? Well, let's take a look at what happened to that pizza you ate for lunch. As you ate those slices, you couldn't help but notice a few greasy spots on the napkin and pockets of oil floating on the pizza itself. All of that was fat—mostly saturated fat, the kind that your body uses to make cholesterol.

As this fat floated through your stomach, it was bombarded by acids in the stomach so strong they could burn a hole in your living room carpet. But as potent as they are, those acids aren't strong enough to break down that saturated fat. In fact, it wasn't until it entered your small intestine that the fat was battered into particles small enough to be absorbed by the bloodstream and transported to the liver. There, about 70 percent of it was made into low-density lipoproteins (LDL), the "bad" cholesterol that over time can clog and damage the arteries in your entire body, especially those to your heart. Fortunately, the liver transformed the remaining 30 percent of saturated fat into high-density lipoprotein (HDL), known as the "good" cholesterol because it helps transport the bad kind out of your system.

DOUBLE TROUBLE

As if that's not bad enough, in addition to the fat, that pizza also contains cholesterol from the milk and meat fat that goes *directly* into your bloodstream after you eat it. So when you ate the pizza, you were, in a way, getting a double doze of cholesterol: from the cholesterol in the pepperoni and cheese and from the fat these two foods contain.

Of course, saturated fat and cholesterol aren't just in pizza. Saturated fat is common in meats and animal by-products such as beef, chicken, lard, butter, sausage, whole milk and cheese. Cholesterol is found in most of those foods, too. In fact, it's hard to find a food high in saturated fat that doesn't have lots of cholesterol. The exceptions are solid and "hydrogenated" shortenings and tropical oils. These vegetable products contain saturated fat but no cholesterol.

Unlike fat, which you often can see, cholesterol is a microscopic, waxy substance that your body uses to make hormones and cell membranes. Sure, you need cholesterol, but your body manufactures all you'll ever need on its own. So what you eat is excess. And where does it go?

It circulates in your bloodstream and accumulates in the arteries and blocks blood flow to the heart. Fortunately, some of the good cholesterol latches onto some of the bad cholesterol and sweeps it out of the body. Unfortunately, there is usually much more bad cholesterol than the good can handle.

TRACKING DOWN THE CULPRIT

Certainly, a small amount of dietary cholesterol and fat probably won't harm you. But what happens to your arteries when you eat a steady diet of foods containing cholesterol and fats?

"Normally, as cholesterol circulates in the blood, it is constantly going in and out of cells in the artery walls," says

Robert DiBianco, M.D., director of cardiology research at Washington Adventist Hospital and associate clinical professor of medicine at the Georgetown University School of Medicine in Washington, D.C. "But when you eat a steady diet of foods high in cholesterol and saturated fat, it can lead to a high concentration of "bad" LDL cholesterol in the blood. When that happens, there is more movement of cholesterol into than out of those cells and the excess cholesterol begins forming plaque deposits on the artery walls."

This is the beginning of a process known as atherosclerosis. As plaque builds up on the artery walls, it chokes off the blood supply. If this occurs in the arteries supplying the heart muscle, the result is angina, a tightness of the chest that indicates severe narrowing of the coronary arteries is taking place. Eventually, if enough plaque accumulates, it can block blood flow to the heart so completely that a heart attack occurs, Dr. DiBianco says. If the plaque buildup occurs in the arteries to the brain, it can result in a stroke.

Plaques are like having several cars double-parked on a street, making it difficult for traffic to pass. As traffic snarls up, the likelihood of an accident increases, explains George L. Blackburn, M.D., Ph.D., associate professor of surgery at Harvard Medical School and chief of the Nutrition/Metabolism Laboratory at the Cancer Research Institute at New England Deaconess Hospital in Boston.

So what do all those traffic jams in the arteries add up to? About 500,000 funerals a year, according to the National Cholesterol Education Program. Statistics show that 1.25 million Americans suffer heart attacks each year, and about one in three of those attacks are fatal. Another 6 million people in America are suffering loss of quality of life from symptoms including angina, cramps and pain in the lower legs, nausea and shortness of breath—particularly after modest physical exertion. All told, nearly 70 percent of adult Americans have some narrowing of their coronary arteries.

IT'S NOT TOO LATE

"Americans are throwing away huge amounts of their lives and spending a fortune on heart disease treatments that they wouldn't need if they took care of themselves," Dr. Blackburn says. "If people, working as a family unit, could be motivated to cut the fat out of their diets and to eat more of the foods that are good for their hearts, they'd be ahead of the game."

There is no question that the American diet needs some fine-tuning, says Dr. Blackburn. And he has plenty of reasons to believe that. Hundreds of studies conducted worldwide in the past 50 years have linked the consumption of fat- and cholesterol-laden foods—mainly highly processed foods and animal foods such as meat, cheese and eggs—to coronary diseases. What's more, many of those same studies are providing powerful evidence that changing what we eat can make an important difference.

In one classic study that began in 1965, researchers examined the dietary habits of more than 10,000 men of Japanese descent, many of whom had adopted an American diet. One group were native Japanese who had immigrated to Hawaii and begun eating the local diet, which is high in saturated fat and cholesterol. A second group were Japanese who had moved to California and adopted a diet that was even richer in saturated fat and cholesterol than that of the Hawaiian group. These two groups of immigrants were compared to a third group of people who lived in Japan and followed their country's traditional diet.

The men who moved to Hawaii and California weighed about ten pounds more, had higher blood cholesterol levels, ate 2½ times more total fat and about 4 times more saturated fat than Japanese men who remained in their native country and ate their native foods. And the researchers found that death from heart disease rose as the amount of saturated fat and cholesterol in the diet increased.

"The death rates from heart disease were lowest in Japan, intermediate in Hawaii and highest in the continental United States," says Millicent Higgins, M.D., associate director for epidemiology and biometry at the National Heart, Lung and Blood Institute in Bethesda, Maryland.

In one ongoing study that began in 1957, researchers have been following the eating and lifestyle habits of 12,763 middle-aged men in seven countries, including Greece, Italy, Japan, Finland and the United States. The men have been examined every five years and assessed for a number of coronary risk factors, including diet, smoking, blood pressure and weight. Among their many findings, the researchers have determined that the men who eat the least amount of saturated fat and cholesterol have a lower risk of developing heart disease compared to other men in the study, says Ancel Keys, Ph.D., of the University of Minnesota School of Public Health in Minneapolis, the lead author of the ongoing study and a pioneer in cholesterol research since 1947.

A study in India also shows the importance of limiting the amount of cholesterol and saturated fat in your diet. In this study, 228 people were asked to eat a low-cholesterol, low-saturated-fat diet that included fewer than 216 milligrams of cholesterol (just one medium-size egg has about 213 milligrams of cholesterol) and just 6 percent of calories from saturated fat daily—basically a vegetarian diet. (A porterhouse steak, by comparison, has 18 percent of calories from saturated fat and 45 percent from total fat.)

The people in the first group were compared to 230 individuals who ate their usual diet, which contained an average of 318 milligrams of cholesterol and 11 percent saturated fat daily. In addition, the higher-fat group consumed twice as much animal protein, nearly 60 percent less fiber, a third less carbohydrates and fewer fruits and vegetables such as grapes, bananas, spinach, radishes and tomatoes.

After one year, the low-fat, low-cholesterol dieters had lower blood pressure and blood sugar levels and had fewer complications of heart disease including arrhythmia (irregular heartbeat), angina pain and heart attack than those who didn't eat a heart-protective diet. Overall, the low-cholesterol, low-fat dieters reduced their risk of heart disease by 32 percent.

In the United States, the famed Framingham Heart Study in Massachusetts also has shown that diet has a great influence on whether you will develop heart disease, says William P. Castelli, M.D., director of the ongoing study that has followed 5,127 men and women for more than 30 years.

"The average American family eats the same bloody stuff night after night, and it's just too rich in cholesterol and fat," Dr. Castelli says. "That's why about 80 percent of us end up with these deposits in our arteries, and about half of us die from that buildup."

SETTING THE TARGET

Based on the evidence, something has to change if heart disease is going to be knocked off the chart as the number one killer in Americans. According to Dr. Castelli, the average American male eats 80 to 100 grams of fat a day and almost 500 milligrams of cholesterol.

As a first step, the American Heart Association and the National Cholesterol Education Program recommended a diet that delivers less than 300 milligrams of cholesterol a day and limits total fat to 30 percent and saturated fat to less than 10 percent of your daily caloric intake.

If you have chronically high blood cholesterol (above 200), then your doctor may recommend that you restrict your consumption of saturated fat and cholesterol even more. Here's why.

The higher your blood cholesterol, the greater your risk of heart disease. And, although some people's bodies naturally produce more cholesterol than others, it's important to remember that the saturated fat and dietary cholesterol we eat also increases the amount of cholesterol in the bloodstream.

THE DIET THAT *REVERSES* HEART DISEASE

It's strict and it includes comprehensive changes in diet and lifestyle, but the regimen prescribed by Dean Ornish, M.D., of the Preventive Medicine Research Institute in Sausalito, California, for his patients has become an important non-surgical breakthrough in combating heart disease.

Research by Dr. Ornish indicates that diet and behavior changes can significantly reverse coronary blockages in just one year. The diet is far more restrictive than the diet recommended by the American Heart Association (AHA), which allows 30 percent of calories from fat and 300 milligrams of cholesterol daily. Instead, Dr. Ornish's diet is vegetarian and permits no caffeine, oils or animal products except for egg whites, nonfat milk and yogurt. It allows less than 10 percent of calories from fat and almost no cholesterol.

The participants are asked to practice an hour's worth of stress-management techniques, such as yoga, daily and to spend about three hours walking a week.

The dramatic result of Dr. Ornish's work was demonstrated in a study comparing 22 men who followed his diet for at least a year to 19 men who followed the guidelines of the AHA. About 82 percent of the people on Dr. Ornish's program had some reversal of their coronary blockages. The reductions were small—averaging about 5 percent—but even small changes can have significant impact on the amount of blood the heart receives, Dr. Ornish says.

Most heart researchers agree that cholesterol becomes a risk when total blood levels are higher than 200, LDL levels go above 130, or HDL levels drop below 35. If your blood cholesterol level is higher than 240, your risk of developing heart disease is four times greater than if it were below 200, according to the National Cholesterol Education Program. Just dropping your cholesterol level by 10

Those who followed the AHA diet didn't experience the striking reversal of the Ornish diet group. Overall, the patients' disease appeared to worsen.

"Dr. Ornish's work is very significant because he has achieved with diet and relaxation the same kind of results other researchers have achieved with powerful cholesterol-lowering drugs," says William P. Castelli, M.D., of the Framingham Heart Study. "But the measures he uses are nontoxic, and you can do them forever."

However, some question if Americans are ready to embrace such a drastic lifestyle change.

"Personally, if I were a young man with coronary heart disease, I would be willing to try the Ornish approach," says Carl Lavie, M.D., of the Ochsner Medical Institution in New Orleans.

Dr. Ornish, author of *Dr. Dean Ornish's Program for Reversing Heart Disease*, thinks many Americans may be willing to choose lifestyle changes as an alternative to bypass surgery or a lifetime of cholesterol-lowering drugs.

"The reason for making changes in diet and lifestyle isn't necessarily to live longer but to live better," he says. "When people realize that the short-term benefits of changing can be so considerable—chest pain often decreases markedly, you feel better, you have more energy—and those benefits often occur within days or a few weeks after changing your lifestyle, then the choices become clearer."

percent should lower your risk of coronary heart disease by 20 percent.

HEART-HEALTHY EATING TIPS

So how do you get started in your efforts to drive down your cholesterol levels and win the war against heart disease? Experts suggest these basic strategies.

Eat less cholesterol. Long before eggs became a staple and fast food became routine, our ancestors ate meals that were naturally low in dietary cholesterol. It's a lesson we need to relearn, Dr. Kay says.

"About 10,000 years ago, when humans were still evolving, they surely didn't eat a bunch of eggs. They ate fruits, nuts, vegetables and occasionally some meat," he says. "This phenomenon of eating two portions of beef every day, two eggs in the morning and a big scoop of ice cream every afternoon is fairly new. Unfortunately, many people think it's a lot easier and more fun to eat three eggs and three slices of bacon than it is to eat a well-balanced, heart-healthy meal."

Avoiding egg yolks and organ meats, such as liver, are two simple ways of slashing the amount of cholesterol in your diet. And since cholesterol is found only in animal foods, you also need to cut back on your consumption of meats and dairy foods.

Shed the fat. Slashing the amount of saturated fat you eat may be your best defense against high blood cholesterol, Dr. Eisenberg says.

"Saturated fat, milligram for milligram, has twice the cholesterol-raising effect as the same amount of dietary cholesterol," he says.

That's because the body easily converts saturated fat into cholesterol, Dr. Eisenberg says. No more than $\frac{1}{10}$ of your total calories should be from saturated fat, common in meats—such as beef and chicken—and dairy products—such as whole milk and cheese.

But the most prudent way to reduce your saturated fat intake is to lower your consumption of *all* fats, Dr. Castelli says. "If you reduce all dietary fat, you automatically knock down saturated fat intake, because about half of the fat we eat is saturated fat."

To get going in the right direction, consider using low-fat alternatives when preparing food. Start substituting 1 percent milk for whole milk, for example. Use low-fat yogurt, buttermilk or evaporated skim milk instead of sour cream, cream or cream cheese.

"There are a lot of imitation and low-fat products that are on the market now," says Andrea Gardiner, R.D., a dietitian specializing in cardiac rehabilitation at the Hospital of the Good Samaritan in Los Angeles. "With careful label reading, you can find products that are fat-free, too. Also you can easily make your own versions at home. For a sour cream substitute, for example, you could mix nonfat yogurt with nonfat cottage cheese in a blender. You should always consider using creative solutions like this."

Whenever possible, use nonfat mayonnaise or mix nonfat yogurt with low-fat mayonnaise when making tuna or chicken salad, she says.

Make the switch. Switching from saturated fats such as butter to monounsaturates such as olive oil or polyunsaturates like corn oil also might help lower your total cholesterol and raise your HDLs.

In a study of 4,903 Italian men and women, researchers concluded that increased consumption of butter was associated with significantly elevated blood pressure and serum cholesterol in men and higher blood sugar levels on both men and women. All three are risk factors for coronary heart disease. But eating more foods made with olive oil and vegetable oil *lowered* those risks in both sexes.

"It looks like olive and other vegetable oils have very similar effects. Olive oil seems to be stronger with regard to blood glucose and blood pressure, while polyunsaturates seem slightly stronger than olive oil with regard to serum cholesterol," says Maurizio Trevisan, M.D., author of the study and an associate professor at the State University of New York at Buffalo School of Medicine and Biomedical Sciences.

"When you're cooking at home, you're always much better off using a liquid oil rather than melting butter, mar-

STARTING OVER

If you want to reduce the cholesterol and fat in your diet, but aren't sure how to begin, this table may give you some ideas.

If You Usually Eat . . .	A Better Choice Is . . .
Butter	Tub or soft margarine
Cakes	Angel food cake
Chocolate	Cocoa
Creamed salad dressing	Oil and vinegar
Fried foods	Broiled, baked or steamed foods
Goose or duck	Chicken or turkey without the skin
Hamburger	Salad or pasta
Ice cream	Sherbet
Mayonnaise	Nonfat mayonnaise or low-fat yogurt
Potato chips	Pretzels or rice cakes
Scalloped potatoes	Rice
Shortening	Unhydrogenated vegetable oil or olive oil
Sour cream	Low-fat yogurt or cottage cheese
Steak	Fish
Toast with butter	Toast with jelly only
Vegetables with butter	Vegetables with herbs, citrus juice
Whole-egg omelet	Three egg whites and one egg yolk
Whole milk or cream	Skim or low-fat milk

garine or shortening because those are solid fats and are more saturated," Gardiner says.

It's important to realize, however, that even though monounsaturates are healthier, they still need to be used sparingly. After all, they're still fats and can easily increase your total fat intake. A rule of thumb: Use no more than one teaspoon in any dish.

Count on the grams. Counting grams is the easiest way to monitor your fat consumption because that's how most food manufacturers label their products.

Most doctors suggest that you should reduce saturated fat in your diet to no more than 10 percent of your total calories. To translate that percentage into grams of fat, take the total number of calories you eat each day and multiply that by 30 percent. That will give you the total number of calories of fat you can eat each day. Then divide by 9 (that's the number of calories in a gram of fat). That will give you the total grams of fat you want in your diet. Finally, divide by 3. That will give the maximum number of grams of saturated fat you can eat each day.

So if you eat 2,000 calories a day, for example, that means you should be eating a maximum of 600 calories of 67 grams of total fat each day. Divide that by 3, and you'll find that you should eat no more than 22 grams of saturated fat daily (that's one-third of your total fat calories).

Knowing the grams of saturated fat allowed in your diet will help plan meals more wisely, Dr. Castelli says. So if you do eat 2,000 calories a day and gobble up 3½ ounces (100 grams) of the fattiest hamburger for lunch, you've just consumed about 20 grams of saturated fat. In other words, you've basically just used up your daily allowance of saturated fat in one meal, Dr. Castelli says. However, if you eat 3½ ounces of select grade hamburger, you'll be getting only 4 grams of saturated fat. "Theoretically, you could have a select grade hamburger for breakfast, lunch and dinner and still have 10 grams of saturated fat to spend that day," Dr. Castelli says.

Lean toward lean meats. Buy the leanest cuts of meat you can, Dr. Castelli advises. Almost half the fat in some cuts of beef, for example, is saturated. So choosing the leanest grades of beef is crucial to maintaining cardiovascular health. Of the three grades of beef, select is your best choice, Dr. Castelli says. Only 10 percent fat by weight, it only has about 4 grams of saturated fat per 3½-ounce serving. (About 28 grams equal an ounce). In comparison, choice beef, the next grade, ranges from 15 to 35 percent fat, and a 3½-ounce serving can have 10 to 15 grams of saturated fat. Prime beef, the fattest grade, is 35 to 40 percent fat by weight and has about 20 grams of saturated fat per 3½ ounces.

One is the healthiest number. To really keep your heart disease risk low, it's probably wise to have no more than one serving of lean meat, fish or poultry a day. "If you eat only one 3½-ounce serving of meat, fish or poultry each day, that means you are eliminating at least two fatty meat meals from your diet," Dr. Kay says. "It's that simple. It's just another easy way of minimizing your fat consumption."

Don't count on alcohol. Is an after-dinner drink a great way to protect your cardiovascular system? "Some studies suggest that people who drink one to two glasses of alcohol a day do slightly better from a cardiovascular standpoint than people who don't drink at all," says Carl Lavie, M.D., co-director of cardiac rehabilitation and prevention at the Ochsner Medical Institution in New Orleans. "But once you get beyond three drinks a day, the risk of heart disease goes way up."

But for many reasons, including the potential risk of alcoholism, doctors are reluctant to advise patients to drink, he says. "There are so many problems associated with alcohol in this country that you really can't recommend that," Dr. Lavie says. "But it is reasonable to tell people who are drinking more than two drinks a day to cut back. It is also reasonable to tell people who are drinking one to two drinks that there is no reason, from a cardiovascular standpoint, to stop doing that."

He suggests that alcohol drinkers limit their consumption to no more than 2 ounces of whiskey; 8 ounces of wine or 24 ounces of beer a day.

ADDING TO SUBTRACT FROM THE RISK

But don't fall into the trap of thinking that eliminating foods from your diet is the only way that you can make a difference. *Adding* some foods to your menu can ensure your heart's health, too.

It does seem like people are always being told to eat less of this or less of that, says Warren Thompson, M.D., an associate professor of internal medicine at the University of Tennessee Graduate School of Medicine at Knoxville. "My feeling is that people shouldn't feel like they're punishing themselves. So I always try to emphasize that people should eat more of certain foods like fruits and vegetables that taste good, are enjoyable to eat and will protect their hearts."

To improve your chances of keeping your arteries clear and your heart pumping for many years to come, try adding a few of these foods to your diet.

If it swims, eat it. Substituting fish for red meat is probably one of your best choices. A serving of cooked Atlantic salmon (one of the fattiest fish) has less than one-third the total fat of the same size serving of broiled ribeye steak. In addition, fish such as mackerel, salmon, tuna and cod all contain high amounts of omega-3 fatty acids, a type of fat that may lower total cholesterol levels, raise HDLs and decrease the risk of heart disease.

Eating fish also helps keep arteries pliable, say researchers at Monash University in Melbourne, Australia. The researchers tested the blood vessels of 53 people and found that folks who ate one or more fish meals a week had more flexible arteries, a signal that their cardiovascular systems were healthier than those of people who ate no fish.

THIS HERB MIGHT BE YOUR ARTERIES' ALLY

So you think eating garlic isn't going to make your heart-throb want to get romantic. But breathtaking findings that this bulb can help ward off coronary disease may give you compelling reasons to persuade your favorite person that snuggling with a garlic lover isn't so bad.

In a study of 40 people with elevated cholesterol levels, readings dropped an average of 21 percent in 20 people taking 900 milligrams of powdered garlic daily for 16 weeks. The cholesterol levels of the 20 people who didn't get garlic only fell 3 percent.

In a larger study, 221 people with high cholesterol were given either 800 milligrams of garlic powder or a look-alike placebo. After four months, those who took garlic pills daily had overall reductions in their cholesterol averaging 12 percent. The placebo group's cholesterol only dropped an average of 3 percent.

In five other studies, garlic also reduced artery-clogging cholesterol, kept blood platelets from clumping (a process that can lead to dangerous clots) and lowered heart attack risk.

But it remains unclear how much garlic is needed to produce a protective effect on the cardiovascular system. In some studies, the equivalent of 7 to 28 cloves of garlic a day were needed to get results.

Another problem is that cooking, drying or steaming

In another small study of 28 South Africans, fatty fish significantly lowered blood cholesterol levels when substituted for red meat.

If eating fish regularly doesn't appeal to you, then you might try taking a fish-oil supplement containing 300 milmay destroy some of the active ingredients—allicin and ajoene—that fend off heart disease.

While it's still too soon to declare garlic a proven therapy, the herb may deserve more prominence in your diet, says Yu-Yan Yeh, Ph.D., associate professor of nutrition at Pennsylvania State University in University Park, who has done preliminary research that shows that garlic can lower cholesterol levels in laboratory rats.

"In general, I think that it is safe to say that if you consume garlic regularly, even just one to two cloves a day, you could be getting some beneficial effects," Dr. Yeh says.

To do that, try mincing garlic and sprinkling it on salads and vegetables, or add it at the very end of preparing pasta sauces.

Garlic also can be served as a side dish. Cut off the tops of the garlic heads to expose all the cloves. Fit the heads snugly in a baking dish. Dot each clove with margarine, then pour about ¼ teaspoon olive oil over each head. Sprinkle with thyme and pepper to taste. Cover and bake at 300° for 30 minutes. Uncover and bake for another hour until the garlic is tender. The husk should be golden brown and the cloves soft enough to squeeze out.

Of course, if you want to take the bite out of heart disease without pungent breath, odorless garlic capsules are available in many drug and health food stores. In general, one to two capsules of dried, odorless garlic powder equal one clove, Dr. Yeh says.

ligrams of omega-3 every day, says William S. Harris, Ph.D., an assistant professor studying dietary fats at the University of Kansas in Kansas City.

"It's better to try to get your omega-3's through your diet than supplements, but you have to live with reality," Dr.

Harris says. "And in reality, many people don't like to eat oily fish."

Health is a thing with feathers. "Poultry is an excellent alternative to red meat," says John Paraskos, M.D., an associate director of cardiovascular medicine and professor of medicine at the University of Massachusetts in Worcester. That's because chicken, turkey and other fowl usually contain fewer calories and less saturated fat than red meat.

To avoid adding unwanted fat to the meal, broil or bake fowl instead of frying it in cooking oils, he says. You can leave the skin on while cooking to help the meat retain moisture, but since the skin is high in fat, it should be removed before eating.

You also should eat dark meat sparingly because it has more fat than white meat, Dr. Paraskos says.

Make room for fiber. Soluble fiber found in certain grains, fruits and vegetables such as oat bran, green peppers, citrus fruits, beans and psyllium seeds may lower blood cholesterol by 10 to 20 percent.

"Soluble fiber is important. It has many beneficial effects," Dr. Lavie says. "Increasing soluble fiber consumption lowers your risk of coronary disease. It probably also decreases cancer risk, particularly for colon cancer."

Soluble fiber dissolves in water, but resists digestion in the gastrointestinal tract. It's still unclear how the process works, but some scientists theorize that as soluble fiber moves through your system, it bonds to bile acid (a digestive fluid that is made with cholesterol) and excretes it from the body. In order to replace those lost bile acids, the liver removes cholesterol from the bloodstream to make more bile.

"Besides that effect, people are probably benefiting in other ways," Dr. Lavie says. "Because soluble fiber is a filler, it satisfies the appetite. It makes people less hungry so they avoid eating foods that are high in saturated fat and cholesterol."

Get a load of oat bran. Of all the fibrous foods, oat bran has clearly been the star. Numerous studies have shown that oat bran significantly lowers serum cholesterol.

In one study of 140 men, researchers found that those who ate two to three ounces of oat bran a day reduced their LDL cholesterol levels 11 to 15 percent in six weeks. In a smaller study, 20 men who ate about four ounces of oat bran daily decreased their total and LDL cholesterol levels by 12 percent in just three weeks.

But while most researchers are convinced that oat bran is an effective way to reduce blood cholesterol, there has been some controversy because of the broad range of results from some studies. A few studies have found that the bran has virtually no effect, while others have shown reductions in blood cholesterol up to 26 percent.

To settle this issue, researchers at the University of Minnesota analyzed 12 previous studies of oat products, including oat bran, conducted since 1985. The researchers concluded that eating a daily dose of three grams of soluble fiber from oat products did cause a modest 2 to 3 percent reduction in blood cholesterol. That's still significant, because every 1 percent drop in blood cholesterol lowers your risk of dying from heart disease by 2 percent. Overall, the Minnesota study backs up the good things that other researchers have been saying about oat bran for a long time.

"If you go off bacon and eggs and substitute any whole-grain cereal with skim milk, you'll lower your cholesterol 6 to 8 percent. That's mainly due to what you took out of your diet," Dr. Castelli says. "But if you eat an oat bran-enriched cereal, you'll drop your cholesterol another 3 to 5 percent. We know that soluble fiber like oat bran does that.

"You'd be hard-pressed to find something else for breakfast that would be such a good first step in a total dietary program of controlling blood fats," he says.

Eat a hill of beans. Not only are beans low in artery-clogging fat, they are a good source of soluble fiber, which may help lower blood cholesterol, says James W. Anderson, M.D., professor of medicine and clinical nutrition at the University of Kentucky College of Medicine in Lexington. To get the heart-saving qualities out of legumes, try eating ½ to 1 cup beans, such as kidney beans, lentils, lima beans or pinto beans, a day. For variety, you can mix beans with rice, pasta or small amounts of chicken, meat or fish.

Pump up on pectin. Pectin, a type of soluble fiber found in apples, oranges and other fruits and vegetables, has lowered serum cholesterol about 8 percent in human studies at the University of Florida College of Medicine in Gainesville.

"It not only helps lower cholesterol levels, it also reduces the risk of coronary heart disease by reducing the amount of atherosclerosis in the arteries," says Frank Robbins, a biological scientist studying the effects of grapefruit pectin in conjunction with James J. Cerda, M.D., a professor of medicine in gastroenterology at the university.

As little as 15 grams of pectin a day—the equivalent of eating two to three grapefruit—might be enough to lower your heart disease risk, Robbins says.

KEEP YOUR ARTERIES "RUST-FREE"

Some researchers suspect that antioxidants such as vitamins C and E and beta-carotene may be an overlooked solution to heart disease.

These vitamins may combat oxidation, the same chemical process that rusts metals and turns butter rancid, which also alters cholesterol in harmful ways inside the body. Once LDL cholesterol is oxidized, cells in the immune system called macrophages ingest it. The macrophages become overloaded with fat globules and are transformed into foam cells. These foam cells collect in artery walls and begin the development of atherosclerosis. Some researchers suspect that this is the point where antioxidant nutrients exert their protective effect.

In the Nurses Health Study of 87,245 women, aged 34 to 59, researchers at Harvard University compared the vitamin intake levels of healthy nurses and those who had suffered heart attacks. The nurses who ate the most beta-carotene (a plant pigment that our bodies convert to vitamin A) had a 22 percent lower risk of heart attack than the nurses who ate the least. Fresh fruits and vegetables such as apricots, carrots, spinach, squash and sweet potatoes provided the beta-carotene. In fact, just one carrot, containing 15 to 20 milligrams of beta-carotene, can make a difference.

In addition, high amounts of vitamin E caused a 34 percent reduction in heart disease risk. Consuming slightly more than 100 I.U. of vitamin E daily could lower heart disease risk, according to the study. Vitamin E is found in nuts and green leafy vegetables. Here are a few simple ways to get more of these antioxidants into your diet.

Swallow the C. Men who consume lots of vitamin C have half the death rate from heart disease of men who don't get as much of the vitamin, says James Enstrom, Ph.D., an epidemiologist at the University of California, Los Angeles, who studied the vitamin consumption of 11,348 men and women. Women who take high doses of vitamin C seem to get less benefit from it than men do, but still have a 25 percent lower death rate from heart disease than women who don't take any. The protective effects of vitamin C appear to kick in at about 50 milligrams. That's equivalent to drinking about four ounces of orange juice a day. The maximum benefit occurred in those people who took about 300 milligrams.

Heavy smokers and people with diabetes probably need to consume about 120 milligrams—about ten ounces of orange juice—each day, says Ishwarlal Jialal, M.D., a researcher studying antioxidants at the University of Texas Southwestern Medical Center in Dallas. That's because these groups tend to have low blood levels of vitamin C and are at higher risk for heart disease.

Get a daily supplement. Denham Harman, M.D., Ph.D., professor emeritus at the University of Nebraska College of Medicine in Omaha and executive director of the American Aging Association, believes that vitamin supplementation is a good way to get the necessary amounts of antioxidants into your diet. "What it comes down to is how much you should take, and I don't think anybody really knows that answer right now," Dr. Harman says. "But what I tell people is to take 500 milligrams of vitamin C two to three times a day and 100 to 200 milligrams of vitamin E daily. I don't know if that will be sufficient. But in all probability, it will be beneficial to the heart and won't be harmful."

TAKING THE EXTRA STEP

For most people, making the dietary changes we've just suggested will be enough to dramatically lower their heart disease risk. But if a person's cholesterol level remains elevated despite making these dietary changes, or there is evidence of heart disease or extensive artery blockage, then a stricter approach may be necessary.

In fact, ongoing work by Dean Ornish, M.D., director of the Preventive Medicine Research Institute in Sausalito, California, indicates that some people with symptoms of atherosclerosis who make dramatic behavioral changes, including adopting a vegetarian diet that limits total dietary fat to less than 10 percent of calories, can reverse dangerous blockages in their coronary arteries.

"Some people still question the connection, but I think if you go on a very vigorous diet that lowers fat consumption to 10 percent of calories and cholesterol intake to less than 50 milligrams a day, you really can reverse atherosclerosis," says Dr. Lavie.

Finally, keep in mind that diet is just one part of a comprehensive plan that includes exercise, stress reduction and smoking cessation to keep your heart healthy. Just walking for 15 minutes at four miles per hour, three times a week, can make a difference.

"It's a matter of how you want to live your life," Dr. Kay says. "If you think it's important to eat junk food, smoke and lounge around, then you can sit back and say, 'Oh well, I'm going to die anyway.' But if you want to lead an active life for many years, you need to exercise, eat healthy foods and stop smoking."

WHAT'S THE SCOOP ON COFFEE?

Does drinking coffee really increase your chances of heart disease, as some scientists once suggested? Probably not, according to research.

Much of the hoopla that swirled around coffee a few years ago was generated by studies conducted in Scandinavia, where coffee is boiled rather than paper-filtered as it is in the United States. In those studies, researchers found that boiled coffee does significantly raise blood cholesterol and increases the likelihood of death from heart disease. "The coffee story is becoming a little clearer. We now know that it's the method of preparation used in Scandinavia that extracts compounds from coffee that are bad for cholesterol levels. Regular coffee, as it's prepared in America, probably does nothing like that," says Alan Chait, M.D., past chairman of the American Heart Association Nutrition Committee.

So a cup or two of coffee a day isn't the heart-stopping hazard some once imagined. "Although large amounts of caffeine can cause arrhythmia [irregular beats] in the upper chambers of your heart, moderate consumption won't give you too much grief," says Thomas Kottke, M.D., a cardiologist at the Mayo Clinic in Rochester, Minnesota.

High-Nutrition Recipes

SPICED CARROTS

Carrots have more going for them than you may suspect—especially in regard to heart health. They're high in soluble fiber, which has been shown to help lower cholesterol. And they're a wonderful source of beta-carotene, which doctors believe may also offer some protection against heart disease. This recipe gives cooked carrots a new, Middle Eastern twist. And it contains both olive oil and garlic, two more foods that may help ward off heart problems. Serve this dish with roast chicken or lemon-broiled fish.

1	pound carrots, thinly cut on the diagonal	½	teaspoon ground cumin Pinch of ground red pepper
3	cloves garlic		
2	tablespoons lemon juice	2	tablespoons minced fresh parsley
2	teaspoons olive oil		

Steam the carrots and garlic for 5 minutes, or until the carrots are just tender. Remove the garlic and set aside. Transfer the carrots to a large no-stick frying pan.

Mash the garlic and place in a cup. Whisk in the lemon juice, oil, cumin and pepper. Pour over the carrots. Toss over medium heat for 2 minutes. Sprinkle with the parsley.

Serves 4
Per serving: *75 calories, 2.6 g. fat (31% of calories), 3.7 g. dietary fiber, 0 mg. cholesterol, 42 mg. sodium*

SEA SALAD

Sardines are among those fish that are high in heart-healthy omega-3 fatty acids. If you're looking for a new way to incorporate them into your diet, this very easy salad should fill the bill. Serve it with crusty, whole-grain rolls. You'll notice that the percent of calories from fat in this salad is high, but that's because practically all the calories come from the beneficial omega-3's and monounsaturated olive oil—the vegetables are very low in calories. Keep in mind that it's the overall level of fat in your diet that's crucial for heart health, not the amount in any single dish.

1 sweet red or yellow pepper, thinly sliced	1 teaspoon Dijon mustard
1 large tomato, seeded and chopped	½ teaspoon dried basil Red and green leaf lettuce, torn into bite-size pieces
1 cup thinly sliced carrots	
½ cup thinly sliced scallions	2 cups alfalfa sprouts
2 tablespoons white-wine vinegar	1 can (3¾ ounces) water-packed sardines, drained and cut into bite-size pieces
1 tablespoon olive oil	

In a large bowl, toss together the peppers, tomatoes, carrots and scallions.

In a cup, combine the vinegar, oil, mustard and basil. Pour over the vegetables and toss to coat.

Line individual dinner plates with the lettuce. Top with the sprouts, then the vegetables. Arrange the sardines on top.

Serves 4
Per serving: *129 calories, 8.6 g. fat (60% of calories), 2.6 g. dietary fiber, 40 mg. cholesterol, 144 mg. sodium*

GINGER-SCENTED MACKEREL

Mackerel is another champ in the omega-3 department. (And don't forget that it's the heart-healthy fats that make this such a super fish, so don't be alarmed by the amount of fat in this dish.) This oriental way of preparing mackerel is so simple you'll want to have it often. Serve it with steamed green beans.

1 **pound mackerel fillet, divided into 4 equal pieces**	1 **tablespoon low-sodium soy sauce**
½ **cup thinly sliced scallions**	1 **tablespoon grated fresh ginger**
¼ **cup minced fresh coriander**	½ **teaspoon ground black pepper**
Juice of 1 lemon or lime	4 **cups hot cooked brown rice**

Coat an 8" × 8" baking dish with no-stick spray. Place the mackerel in a single layer in the dish.

In a small bowl, combine the scallions, coriander, lemon or lime juice, soy sauce, ginger and pepper. Spoon over the fish.

Cover the dish tightly with foil. Bake at 450° for 20 minutes, or until the fish flakes easily with a fork. Serve with the rice.

Serves 4
Per serving: *481 calories, 17.7 g. fat (33% of calories), 4.8 g. dietary fiber, 80 mg. cholesterol, 265 mg. sodium*

CREAMY MASHED POTATOES

Here's a way to get lots of garlic into your diet. But don't fret that the generous amount will overwhelm the rest of your meal. Parboiling tames garlic's flavor, so it blends in nicely with the mashed potatoes.

2   **heads garlic (about 30 cloves), unpeeled**

2   **pounds baking potatoes, peeled and cut into 1" cubes**

1   **cup buttermilk**

2   **tablespoons minced fresh parsley**

2   **tablespoons butter-flavored sprinkles**

½   **teaspoon ground black pepper**

Separate the cloves and drop into boiling water. Boil for 2 minutes. Drain and slip off the peels.

Place potatoes in a 3-quart saucepan and cover with cold water. Add the garlic. Bring to a boil and cook for 15 minutes, or until the potatoes are tender. Drain, then return the vegetables to the pan and stir over medium heat for 2 minutes to evaporate excess moisture.

Using a food mill or potato masher, mash the potatoes and garlic. Beat in the buttermilk, parsley, butter-flavored sprinkles and pepper.

Serves 4
Per serving: *214 calories, 0.9 g. fat (4% of calories), 2 g. dietary fiber, 2 mg. cholesterol, 181 mg. sodium*

CHAPTER 22

Energy and Performance

Choosing the Right Fuel

There he was, fitness and nutrition director for SportsMind, a Seattle-based company charged with boosting the performance of employees at Fortune 500 firms—and some of Larry Burback's charges were falling asleep in class. The rigors of lectures, obstacle courses and assorted team-building exercises were just too physically demanding for those who had tried to re-energize at lunch with a burger, fries and a coffee chaser.

But then SportsMind stopped merely talking about the importance of nutrition during its training sessions and began serving chicken fajitas, pita sandwiches stuffed with turkey, vegetarian lasagna and other low-fat meals and snacks.

They're not nodding off now. In fact, says SportsMind founder Chris Majer, the executives often report *increased* energy—even before completing the course. "It's a fairly common experience for them to tell us that their energy has been enhanced."

You may not be a captain of industry, but if you're like most of us, your ship of state could probably use a little extra steam.

In fact, having enough get-up-and-go just to get through the day—without feeling like you've run a grueling marathon—would probably make you happier than winning a gold medal.

Fortunately, experts say that if you're willing to feed your body the right fuel at the right time while including a moderate amount of exercise in your daily routine, you're on your way to the winner's circle.

For more proof, look no further than the role of nutrition in competitive athletics. "If you look at an athlete competing against another athlete of the same age, equal ability and equal training, at that point, diet can make a 100 percent difference in who claims the victory," says Ann Grandjean, Ed.D., chief nutrition consultant for the U.S. Olympic Committee.

Remember, your quest for more energy doesn't have to be a heroic struggle. The right nutritional choices can help boost stamina and make you a better performer at home, at the office or in the gym.

Energy Essentials

A crowd packed elbow-to-elbow at a buffet table is evidence enough that many people live to eat. But actually, we're supposed to eat to live. Although your body can produce some of the chemicals needed to keep you healthy, it's your mouth's sometimes-delicious job to supply what are called essential nutrients. Among them: carbohydrates, protein, vitamins, minerals—even some fat.

You've probably seen essential nutrients listed on cereal boxes and can labels under such assumed names as the U.S. Recommended Daily Allowance. But there's no secret about their task. Essential nutrients help promote growth and repair of skin and internal organs, regulate critical body processes, and—equally important—boost your energy.

When you're energetic enough to vacuum the rug, wash the windows, do the laundry and cook dinner as a warm-up for an evening of transmission repair, you've supplied your body with just the right mixture of these nutrients: Roughly 60 percent carbohydrates, 25 percent fat and 15 percent protein, experts say.

But when you can't even get yourself into first gear, you may be suffering the consequences of any number of energy-sapping eating sins, according to Liz Applegate, Ph.D., sports nutrition columnist for *Runner's World* magazine and author of *Power Foods*. Perhaps the worst: Missing a meal and then trying to compensate with a sugary snack.

"Any time you deprive your body of the fuel you need, you're setting yourself up for a fall," Dr. Applegate says. "And if you love sugary things, you're better off eating them after a meal. That way, your body gets the important nutrients instead of only empty calories from sugar." Or better yet, Dr. Applegate says, turn your sweet tooth into a craving for the energizer of the sports world—complex carbohydrates.

STAMINA FROM STARCH

The days of starch-bashing are definitely over. Elite athletes and weekend warriors have known the energy-boosting benefits of complex carbohydrates for years.

But the merits of carbs actually came to light in the 1930s, says William Fink, assistant to the director of the Human Performance Laboratory at Ball State University in Muncie, Indiana.

While breakthroughs were occurring in chemistry, physics and biology, two Swedish researchers studying amateur athletes like cyclists and skiers pushed exercise physiology to the edge of a new frontier by simply adding a little starch.

During their experiment, some athletes were fed potatoes and bread, foods loaded with carbohydrates; others were fed low-carbohydrate fare. Later, both groups were required to ride a bicycle to exhaustion. The results, repeated hundreds of times since that first test, were astonishing: The athletes

WHERE ARE THE CARBOHYDRATES?

If you're a moderately active male who weighs 150 pounds, you need to consume about 350 grams of carbohydrates each day. A variety of foods and their carbohydrate values are listed below.

Food	Portion	Carbohydrates (g.)
Raisins	1 cup	114.8
Dates	10	61.0
Potato, baked	1	51.0
Peanut butter and jelly sandwich	1	44.6
Spaghetti	1 cup	39.7
Bagel	1	31.0
English muffin	1	30.0
Apple juice	1 cup	29.0
Apple	1	21.1
Roll	1	19.6
Whole-wheat bread	1 slice	13.8
Low-fat milk	1 cup	11.7
Graham cracker	1	10.4
Saltine crackers	5	10.2
Carrot	1 med.	7.3
Spinach	½ cup	3.4
Coffee	¾ cup	0.7
Egg	1	0.6
American cheese	1 oz.	0.5
Diet cola	1½ cups	0.4

who ate the high-carbohydrate foods rode significantly longer than their counterparts, Fink says.

But it wasn't until later that scientists learned *why* carbohydrates boosted athletic endurance. And why complex carbohydrates like pasta, potatoes and bagels provide a more even-burning fuel than simple carbohydrates like jelly beans and sugary soft drinks.

Just as your fuel choices at the pump determine whether your car will be burning regular or premium gas, your food choices at the table determine whether you'll be getting the important nutrients your body needs for better performance, such as fiber, minerals, vitamins and complex carbohydrates, Dr. Applegate says.

Complex-carbohydrate foods, such as whole-wheat bread, pasta, grains, rice, vegetables and beans, are packed with nutrients and fiber.

Simple carbohydrate foods, such as candy, cookies, honey, presweetened cereals and soft drinks, are generally low in fiber and nutritional value.

The body burns both kinds of carbohydrates for energy. Simple carbohydrates are metabolized rapidly. Most complex carbohydrates contain fiber and pulp and take longer to break down into glucose, providing even, longer-lasting energy.

Some of the digested carbohydrates are recombined to form glycogen, which is stored in your liver and muscles as a reserve energy source that can be called upon for additional glucose as needed during a workout. Your brain is powered almost exclusively by glucose.

If you're engaged in moderate or intense athletic activity—running or bicycling, for example—your muscles' glycogen stores will be depleted in about an hour or two. Through such techniques as carbo-loading, however, an athlete can significantly increase the body's ability to store glycogen and, as a result, improve endurance.

You don't have to be a triathlete to benefit from complex carbohydrates. One of the most promising findings linking food and energy levels in regular folks came from a study at the University of California at Los Angeles. After nearly a month of eating a high-carbohydrate, low-fat diet—lots of bran, rice and vegetables and a little fish or fowl—and walk-

PASTA: THE PRE-RACE FAVORITE

Here's a fact to keep in mind next time you feel pressured preparing a spaghetti dinner for your family. The athletes at the U.S. Olympic Training Center in Colorado Springs eat more than $^1/_2$ *million* pounds of pasta a year, according to Terri Moreman, food service manager for the U.S. Olympic team.

The reason, in part: carbo-loading. Research shows that by stuffing themselves with starchy, high-carbohydrate foods like pasta each day for two to three days before an endurance event, athletes can essentially supercharge their bodies with energy to levels roughly twice those of a normal person. First developed in the late 1960s and early 1970s, carbo-loading is popular today with marathon and distance runners, cross-country skiers, cyclists and triathletes.

Before the technique was perfected, researchers thought it was necessary for athletes to consume a low-carbohydrate diet for three days before carbo-loading. The idea behind first dropping the carbs: Depleting the body of glycogen would make it hungry for even more. The unintended result: Athletes with low blood glucose levels were irritable and unable to train.

However, research by William Sherman, Ph.D., of the Exercise Physiology Laboratory at Ohio State University in Columbus, showed that three days of eating a moderate amount of carbohydrates prior to loading worked just as well as depletion—and without the side effects.

Today, endurance athletes are encouraged to rest two to three days before the event while consuming eight to ten grams of carbohydrates daily for each kilogram (2.2 pounds) of body weight. And that's the equivalent of a lot of pasta—roughly a 2-pound plateful.

ing twice a day, the participants—all in their seventies—significantly improved their performance on a treadmill, according to James Barnard, Ph.D., vice chairman of the Department of Physiological Science at UCLA. His conclusion: "People can significantly improve their work and health by switching to a high-complex-carbohydrate, low-fat diet and undertaking a walking program."

There's only one side effect associated with eating lots of carbohydrates. Research has shown that they may have a calming or relaxing effect in some people.

DON'T FORGET THE PROTEIN

A small amount of protein eaten with your carbohydrates could be just what the doctor ordered to prevent any carbohydrate calming tendencies that might occur and help keep mental performance at its peak, according to brain researchers Judith Wurtman, Ph.D., at the Massachusetts Institute of Technology.

The production of three important chemical neurotransmitters in the brain—serotonin, dopamine and norepinephrine—is influenced by the foods we eat, says Dr. Wurtman, in her book, *Managing Your Mind and Mood through Food*. Dopamine and norepinephrine help keep our mental performance up to speed. Serotonin, a calming chemical, makes us relax.

Eating protein prompts the creation of dopamine and norepinephrine, which keeps you more alert, Dr. Wurtman's research shows. Eating carbohydrates, though, sparks creation of serotonin—making you more relaxed.

The ideal interaction between the physical performance benefits of carbohydrates and mental performance benefits of protein is activated by this simple technique: Include three to four ounces of protein at lunch or dinner. The trick, Dr. Wurtman says, is to have several bites of protein with the carbohydrates.

Some good sources of protein, according to Dr. Wurtman, are shellfish, fish, chicken, veal, very lean beef, low-fat cottage cheese, skim or low-fat milk, low-fat yogurt, dried peas and beans, lentils and tofu.

FAT'S ROLE IN FATIGUE

For an essential nutrient, fat has a terrible reputation. The problem is, we eat way too much fat for our own good. On the average, Americans get 37 percent of their calories from fat. Think of it: Fat accounts for over a third of what we put in our mouths—while we only need roughly 2 percent to survive.

While the health problems associated with fat are well known, researchers are only beginning to understand what effect fat has on our energy levels.

There's strong evidence to suggest that high-fat meals slow digestion. As a result, you may feel sluggish, says Judith Hallfrisch, Ph.D., research leader for the Carbohydrate Nutrition Laboratory at the U.S. Department of Agriculture's (USDA) Human Nutrition Research Center in Beltsville, Maryland.

Once digested, some of the fat makes its way into the blood, actually making it thicker. According to Dr. Barnard, thicker blood slows circulation, reducing the amount of oxygen delivered by the blood to the rest of the body. Think of it as a raging river reduced to a slow-moving stream. Does less oxygen mean less energy? Could be, says Dr. Barnard. "That may be one of the reasons people are so lethargic in this country," he says.

But a study conducted by the Pennington Biomedical Research Center, a division of Louisiana State University in Baton Rouge, perhaps sheds the most light on the fat/energy debate. Researchers studying the effects of dietary fat on the energy levels of 44 women discovered that those who were getting fatter actually became less active after putting on the weight. "It appears to be a chain reaction," says Don

EATING FOR ENERGY MADE EASY

To ensure fuel for your busy day, sports nutrition columnist and author Liz Applegate offers these top ten eating tips.

1. Begin with breakfast. Skipping breakfast can undercut reading skills, memory and the ability to concentrate. Children who miss breakfast, research shows, have poorer school performance.

2. Carb-up. Complex carbohydrates such as beans, whole grains and vegetables, start to enter your system almost immediately, but because they break down slowly, they provide a steady stream of energy.

3. Cut the caffeine. Not only can caffeine let you down after an initial surge of activity during the day, but if you consume too much, you might even have trouble falling asleep at night.

4. Lunch lightly. Mental performance tests scores were lower for subjects fed over 1,000 calories at lunchtime. Remember to eat slowly; it takes 20 minutes for your brain to get the message that your stomach is full.

5. Schedule mini-meals. Eat at least a little something every three to four hours to keep energy flowing. Snack-

Williamson, Ph.D., director of the Psychological Service Center at Louisiana State University.

In any case, the U.S. Army isn't taking any chances. Army officials have enlisted the aid of experts at Pennington to slash fat, cholesterol and sodium from the menus of soldiers stationed at forts and garrisons across the country, according to Catherine Champagne, Ph.D., Pennington's assistant professor of research. "I think they feel that if the soldiers are in better shape, they'll get more out of them," Dr. Champagne says. "A healthier person is a more productive person."

ing throughout the day will give you the fuel you need to keep going, but only if you choose healthy items such as sport bars, rice cakes, plain popcorn, unsalted pretzels and muffins and bagels without butter.

6. Pull your sweet tooth. Or at least wait until the end of your meal to indulge. That way, normally fast-burning simple carbohydrates will mix with what's already in your stomach and be digested more slowly.

7. Pump up your protein. Carbohydrates are a great energy source but you also need some protein to increase alertness. Chicken, fish, and low-fat cottage cheese are good sources.

8. Replace a missed meal. If you do have to skip a meal, don't hold off until the next one to make up for the lost calories. Try a high-carb snack containing 200 to 300 calories, such as a sport bar, a bagel with fruit, or nonfat yogurt with pretzels.

9. Set your watch. Consistency pays. Eating frequently, every three hours or so, can keep energy levels up and prevent you from overeating.

10. In case of hunger, break glass. Always keep some emergency high-carb snacks on hand.

FIVE-MEAL-A-DAY PLAN

Before you get your own marching orders, make sure you've made plans to provide the food you need to fuel your day. And make sure you get that food at regular intervals. Skipping meals is a lot like writing your mind and body a bad check. And, boy, do they bounce! Your body is forced to rely on insufficient reserves of glycogen in the liver and muscles to fuel your activity, leaving you hungry, tired, and sapped of brain power, Dr. Applegate says. If you skip breakfast, for example, you're likely to concentrate less effectively in the late morning, work or study less efficiently, and then binge at lunch, she says. The experts who were interviewed all favored the idea of eating at least five times a day—even if some of those "meals" are quite small.

Breakfast. You want to use this opportunity to get your day off to a power start. Executives participating in SportsMind's early-morning training sessions fuel up on oatmeal, pancakes, fruit and fruit juices, and potatoes. Noticeably absent; runny eggs and high-fat bacon or sausage. "They're not going to get any of that stuff here," says SportsMind's Burback. If you're in a hurry, Dr. Applegate recommends a small stick of low-fat string cheese, a whole-wheat bagel and a can of orange-pineapple juice. "Whether you eat it in the car or while you're getting dressed, it doesn't matter," she says. "Just make sure you eat something good for you."

Midmorning snack. Eating something light at this point can help keep your performance at a peak until lunchtime. An apple is a common midmorning snack for Dr. Barnard. "I keep the apple machines here at UCLA in business," he says. Dr. Grandjean prefers cantaloupe.

Lunch. The idea here is to keep it lean and include some protein to heighten mental performance. Dr. Applegate suggests a chicken sandwich, along with whole-grain crackers and fruit. Chicken fajitas, pita-bread turkey sandwiches and soup are common lunch entrées at SportsMind, says Bruback.

Midafternoon snack. A modest repast here helps ensure against any post-3:00 P.M. droop. Midafternoon snacks range from Dr. Grandjean's yogurt to Dr. Applegate's sport bars. Also popular with our crew of experts: Rice cakes, bagels, muffins, hard pretzels, even sports drinks.

Dinner. Depending on what you've eaten earlier in the day, supper may be your main meal—or something less. In any case, the goal is the same: power for your evening activities. Dr. Barnard indulges in lean chicken or beef, while SportsMind serves vegetarian lasagna. Dr. Grandjean often restricts this meal to cereal with 1 percent milk.

DECISIONS, DECISIONS

Next time you have a choice between a diet soda and a chocolate bar, choose candy if you have an afternoon of pencil pushing planned. But yogurt would be even better.

That's the finding of a study at Tufts University in Boston that measured the mental performance ability of college men fed an afternoon snack of either diet soda, chocolate or fruit-flavored yogurt.

"The basic conclusion is that a calorie snack in the late afternoon had a beneficial effect on memory tasks and on the ability to pay attention," according to Robin Kanarek, Ph.D., professor of psychology and author of the study.

The men solved significantly more math problems in less time an hour after eating yogurt than they did after eating candy or drinking diet soda. Their visual reaction time was also better after eating either the yogurt or the candy, Dr. Kanarek says.

ENERGY ROBBERS

When a dawn-to-dusk schedule puts your dining in doubt, don't put your energy at further risk with the wrong kind of quick pick-me-up. Some energy boosters can actually backfire, becoming energy robbers that steal your spunk in the long run. In other cases, shortfalls of key nutrients can put the brakes on your go-power even more insidiously.

Caffeine. A proven short-term eye-opener, caffeine has even been found to enhance endurance in some athletes, Dr. Applegate says.

But the more coffee you drink over time, the more you'll need to just keep you going, let alone give you a boost, according to Dr. Applegate. Two cups a day isn't bad, she says. Once you're making hourly pilgrimages to the percolator, though, you know its time to cut back.

"Caffeine for a lot of people really is an energy robber because they become dependent on it," she says. "They make their day around various cups of coffee."

Just stopping what you're doing to fetch a cup cuts productivity. And many heavy coffee drinkers complain of such problems as anxiety, irregular heartbeat, insomnia, shaking and nervousness.

Sugar. It does have a reputation as a short-term energy booster. But turning to sugary snacks like cookies, cake and candy bars when your go-power sags isn't a wise move, says Dr. Applegate.

"The concern is that these high-sugar foods, which are devoid of important nutrients, like B vitamins and fiber, will displace more nutritious foods from your diet. So in that sense they rob you of what you could have had," says Dr. Applegate.

By choosing a snack with less sugar and more complex carbohydrates—carrot sticks, for instance—you'll gain the benefit of extra nutrients. If the urge to splurge on something sweet is still too great, compromise, says Dr. Applegate.

"When eating a high-sugar food like candy or cookies, it's best to moderate the amount and throw in something additional that will enhance performance like a muffin or a bagel," she says.

Nutritional deficiencies. Fatigue can also be the result of things that we fail to do, like not getting enough vitamins and minerals. For example, thiamine—a B vitamin found in breads, cereals and beans—is essential for energy. Without enough, you may feel lethargic and lose your appetite, experts say.

On the mineral front, iron deficiency can lead to anemia and corresponding fatigue, weakness, irritability and shortness of breath.

"At least 10 percent of the female population is iron deficient, and 60 to 80 percent have reduced iron stores. That's pretty scary. That tells you that there are lots of people walking around with marginal iron status," Dr. Applegate says.

POWERING UP WITH SPORTS DRINKS

Drinking and athletics rarely go together—unless you're talking about sports drinks. Once limited to Gatorade, no fewer than a half-dozen sports drinks are now common in America's locker rooms.

Amateur athletes and researchers have apparently made the same discovery: A sports drink made with the right proportion of carbohydrate (about 6 percent) moves into the bloodstream as quickly as plain water—and does a better job of enhancing energy.

And it may even be better than carbo-loading at giving a pre-race boost. Researchers from Ohio State University, Virginia Military Institute and the University of Wisconsin working together discovered that pre-race loading with a sports drink containing maltodextrin, also known as glucose polymer, helped endurance runners perform as well as those who feasted on precompetition meals of pasta—with less stomach discomfort.

Among the chief nutritional causes of iron deficiency: cutting back on meat (a superior iron source). In addition, runners, menstruating women and pregnant women are all susceptible to iron deficiency. Runners may lose extra iron when they sweat in large amounts. Menstruating women lose iron along with blood. And during pregnancy, a woman's body is programmed to put her baby's iron needs ahead of her own. Most women need 15 milligrams of iron a day (30 milligrams during pregnancy), men require just 10.

To pump up your iron, eat lean beef and other low-fat cuts of meat as well as enriched or whole-grain cereals. The caffeine in coffee and tea interferes with iron absorption, so it's best to avoid them. Instead, have a glass of orange juice. The vitamin C in citrus fruits helps iron absorption. Cooking in a cast-iron skillet can also boost your iron intake.

Whatever approach you develop to maximize your energy level, avoid what some executives have done. "They seem to have a fairly high level of nutritional knowledge," Sports-Mind's Majer says, "but they are relatively poor at acting on what they know."

High-Nutrition Recipes

POACHED SALMON WITH POTATO PANCAKES

When you need a steady boost of energy, combine some protein and complex carbohydrates. In this recipe, the salmon supplies the protein, and the pancakes kick in carbohydrates from the potatoes and apples they contain. This is a good way to use up leftover baked potatoes. You'll notice that the percent of calories from fat is a little high, but that's because salmon is a very good source of heart-healthy monounsaturated fat. When you combine the fish and pancakes with low-fat side dishes, the total percent for the meal will be reduced.

2	tablespoons lemon juice	1	tart green apple, peeled and cored
½	teaspoon ground black pepper	¼	cup fat-free egg substitute
4	salmon steaks (about 5 ounces each)	1	small onion, minced or shredded
2	large cold baked potatoes, peeled		

| 2 tablespoons grated
Parmesan cheese
½ teaspoon dried tarragon
Pinch of grated nutmeg
or crushed caraway seeds | 1 teaspoon olive oil
1 cup mild or medium
chunky salsa |

In a 8" × 8" glass baking dish, mix the lemon juice and pepper. Add the salmon and turn to coat both sides. Set aside.

Coarsely shred the potatoes into a large bowl. Then shred the apple into the bowl. Stir in the egg, onions, Parmesan, tarragon and nutmeg or caraway. Form the mixture into 8 flat pancakes about ½" thick.

Coat a broiler rack with no-stick spray. Add the salmon steaks. Broil about 4" from the heat for 5 minutes. Flip and broil for 5 to 7 minutes more, or until cooked through.

While the salmon is cooking, heat ½ teaspoon of the oil in a large no-stick frying pan over medium heat. Add 4 of the pancakes and sauté until browned on both sides. Repeat with the remaining oil and pancakes. Serve with the salmon and salsa.

Serves 4
Tip: *Baked potatoes are easier to shred if they're cold. If you don't have any leftovers, bake potatoes in the microwave then chill for at least 30 minutes.*

Per serving: *332 calories, 12.3 g. fat (33% of calories), 2.8 g. dietary fiber, 34 mg. cholesterol, 366 mg. sodium*

TURKEY PITA SANDWICHES

A turkey sandwich pairs high-quality protein with complex carbohydrate-rich bread. If you use pita bread, the sandwich will be nicely portable—take a half sandwich along to work for a midmorning energy boost.

2 cups diced or shredded cooked turkey breast	¼ teaspoon ground black pepper
½ cup diced sweet red peppers	½ cup fat-free mayonnaise
½ cup diced carrots	¼ cup nonfat yogurt
¼ teaspoon dried thyme	4 whole-wheat pitas, halved
	1½ cups alfalfa sprouts

In a large bowl, combine the turkey, peppers, carrots, thyme and black pepper. Stir in the mayonnaise and yogurt.

Spoon into the pita pockets. Top each half sandwich with sprouts.

Serves 4
Per serving: *260 calories, 3 g. fat (11% of calories), 1.5 g. dietary fiber, 49 mg. cholesterol, 656 mg. sodium*

CHAPTER 23

Staying Younger Longer

Anti-Aging Nutrients

Imagine old age without arthritis, cataracts, osteoporosis and memory loss. Imagine being able to stave off cancer and heart disease indefinitely. You may not need to have a rich imagination to picture a healthy old age. You may be able to live it.

Welcome to nutrition's "brave new world." Ongoing research, much of it done at the U.S. Department of Agriculture's (USDA) Human Nutrition Research Center on Aging at Tufts University in Boston, may yet make it possible to grow old gracefully, without growing chronically ill and infirm. The Human Nutrition Research Center is the only research center in the country whose sole purpose is to study the relationship between nutrition and the aging process.

Through proper diet—with the right amounts and kinds of nutrients—we may be able to remain healthy throughout the life that medical research and technology is prolonging.

YOUTH-FULL NUTRIENTS

Research on the aging process—like that coming out of the U.S. Department of Agriculture's Human Nutrition Research Center on Aging at Tufts University in Boston—suggests that maximizing the nutritional quality of your diet may slow down or prevent age-related problems that many people think are inevitable. The following are top food sources of key nutrients that have shown promise in anti-aging research. (Since a number of these nutrients are destroyed by light and air, store foods in airtight containers and avoid light exposure. Also cook foods for as short a time and in as little water as possible.)

Vitamin E. (RDA: 10 milligrams for men; 8 milligrams for women) Good sources: wheat germ, peanut butter, almonds, filbert nuts, sunflower seeds, shrimp and vegetable oils. Green leafy vegetables also supply vitamin E.

Vitamin C. (RDA: 60 milligrams for men and women) Good sources: citrus fruits and juices, strawberries, red and green peppers, broccoli, cantaloupe and fortified juices. Also, potatoes (white and sweet), mangoes, tomatoes and tomato juice, watermelon, honeydew, brussels sprouts, snow peas and cauliflower.

No Magic Bullet

With everyone looking for an easy answer, how close are we to an anti-aging supplement? "I wish I could say, 'We're almost there,' but I don't think we'll ever find a single magic bullet. Life is more complicated," says Jeffrey Blumberg, Ph.D., associate director of the research center and a leading authority on aging and nutrition.

"However, I must say vitamins E and B_6 are showing a lot of promise in our anti-aging research. We have done

Beta-carotene. (RDA: none) Good sources: carrots, winter squash, pumpkin, sweet potatoes, dark green vegetables (like spinach, kale and broccoli), apricots, cantaloupe, mangoes and peaches.

Vitamin B$_6$. (RDA: 2 milligrams for men; 1.6 milligrams for women) Good sources: chicken, fish, lean pork and eggs. Also, whole-grain rice, soybeans, oats, whole-wheat products, peanuts, bananas, plantains and walnuts.

Vitamin B$_{12}$. (RDA: 2 micrograms for men and women) Good sources: lean meats and fish. Also, milk products and eggs.

Folate. (RDA: 200 micrograms for men; 180 micrograms for women) Good sources: legumes, such as lentils, kidney beans and black-eyed peas; citrus fruit; whole-grain products and vegetables, particularly spinach.

Calcium. (RDA: 800 milligrams for men and women) Good sources: dairy products, broccoli, kale, collards and sardines.

Note: Fortified cereals may provide fair amounts of some or all of these nutrients. Check the labels, since products vary.

some exciting studies with these two nutrients; it appears that they affect the health of the immune system. Generally, immunity declines somewhat as we get older, making us more susceptible to bacterial and viral infections as well as certain diseases most common among the elderly, like cancer, arthritis and heart disease.

"Several studies have shown that certain nutrients may slow or prevent the decline in immunity," says Dr. Blumberg. "Our most striking work in this area was with vitamin E supplements in older people. We found that high doses markedly improved certain tests of immune function." For example, when they did a skin-patch test exposing the skin to certain toxins, the person normally would have reacted with a red swelling (caused when the immune system increases its output of white blood cells that surround and destroy the toxin). The reaction is an indication that the immune system is responding and fighting the antigen. "In older people, we found this response didn't occur because their immune systems are less vigorous," he says. "However, after giving older people vitamin E supplements, their response to the skin patch test was like that of younger people."

Researchers found that vitamin B_6 might play a role in the proper functioning of the immune system, too. Robert M. Russell, M.D., professor of medicine at Tufts Medical School, and Simin Meydani, Ph.D., of Tufts School of Nutrition, discovered that when healthy elderly people had vitamin B_6 almost completely taken out of their diets, their immune response went down, as expected. What wasn't anticipated was the finding that the amount of vitamin B_6 needed to restore immune function was much higher than the Recommended Dietary Allowance (RDA) of about two milligrams. And when the study participants were given higher than the RDA levels, their immune function was even better than it was before the study started! A word of caution, however: Vitamin B_6 can be toxic at high doses.

OLDER PEOPLE ARE SPECIAL

The Tufts findings suggest that the RDA for certain vitamins might not be high enough to put the brakes on the illnesses that accompany aging. "I believe that, for some nutrients, the RDAs should probably be increased as we age," Dr. Blumberg says. "In other cases, however, the RDAs may need to be lowered for older adults since the need for certain nutrients seems to decrease as we age."

Remember that the RDAs are nutritional guidelines designed to help prevent deficiency symptoms in the average healthy person. But there is a growing number of studies that suggest that the RDAs are not really appropriate or sensitive to the changing nutritional needs of aging adults. Nor are they focused on our most important public health objectives—preventing chronic diseases like cancer and heart disease.

"In most cases, the RDAs are extrapolations based on studies of younger people," Dr. Blumberg says. "If you look at the current RDAs, you'll see that although there are special amounts for children and young adults, there really aren't special amounts for people over age 51. But we're finding that the needs of younger adults are not the same as those of people in their sixties, seventies and eighties.

"Take the vitamin B_6 study as an example. While it was only a preliminary study, it does suggest the need for vitamin B_6 may increase with age and even higher amounts of vitamin B_6 might prevent or delay age-related changes in the immune system. More research needs to be done, however, before we can make any specific recommendations."

THE WEAR-AND-TEAR FIGHTERS

Certain nutrients, called antioxidants, have been shown to slow down the deterioration that accompanies aging. These nutrients, which include vitamins E and C and beta-carotene, may slow down or prevent damage from chemicals called free radicals. Free radicals occur naturally, for instance, when the fat and proteins you eat interact with the oxygen in your body to form toxic compounds. When there are too many free radicals, they can attack parts of your body's cells, like cell membranes, causing them to break down.

"There is a theory that aging is the result of accumulated damage from free-radical reactions, Dr. Blumberg says. "Fortunately, Mother Nature has provided a natural way to cope with free radicals, in the form of these antioxidants. Antioxidants help inactivate free radicals and prevent them from attacking cells. Each one seems to work in a different way to counteract free-radical damage, so they're all important."

Even if free-radical reactions don't cause aging per se, a growing body of evidence suggests they are involved in immune-function decline as well as in causing common age-related diseases, including heart disease and cancer. Based on experimental studies, some researchers believe antioxidants may help prevent these ailments.

As a case in point, a Harvard Medical School study revealed that 333 men with heart disease who were given beta-carotene supplements for an average of six years had fewer heart attacks and heart-related deaths than did men not given the supplements.

Researchers speculate that there may be a way to get a jump on stalling the aging process by increasing our intake of certain nutrients while in middle age. "My feeling is that if we can retard or reverse a phenomenon like the decline in immunity with nutritional intervention in older adults, then it's reasonable to speculate that we can slow age-related changes by having a relatively high intake of these nutrients in the middle years," Dr. Blumberg says. "Since research in this area is still in early stages, however, it will be years before we know whether certain vitamins—and what amounts—slow aging. We do know changes in the immune system—and in nutrient needs—are gradual. So I think it makes sense to pay special attention to your diet, increasing intake of nutritional foods, before you reach old age."

HOW TO GET MORE FROM LESS

With weight control a growing concern for many of us as we grow older, the question is: How do we eat more foods without consuming more calories?

Make the most of every mouthful. The most obvious way is to focus on foods that contain the greatest concentration of nutrients with the least amount of calories and fat. Most fresh fruits and vegetables, whole grains, lean meats and fish and low-fat or nonfat dairy products do that. Don't waste your calories on sugary soft drinks, sweet confections or alcohol—the so-called empty-calorie foods.

Burn more to eat more. Exercise can also help. By virtue of the fact that you're burning off more calories, you can eat more food than someone who doesn't exercise. When you eat more food, you have a better chance of getting more vitamins and minerals. Exercise can also optimize the way the body handles certain nutrients. "Calcium, for instance, seems to be incorporated into bone more efficiently if you exercise regularly," Dr. Blumberg says.

Consider extra vitamin E. Getting adequate amounts of vitamin E and other fat-soluble vitamins, which are found in polyunsaturated fats, can be difficult on a low-fat diet. "This is a major problem," Dr. Blumberg says. "Not only are many health-conscious people cutting back on fats of all types, but the polyunsaturated fats that are on the market tend to have less vitamin E than they used to because of processing methods. In fact, a study published in the *Journal of the Canadian Dietetic Association* indicated that people who went from a diet containing more than 30 percent fat calories to one providing less fat experienced a drop in vitamin E intake that placed them well below RDA levels. Even RDA amounts may not be enough to optimize immune function as we grow older. This may be one case when supplementation may be in order. Many vitamin E researchers suggest supplements of 100 to 400 I.U. per day; however, there aren't enough studies yet to be more specific than that."

CAN YOU BE TOO THIN?

Some newspaper reports have suggested that being underweight may actually prolong life. But Dr Blumberg isn't convinced. "As far as longevity is concerned, I don't think that there's much sound evidence that being underweight prolongs human life. Yes, numerous studies in rats and mice show that animals fed diets that are deficient in calories but adequate in protein, vitamins and minerals tend to live longer than animals fed normal diets. The problem is that these studies have only been done in animals that have very short life spans, and the findings may or may not apply to humans. We'll have a better answer years from now when ongoing studies in monkeys (which have much longer life spans and are biologically more like people) are completed by the National Institute on Aging (NIA)."

In the meantime, Dr. Blumberg doesn't recommend cutting back on calories if you're trying to stay younger longer. "I don't recommend caloric restriction because it's very experimental," he says. "Animals in caloric restriction studies are 'undernourished, but not malnourished.' They're on carefully planned diets that assure the animals are getting the right nutrients. People who try this on their own could easily become malnourished. I've already pointed out how important it is to have a nutrient-rich diet if you want to slow aging. That becomes much tougher if you cut way back on calories."

That doesn't mean, though, that it's okay to get fat as you grow older. "We're not talking about becoming obese," Dr. Blumberg explains. "This just suggests that maybe it's good to have a little fat reserve when you're older so that if you do develop some sort of disease, you have something to draw upon. Being a little heavier may also act as a hedge against the natural decline in appetite that tends to occur as we age. I'd say that if you were not overweight when you were younger, then you certainly shouldn't panic if you weigh up to 5 percent more than your youthful weight during middle age."

No matter what you weigh, your goal should be to keep up your muscle tissue by exercising. Since muscle tissue burns fat but fat tissue doesn't, that should help boost your

---

FIVE STEPS TO AN ANTI-AGING DIET

1. Decrease fat to less than 30 percent of your overall calorie intake.

2. Increase fiber to between 20 and 35 grams a day.

3. Eat foods rich in the antioxidants—vitamins E and C and beta-carotene.

4. Consume low-fat foods high in calcium.

5. Take a multivitamin/mineral supplement to ensure you're getting at least the Recommended Dietary Allowances.

---

calorie requirement. Thus, if you're exercising, you can afford more calories.

William J. Evans, Ph.D., chief of the Human Physiology Laboratory at Tufts, and his coworkers have done a series of studies to examine the impact of fairly intensive exercise training—involving a combination of activities like bicycling, walking and weight lifting—on people of various ages. "Not surprising, they found that people who exercised more were the most physically fit—whether they were young or as old as 90. What came as a surprise was the finding that the extent to which exercise helped a person maintain muscle mass seemed to depend on how "nutritionally fit" he or she was.

The researchers put people on an exercise program and gave them a liquid supplement containing a variety of vitamins and minerals as well as protein. They found that this regimen seemed to increase both muscle mass and strength in older people, but made no difference in young adults. "Since the supplement contained many different nutrients, we don't know which one or ones might have been responsible for the improvement," Dr. Blumberg comments. "But the fact that the participants were all eating pretty well balanced diets indicates that getting extra amounts of one or more nutrients might optimize the effect of exercise in middle-aged and older adults."

KEEPING THE MIND SHARP

There's also evidence that good nutrition might be able to keep our brains as healthy as our aging bodies. That's encouraging because many people fear the loss of mental acuity more than they fear some of the killer diseases.

"There's some exciting research going on aimed at keeping the brain young," Dr. Blumberg says. "For a long time we've known that people who are seriously deficient in B vitamins start to develop mental or cognitive troubles as well as other problems, such as anemia. But we now have sophisticated new tests that tell us when people are just borderline-deficient—when they show no outward or obvious signs of deficiency—in vitamins B_6, B_{12} and folate."

When someone is borderline-deficient in any of these nutrients, levels of an amino acid called homocysteine become elevated. "There's evidence that a small but significant number of elderly people have elevated homocysteine levels that return to normal when the mild deficiencies are corrected with B-vitamin supplements," says Dr. Blumberg. "Not only that, but preliminary studies suggest some people show improvement in memory and learning ability after B supplementation."

So what does this mean for younger people who want to stay sharp into a ripe old age? "Based on the limited evidence we have, I'd say that changes in cognitive function are gradual," Dr. Blumberg explains. "So you want to make sure that your diet is rich in these three nutrients—vitamins B_6, B_{12} and folate—because they seem to be particularly vulnerable to the aging process. I don't mean to imply, however, that taking B vitamins will prevent or reverse all cognitive changes related to aging."

Conserving Your Vision—And More

Speaking of keeping sharp, what about the eyes? Is there any dietary way to preserve your vision as you grow older?

Most people don't realize that cataracts afflict virtually everyone who lives long enough. The process, which results in loss of transparency of the lens of the eye and eventual loss of vision, usually starts around age 60. Cataracts can be easily corrected with surgery, but who wants to go through the trouble and expense if you can avoid it?

"Since we now know that cataracts develop because of free radical damage to the lens—for example, as a result of exposure to ultraviolet light from the sun—it makes sense that antioxidants would play a protective role," says Dr. Blumberg. Indeed, studies of older people by Paul F. Jacques, D.Sc., an epidemiologist at Tufts, showed that those with higher blood and dietary levels of vitamins E, C and beta-carotene had the lowest incidence of cataracts. But Dr. Blumberg points out there are no guarantees: I want to stress that this refers to a reduction in risk—some people who had high antioxidant levels also had cataracts. It may be that these people had more exposure to UV light when they were younger.

So what's the bottom line for people who want to do everything in their power to put the brakes on aging through nutrition? "In essence, eating a super high quality diet is crucial if you want to do all you can to stay young longer," Dr. Blumberg says. "It's especially important to key in on good food sources of vitamins E, C and beta-carotene. It's interesting that it keeps coming back to these antioxidants—whether we're talking about immune function, cardiovascular disease or cataracts. I'd work on eating good sources of B vitamins and folate as well. In addition, I'd go so far as to advise people who want to take steps to slow down the aging process to take a daily multivitamin/mineral supplement."

Research so far suggests that if you're an older adult, you should take a multivitamin/mineral supplement formulated at one to two times the RDA levels, plus eat a diverse diet low in fat and high in fiber. The idea behind this is that then you can die "young"—as late as possible.

CHAPTER 24

Cancer Prevention

It Starts on Your Plate

"**I give** up! Everything causes cancer!" Each time we read about a new cancer-causing substance in our diets we may react that way—feeling like it's hopeless. We might as well go ahead and eat, drink and be merry, we tell ourselves, because we all know what's next, and it's no fun at all.

But the truth is, not everything we eat or drink causes cancer. As researchers find out more about the things that cause cancer, they are also discovering foods and substances in foods that help to *prevent* cancer. In fact, some foods may be so good at discouraging cancer that the suspected beneficial components in these foods are being studied as potential anti-cancer *drugs*.

"In many cases, the foods that cut our risk for developing cancer are the same ones that protect us from other big killers—heart disease, diabetes and stroke," says Daniel Nixon, M.D., the American Cancer Society's vice president for detection and treatment. These foods, part of an all-around healthy diet, include fruits and vegetables, whose grains, beans, low-fat dairy products, fish and lean meats.

HOLD THE HAM

Baked ham with honey mustard. Beef jerky. Franks at the ballgame. Your idea of a treat? Better make it an occasional one.

Both the National Cancer Institute and the American Cancer Society suggest you limit your intake of salt-cured, smoked and nitrite-preserved foods such as ham, hot dogs, bacon and some varieties of sausage, cold cuts and fish. These foods contain a number of compounds chemically similar to the carcinogenic tars present in tobacco smoke. In population studies, people whose diet is top-heavy with such foods are more likely than normal to develop stomach or throat cancer.

What's considered a safe amount of these foods to be eating? "No one knows for sure, but if you consume a serving of something from this group once a week or less you're probably within a safe range," says Daniel Nixon, M.D., of the American Cancer Society.

LOOKING FOR CLUES

So far, much of what we know about food and cancer comes from population studies. These studies evaluate the health and eating habits of large groups of people. Some follow groups over many years to see who develops cancer; others look at people who already have cancer and work backward, asking questions about dietary habits in the past or analyzing nutrient levels in blood samples taken earlier. Both look for associations between what people eat, or don't eat, and the kinds of cancer they develop.

"It's these types of studies that have suggested that certain types of fruits and vegetables may help protect against mouth and throat cancer, for instance, or that point an accusing finger at high-fat diets when it comes to colon cancer," Dr. Nixon says.

Such studies lead researchers to estimate that about 35 percent of all cancer deaths are related to diet, and another 5 percent to alcohol consumption. That's an impressive percentage. It means that what we put in our stomachs may account for more cancer deaths than pollution, tobacco and occupational exposure to chemicals *combined*. And some types of cancer may have an even stronger dinner-plate connection. Some researchers believe that most cases of colon cancer and breast cancer may be food-linked.

THE KEY DIETARY FACTORS

Exactly what foods are cancer researchers most interested in, and why?

Fats. A high-fat diet seems to work in a number of ways to increase the risk of colon, pancreatic, breast, prostate and most likely other cancers. "A high-fat diet in general, and polyunsaturated fats specifically, are implicated," says Leonard Cohen, Ph.D., head of the Section of Nutritional Endocrinology at the American Health Foundation in Valhalla, New York. Monounsaturated fats (found in olive, peanut and canola oil) seem to be neutral, Dr. Cohen says. They neither promote nor protect. And fish oils seem to have a protective effect. But researchers don't know just why this is so.

Fiber. A low-fiber diet seems to promote colon and rectal cancer and may also contribute to the development of breast cancer, Dr. Cohen says. Populations eating high-fiber diets show reduced breast and colon cancer rates, and in animals, high-fiber diets are associated with decreased tumor development.

Fruits and vegetables. Diets low in fruits and vegetables have been associated with increased risk for colon, breast, prostate and other types of cancer. "Fruits and vegetables contain a multitude of possible cancer-preventing vitamins, minerals, fibers and other compounds," Dr. Nixon says.

Dairy products. A calcium-rich diet has been tentatively linked with reduced risk of colon cancer. Vitamins A and D in milk and other foods also seem to promote normal cell growth, experts say.

With those general points in mind, let's take a more detailed look at several specific cancer sites.

COLON CANCER

We'll start with colon cancer, which most researchers agree has the best evidence backing up its nutritional connection. Your colon is directly exposed to the consequences of a poor diet. Too much fat, especially saturated fat from animal foods, and not enough fiber from foods like whole grains, beans, fruits and vegetables, have made colon and rectal cancer all too common these days. Most population and animal studies show that diets high in fat and low in fiber increase the risk for colon cancer.

One study, by researchers at Harvard University, found that people who normally ate beef, pork or lamb every day could halve their risk of colon cancer by eating red meat just once a week and substituting fish or chicken on other days. Fat itself isn't carcinogenic, scientists say. But it sets off a chain reaction in the digestive system that can produce cancer-causing substances.

The typical American diet dishes out almost 40 percent of its calories from fat, or about 67 to 89 grams of fat a day. The current National Cancer Institute recommendation is to reduce fat intake to no more than 30 percent of calories. "An increasing number of researchers, though, believe an optimum cancer-protecting level is closer to 20 to 25 percent of calories," Dr. Cohen says. That translates to just 33 to 56 grams of fat a day, based on a daily intake of 1,500 to 2,000 calories.

A Bulking Effect

Fiber helps prevent colon cancer in several ways. It bulks up the stool, increases acidity in the colon and creates an environment that reduces the concentration of potential carcinogens. "And it may have other whole-body effects, such as reducing blood levels of hormones like estrogen, which could mean it can also fight breast cancer," Dr. Cohen says.

Some studies suggest that wheat bran and rye bran are most effective at reducing cancer risks. "Most cancer experts say that simply eating more fiber-rich foods—grains, legumes, fruits and vegetables—is the most important thing to do," says Moshe Shike, M.D., director of clinical nutrition at Memorial Sloan-Kettering Cancer Center in New York City. Dr. Shike is also director of the hospital's Diet Colon Polyp Prevention Program.

The average American consumes just 11 to 12 grams of dietary fiber a day. But you'll be well on your way toward the 20 to 30 grams recommended by the National Cancer Institute if you eat a bowl of high-fiber cereal, three slices of whole-grain bread, four servings of fresh vegetables and two pieces of fruit a day, says Abby Block, R.D., coordinator of clinical nutrition research at Memorial Sloan-Kettering. (Check the label on the cereal; it must provide at least 9 grams of fiber per serving to be considered high-fiber, Bloch advises.)

A Role for Calcium?

Some evidence also shows that certain vitamins and minerals may help protect against colon cancer. Calcium seems to be the most promising of these. A few studies link higher levels of calcium intake with a lower rate of colon cancer.

Like fiber, calcium seems to bind bile acids, which prevents them from irritating the colon wall. And it may help normalize growth and development of the cells lining the colon wall. Research indicates that a daily calcium intake of

1,200 milligrams or more is linked to decreased colon cancer risk.

"For right now, though, I'd say it's important to simply get the Recommended Dietary Allowance (RDA) of calcium—800 milligrams," says Dr. Shike. About one-third of all men and more than half of all women in the United States get less than 70 percent of the RDA for calcium, studies show.

THE CABBAGE CONNECTION

Diets rich in fruits and vegetables may halve your risk for colon cancer, according to several studies. "It's true that fruits and vegetables are markers for a low-fat, high-fiber diet, but it's probably more than that, because we know that fruits and vegetables are also very good sources of the dietary antioxidants," says Jeffrey Blumberg, Ph.D., who in addition to being the associate director of the U.S. Department of Agriculture's (USDA) Human Nutrition Research Center on Aging at Tufts University in Boston, also heads the Antioxidants Research Laboratory there. Antioxidants are substances that help block the formation of harmful oxygen breakdown products in the body.

In both animal and population studies there seems to be an independent protective effect for the antioxidants, Dr. Blumberg says. "Across the normal range of intake of fats and fibers—high or low—increasing intakes of the antioxidants provides additional cancer protection."

Vitamins E and C are two antioxidants that may play a direct role in neutralizing cancer-promoting nitrosamines in the stomach, Dr. Blumberg says. Nitrosamines are produced during the digestion of nitrates and nitrites, compounds found in especially high concentration in preserved meats.

How many servings of fruits and vegetables do *you* eat in a day? (Catsup doesn't count.) Try keeping track for a few days. If you are like a lot of people, you are lucky if you come anywhere near the five daily fruit or vegetable servings that would move you into the recommended consumption range. One survey of nearly 12,000 consumers found that only 9 percent met the USDA guidelines recommending five servings of vegetables and fruit a day.

BREAST CANCER

High-fat diets have also been implicated in the case of breast cancer, and in animal studies, the connection is particularly strong, Dr. Cohen says. (Some population studies find little linkage between breast cancer rates and levels of dietary fat, apparently because *all* the people in the study—even those eating the least fat—have a relatively high-fat diet—30 percent fat or more, Dr. Cohen says.)

Researchers are making the same tentative recommendations regarding breast cancer as they are for colon cancer: reduce your fat intake down to 20 to 25 percent of calories.

"We believe that cut would result in a significant decrease in the breast cancer rate," Dr. Cohen says. "We've seen in animals that there doesn't seem to be a continuum of gradually decreasing risk between fat intake and breast cancer. Instead, there seems to be a point somewhere—we don't know exactly where—between 25 and 30 percent of calories or lower, where the promoting effect of fat switches on."

TAMING ESTROGEN

Fiber—wheat bran in particular—seems to play a special protective role in breast cancer. How? High-fat diets appear to raise blood levels of estrogen, a female hormone that stimulates breast cell growth and may contribute to the development of breast cancer. Fiber reduces blood levels of estrogen, even in the face of a high-fat diet, researchers at the American Health Foundation have found.

"And in animals, when you combine a low-fat diet with a diet high in wheat bran, you reduce the rate of mammary

COULD A CLOVE A DAY KEEP CANCER AT BAY?

For folk healers around the world, garlic is a revered remedy for everything from intestinal parasites to heart disease.

And evidence that this odiferous globe may also fight cancer has been mounting steadily. Two studies found reduced rates of stomach cancer, and another showed reduced rates of colorectal cancer in people who indulged liberally in garlic-laden foods. Another found that rats that ate the equivalent of about 20 cloves of garlic a day had a marked decrease in mammary cancer.

The sulfur-containing substances that give garlic its pungent, elevator-clearing aroma are also what probably give it its anticarcinogenic activity, says Daniel Nixon, M.D., of the American Cancer Society. These compounds may inhibit the body's production of harmful biochemicals; they may also enhance immune system function so that carcinogens can be intercepted before they can damage cells, Dr. Nixon explains. "And some components of garlic may also have the potential to stimulate the liver to clear toxins out of the body," he says.

Both raw and cooked garlic may have beneficial effects, although the raw may be somewhat more potent. No one knows how much you'd need to eat to see a protective effect. And little cancer-related research has been done with deodorized garlic extracts available at health food stores, Dr. Nixon says.

If you like garlic, indulge in good health. (And invite your friends to join you. If they're eating it, too, they'll never notice *your* breath.) One serving suggestion: Roast whole cloves, then squeeze the insides onto toasted Italian bread lightly brushed with olive oil and fresh rosemary. Enjoy!

cancer even further than you do with a low-fat diet alone," Dr. Cohen says. Here again, the suggestion is to double your fiber intake, to about 30 grams a day.

Diets high in fruits and vegetables also seem protective against breast cancer. Such diets are naturally low in fat and high in fiber. And there are also potentially protective constituents in these foods, says Dr. Blumberg.

Vitamins C, E and A and beta-carotene (a vitamin-A precursor found in many fruits and vegetables) and selenium (a trace mineral found in grains and seafoods) may all play a role. "Low intake of any one of these nutrients has been associated with higher rates of breast cancer," Dr. Blumberg says. "The link so far is strongest for beta-carotene and vitamin C and weakest for vitamin E, even though pharmacological doses of vitamin E have been used to treat fibrocystic breast disease, and there has been some success along those lines."

In one study, breast cancer risk was almost twice as high in women eating the fewest carotene-rich foods, compared with women eating lots of those foods. (The low beta-carotene group ate less of the following: tomato juice, vegetable juice cocktail, tomatoes, corn, asparagus, strawberries, apples, grapefruit, lemons and limes.) The risk appeared to drop off significantly once women reached a beta-carotene intake of more than 5,824 I.U. per day, the researchers note.

LUNG CANCER

In population studies, one category of nutrient stands out as being consistently associated with reduced rates of lung cancer: It's the carotenoids (including beta-carotene)—the pigments found in green leafy vegetables such as kale and yellow and orange fruits and vegetables such as carrots and cantaloupe.

Other nutrients—vitamins A, E and C and selenium—may also cut your risk for lung cancer, but in population

EASY DOES IT WITH ALCOHOL

Do alcoholic beverages cause cancer? Scientists can't say for sure. Studies do consistently show that people considered "heavy drinkers" (more than one or two drinks daily) have higher than normal rates of cancer of the mouth and throat. Heavy drinking has been less strongly linked with cancer of the esophagus, stomach, pancreas and liver. (Some studies show an association; others don't.) "Since heavy drinkers have notoriously poor eating habits and often smoke cigarettes, it's hard to say exactly what's causing what," says Clark Heath, M.D., the American Cancer Society's vice president for epidemiology and statistics.

If alcohol does promote cancer, it may do so by compromising the liver's ability to detoxify potential cancer-causing substances, by irritating the mouth and throat in a way that makes them more susceptible to cancer or by carrying cancer-causing substances produced during distillation. (Darker liquors, such as rum, bourbon and scotch are more likely culprits here.)

"When it comes to moderate or light drinking, the picture is even murkier," Dr. Heath says. One well-publicized study by Harvard researchers showed an increase in breast cancer in women who had even a few drinks a week. But while most researchers agree that the more a woman drinks, the greater her risk for breast cancer, many say that for the average woman drinking alcohol in moderate amounts (one drink or less a day), that risk is so small there's no need to stop drinking. "And risks for other cancers with light to moderate drinking seem small, too," Dr. Heath says.

What's a safe ceiling? According to the American Institute for Cancer Research, under no circumstances should you drink more than 1.5 ounces of pure alcohol a day. You'd get that amount in two 12-ounce beers, 8 ounces of table wine or two shots of straight spirits.

A REASON TO DRINK GREEN TEA?

Could an Eastern passion for green tea be one reason Japanese men can smoke more than American men but still have lower rates of lung cancer? Researchers studying the tea think it may.

In one study, consumption of green tea cut the lung cancer rate by 45 percent in mice exposed to one of the most potent cancer-causing components in cigarette smoke. Other studies in animals suggest that drinking green tea could cut the rates of stomach and liver cancer as well.

"Many constituents in green tea are capable of blocking cell mutations which could set the stage for cancer," says Chi-Tang Ho, Ph.D., professor of food sciences at Rutgers University in New Brunswick, New Jersey. "The tea contains a wide variety of antioxidant compounds that have demonstrated significant cancer-preventive activity in animals."

Green tea is made from the same plant as the black tea commonly used in western countries. But the leaves undergo less processing. (Black tea is known to contain much lower amounts of certain protective antioxidants than green tea.)

Many Japanese researchers are encouraging people to drink up and live long. American researchers say one or two cups of green tea a day won't hurt you, but that more research is needed to confirm any health benefits—or risks.

studies, these nutrients are less consistently associated with reduced rates of lung cancer than are carotenoids, says Jerry McLarty, Ph.D., of the Department of Epidemiology and Biomathematics at the University of Texas Health Science Center at Tyler.

Dr. McLarty is directing a clinical trial using beta-carotene and vitamin A (retinol) in a group of people at up to 100 times the normal risk for lung cancer—smokers who have been exposed to asbestos. The study will see whether large amounts of these nutrients (equivalent to several pounds of carrots a day) reduce these men's risk. Several other studies using varying doses of these nutrients are being conducted around the country.

"We realistically should expect that some of these trials won't come up with positive results, but that doesn't mean the idea isn't a good one," Dr. McLarty says. "One of the problems all of us have had to face is that we don't know how much of these nutrients to give and how long to give them. We know that years of the right kind of diet has been shown to protect people, but can you overcome a lifetime of asbestos exposure and cigarette smoking with just a short period of supplementation, even at fairly high levels? We don't know."

Until results are in, "we can only recommend what we know—diets that are high in fruits and vegetables." And no dietary changes reduce your risk of lung cancer as much as not smoking, Dr. McLarty emphasizes. "Smoking increases your risk tenfold. With these nutrients, at best, we may be able to cut that risk in half."

Cancer-Proofing Your Diet

So, to sum up, what overall strategies can you take to minimize your risk of developing cancer?

Carve away fat. Cut a quarter, a third or even half of the fat calories in your diet. "Cutting down on total fat should be your main concern, and you may also want to cut back on polyunsaturated fats," says Bloch.

Try substituting broiled fish, skinned chicken breasts, ground turkey burgers or a vegetarian main dish for red meat.

And when you do eat red meat, reduce your serving size to about three ounces (about the size of a deck of cards.) Switch to 1 percent fat or nonfat milk. Sauté foods in fruit juice or vegetable stock instead of oil or butter. Use reduced fat or nonfat versions of cheeses, salad dressings, mayonnaise, ice cream, yogurt and sour cream. Use nonfat butter-flavored sprinkles such as Butter Buds instead of the real thing.

Fill up on fiber. Many cancer prevention specialists believe we would do well to double our average fiber intake to 30 grams or more a day. To do that, you need to eat high-fiber foods throughout the day: Eating three or four servings of whole grains and beans and five servings of fruits and vegetables a day will provide plenty of fiber. "If you've been on a low-fiber diet, avoid intestinal problems by increasing fiber intake gradually," Block says. "Your system needs time to get used to handling and processing fiber."

Bran cereals (nine or more grams per serving) and beans (with up to seven grams) are significantly higher in fiber than other food sources. A slice of whole-wheat bread has about two grams of fiber, and so does a serving of broccoli. Most fruits and vegetables have two to four grams of fiber per serving.

Fruits highest in fiber are dried figs, peaches and apricots; prunes; raisins; kiwi; pears (with skin); rapsberries; oranges; blackberries and apples (with skin). Vegetables highest in fiber are artichokes, brussels sprouts, potatoes (with skin), corn, peas, carrots and sweet potatoes. Real rye bread, usually found in delicatessens, is also high in fiber. So are most rye biscuits or wafers.

Go for the orange, green and red. Dark leafy greens and orange, red or yellow fruits and vegetables are generally rich sources of carotenoids, including beta-carotene, Bloch says. Top choices: sweet peppers, carrots, winter squash, pumpkin, sweet potatoes, spinach, kale, broccoli, apricots, cantaloupe, mangoes and peaches. Hold the iceberg lettuce; it's mostly water and doesn't have much beta-carotene or fiber. Other good leafy greens are romaine, buttercup or red sail lettuce; radicchio; endive and collard or mustard greens.

Crunch on the cruciferous crowd. Broccoli, cauliflower, cabbage, bok choy, brussels sprouts, rutabaga, watercress and some of the new hybrids like broccoflower and orange cauliflower are all in this group. These vegetables contain high levels of indole gluosinolates (indoles for short), compounds that appear to have a variety of cancer-fighting talents. They seem to block carcinogenic changes in the colon and other organs.

For maximum indoles, eat them raw. Or make low-fat coleslaw, borscht, ground-turkey-and-rice-stuffed cabbage rolls or an apple-cabbage side dish.

Bone up on calcium. Eat a cup of low-fat or nonfat yogurt, with 452 milligrams of calcium. Drink a glass of skim milk, with 302 milligrams of calcium per cup. Stock up on sardines. One can of Atlantic sardines offers 351 milligrams of calcium, plus 1.4 grams of omega-3 fatty acids, which may have their own anti-cancer talents.

Add antioxidants. Vitamins E and C, beta-carotene and the trace mineral selenium, are antioxidant nutrients. They help to protect cells from membrane and chromosome damage that can lead to cancer, Dr. Blumberg explains. They may also neutralize some carcinogens you may eat, inhale or produce in your body.

Vitamin E is found in almonds, sunflower seeds, wheat germ, peanut butter, filbert nuts, shrimp and vegetable oils. "These foods are all high in fat, though, so don't go overboard eating them," Bloch points out. Citrus fruits and juices, strawberries, red and green peppers, broccoli, cantaloupe and fortified juices are all great sources of vitamin C. Orange and yellow vegetables and fruits are good sources of beta-carotene. Sources of selenium include fish and shellfish (tuna, salmon, oysters, shrimp) and Brazil nuts. Whole grains can be a good source if they're grown in selenium-rich soil. Grains grown in the United States are generally good sources of selenium, Bloch says.

Go easy on smoked foods. Salt-cured, smoked and nitrite-preserved foods like hams, hot dogs and bacon contain compounds similar to the carcinogenic tars in tobacco smoke. In population studies, these foods are associated with a rise in throat and stomach cancers. "Eat these foods only on special occasions," Bloch suggests.

Put a ceiling on the hard stuff. Never drink alcohol when you're thirsty. Start with water or juice to satisfy your thirst. "Dietize" any alcohol you do consume by ordering diluted drinks such as wine spritzers (wine mixed with sparkling water and ice.) At parties, eat before you drink and while you're drinking to help limit the amount you drink. Don't allow your drinks to be continually "freshened up" with alcohol. It's an easy way to drink more than you planned.

High-Nutrition Recipes

OVEN-ROASTED TOMATO SOUP

When the American Cancer Society geared up for its third annual Great American Food Fight against Cancer, it enlisted the help of top chefs—professionals who could create truly delicious recipes that people would enjoy. One of the chefs was Victor Gielisse, owner of the acclaimed Actuelle restaurant in Dallas. Among his culinary creations were the following recipes. This unusual tomato soup could be a wonderful first course or a light lunch.

20 Italian plum tomatoes	1 teaspoon ground cumin
1 teaspoon canola oil	1 teaspoon ground
1 tablespoon minced fresh parsley	coriander
1 teaspoon dried basil	½ teaspoon ground black pepper
1 teaspoon dried tarragon	1 teaspoon chopped fresh coriander
4 cups defatted chicken stock	

With a small sharp knife, lightly score the peel on each tomato. Halve lengthwise and scoop out the seeds. Place the tomatoes, cut side down, on a baking sheet. Rub with the oil and sprinkle with the parsley, basil and tarragon. Bake at 250° for 1½ to 2 hours, or until softened.

Puree the tomatoes in a blender or food processor. Transfer to a 3-quart saucepan. Add the stock and bring to a boil over high heat. Stir in the cumin, ground coriander and pepper.

Ladle the soup into bowls and garnish each serving with fresh coriander.

Serves 6
Per serving: *57 calories, 2.2 g. fat (34% of calories), 1.4 g. dietary fiber, 0 mg. cholesterol, 64 mg. sodium*

PAN-SEARED LAMB

Although this individual recipe gets a fairly high percent of its calories from fat, the actual grams of fat are reasonable for a red-meat dish. And serving it with Tuscan Beans (page 458) brings the figure down to 30 percent.

1 pound lamb loin, trimmed of all visible fat	½ teaspoon red-pepper flakes
2 tablespoons canola oil	½ teaspoon ground black pepper
1 teaspoon minced garlic	¼ teaspoon dried thyme
1 teaspoon minced shallots or onions	¼ teaspoon dried basil
1 teaspoon mustard seeds	

With a sharp knife, cut the lamb crosswise into 6 medallions. In a 9" × 13" baking dish, combine the oil, garlic, shallots or onions, mustard seeds, red-pepper flakes, black pepper, thyme and basil. Add the lamb and turn to coat both sides. Cover, refrigerate and allow to marinate for 2 hours.

Preheat the oven to 375°. Heat a large no-stick frying pan over medium-high heat until hot. Add the lamb and sear on both sides until golden brown. Transfer to a baking dish and bake for 6 to 10 minutes, or until just cooked through.

Transfer to a platter. Cover and chill. To serve, cut into very thin slices.

Serves 6
Per serving: *149 calories, 9.2 g. fat (56% of calories), 0.1 g. dietary fiber, 53 mg. cholesterol, 59 mg. sodium*

RIGATONI IN MUSHROOM BROTH

You may serve this as a soup or as a "brothy" main dish. Chef Gielisse likes a mixture of mushrooms, including porcinis, shiitakes and morels, but you may use whatever kind you prefer. For variety, you may add some protein such as cooked chicken, turkey or seafood.

1 **pound rigatoni or other tubular pasta**	1 **tomato, seeded and finely diced**
1 **red onion, thinly sliced**	2 **tablespoons sherry extract (optional)**
1 **tablespoon minced shallots**	3 **tablespoons chopped fresh basil**
1 **teaspoon minced garlic**	¼ **teaspoon ground black pepper**
2 **tablespoons canola oil**	
¾ **cup finely diced mushrooms**	3 **tablespoons grated Parmesan cheese**
4 **cups defatted chicken stock**	

Cook the pasta in a large pot of boiling water until just tender. Drain and set aside.

In a 3-quart saucepan over medium-high heat, sauté the onions, shallots and garlic in the oil for 2 minutes. Add the mushrooms and sauté for 5 minutes.

Stir in the stock, tomatoes and sherry extract, if desired; bring to a boil, stirring often. Reduce the heat to low and simmer for 5 minutes. Add the basil and pepper. Stir in the pasta and heat through.

To serve, ladle into soup plates. Sprinkle with the Parmesan.

Serves 6
Per serving: *378 calories, 7.8 g. fat (19% of calories), 1.9 g. dietary fiber, 2 mg. cholesterol, 121 mg. sodium*

TUSCAN BEANS

Fiber has been shown to help prevent various types of cancer, especially those of the digestive tract. Beans are loaded with fiber, so including them in your diet makes plenty of sense. This salad can be made ahead and marinated overnight. If you neglected to presoak the beans, you may take this shortcut: Place them in a 2½-quart glass casserole and cover generously with cold water. Microwave on high for 15 minutes. Stir, cover and let stand until the beans have swelled up, about 15 minutes. Drain and proceed with your recipe.

18 ounces small white dried beans, soaked overnight	2 tablespoons minced fresh parsley
1 large carrot, diced	½ cup rice-wine vinegar
1 celery stalk, diced	3 tablespoons olive oil
1 red onion, diced	¼ teaspoon ground black pepper
¼ cup diced green, sweet red or yellow peppers	
2 tablespoons snipped chives	

Drain the beans. Cook in fresh water until tender, about 1 hour. Drain and rinse with cold water. Cover and refrigerate until well chilled.

In a large bowl, combine the beans, carrots, celery, onions, peppers, chives and parsley.

In a small bowl, whisk together the vinegar, oil and pepper. Pour over the bean mixture and toss to combine. Let marinate at room temperature for 2 hours before serving.

Serves 6
Per serving: *364 calories, 7.9 g. fat (20% of calories), 8.8 g. dietary fiber, 0 mg. cholesterol, 22 mg. sodium*

CHAPTER 25

Sex and Reproduction

The Dietary Factor

Who'd ever think that the orange juice you toss down at breakfast or the grilled chicken breast you sink your teeth into at lunch has anything to do with your sex life?

That's right. Your *sex life*.

It only makes sense that what you eat has an impact on your sexual self. Your reproductive system depends on good nutrition to function optimally, just as the rest of your body does.

Hormone-producing glands like the ovaries and testes slow down or shut down if the proper building materials—protein, fat, certain vitamins and minerals—aren't available in needed amounts. Some areas with high cell turnover, such as the cervix and testes, show signs of abnormal or slowed cell growth when they're low on nutrients like folate or zinc.

In fact, several aspects of reproduction—from sex drive to fertility to delivering a healthy baby—may depend on adequate nutritional status.

CAN FAT KILL ROMANCE?

A steady diet of cheeseburgers, french fries, cheesecake and other fatty foods may leave some men uninterested in sex. That, at least, is what researchers are theorizing after their study suggested that fatty meals may actually curb the production of testosterone, a hormone that can influence sex drive.

Four hours after serving fatty shakes to a group of eight men, the researcher saw the men's blood levels of testosterone decrease by 30 percent. When the men drank a low-fat drink of carbohydrates and protein or a nonnutritive drink instead, this sex hormone was unaffected.

"We looked only at the immediate result of one high-fat meal, though it may be hypothesized that after some time a high-fat diet could lower testosterone and weaken a man's sex drive," says A. Wayne Meikle, M.D., professor in the Division of Endoctrinology and Metabolism at the University of Utah in Salt Lake City.

Testosterone levels can also affect a woman's sex drive, but this study only looked at men.

BOY MEETS GIRL

For all the time and trouble we go through to prevent it, you'd think pregnancy would happen naturally if we just let it. For most couples, that's the case.

But about one of every six couples has trouble conceiving. They have tried, without success, for a year or more, to produce a baby. Often the problem can be disgnosed and corrected. But sometimes the problem is not so obvious and seems to be related to hormonal or metabolic imbalances. That's where it might pay to see if your eating habits and lifestyle are thwarting your chances for parenthood, experts say.

TURN-ON FOODS?

How about a nice steaming bowl of sea slug soup? Some ginseng tea? A plate of raw oysters?

For centuries, people around the world have turned to these and other foods, herbs and concoctions in an attempt to fuel sexual desire and perk up performance. But do they really work?

Overblown claims and lack of proof led the Food and Drug Administration in 1990 to prohibit interstate sales of any over-the-counter product that claims to act as an aphrodisiac or to restore sexual vigor. In this government agency's eyes, there's no such thing.

But some think a few of these foods may actually have something going for them.

Oysters and other shellfish, which have long been considered to have aphrodisiac properties in many cultures, are a rich source of zinc, which plays a major role in male testosterone production. For man lacking this mineral, oysters might indeed be fuel for love.

Ginseng, a plant whose gnarled root is dried, ground and powdered, has a 5,000-year-old reputation as a cure-all. Some studies report ginseng steps up mating behavior in rats, but its effects on humans have not been proven.

Yohimbine, which is really a chemical, not a food, is derived from the bark of the African yohimbe tree. It has a long history as a "love potion"and is now used as a prescription drug to treat male impotence. Just how it works isn't understood. Some investigators think it acts directly on the central nervous system, others through complex hormonal pathways. In studies, it has consistently im-

Stress, alcohol and cigarettes are well-known monkey wrenches when it comes to making babies, for both men and women. Improper nutrition has long been recognized as a

proved symptoms in about one-third of men with physical or psychological impotence.

Many reputed aphrodisiacs, however, probably operate only by power of suggestion, if at all. "If you believe a particular food or herb is going to work, it may just work for you," says University of Florida anthropologist George Armelagos. And the rarer and more expensive the food, the more powerful its suggestive force. Whole species of animals (like rhinos and sea turtles) have been hunted to near-extinction just for their horns, penises or sex glands, says Armelagos, coauthor of *Consuming Passions*.

Some health food stores carry both male and female "formulas" that imply that they can improve sexual performance. These products have a variety of ingredients, including vitamins, minerals and herbs. The male potency versions may include yohimbine, ginkgo (added for its alleged ability to increase peripheral vascular circulation) and saw palmetto (a palm used in European herbal remedies for prostate problems).

"In small amounts, these products are unlikely to hurt you," says William J. Keller, Ph.D., head of the Division of Medicinal Chemistry and Pharmaceutics at Northeast Louisiana University's School of Pharmacy in Monroe.

But as with any other product, it's important to read the label and understand what's in the product, Dr. Keller says. "One potential danger is that, by relying on an over-the-counter remedy to treat your symptoms, you may be neglecting a problem that needs medical treatment," he says. "Impotence can be an early sign of diabetes or peripheral vascular disease. And lack of sexual desire can be cause by depression. Both symptoms are frequent side effects of certain prescription medicines."

factor in infertility, too, but when it comes to understanding the details, "We know more about cows than we do humans," says Earl Dawson, Ph.D., associate professor of obstetrics and gynecology at the University of Texas Medical School at Galveston.

In men, infertility sometimes means that sperm are too few, too slow or downright defective, Dr. Dawson explains.

Several different nutrients have been recommended over the years to improve a man's "batting average." Two of the more commonly recommended—zinc and vitamin C—are both highly concentrated in semen and play an important role in male sexual functioning.

Ask your doctor to check your zinc status. "We proved long ago that zinc deficiency prevents or delays sexual maturation in men," says Ananda Prasad, M.D., Ph.D., professor of medicine at Wayne State University in Detroit and a leading researcher on the health effects of zinc. "It's also known that, in adult men, zinc deficiency leads to reduced levels of testosterone, the main male hormone." Low testosterone levels lead to impaired fertility.

In one study, Dr. Prasad and colleagues found that men on diets deliberately made low in zinc had significant drops in testosterone levels and in sperm count. When the men's zinc intake was restored to levels on a par with the Recommended Dietary Allowance (RDA), both the testosterone levels and sperm count slowly came back to normal in 6 to 12 months.

Since low sperm counts can be caused by many things, Dr. Prasad doesn't routinely recommend zinc supplements as a quick fix for male infertility. "But if a man is zinc deficient and has low testosterone levels, he may benefit from additional zinc," Dr. Prasad says.

The RDA for zinc, 15 milligrams, is thought to be more than adequate to keep up zinc stores in healthy young men. In one study, though, people who got only 10 milligrams a day showed blood zinc levels dropping by 1 to 2 milligrams a day. Most people get 10 to 15 milligrams of zinc a day, studies show. Try oysters, wheat germ, pumpkin seeds, beef, lamb and shiitake mushrooms for good amounts of zinc.

Keep sperm moving with vitamin C. Vitamin C plays a much different role in male fertility. It maintains sperm function.

A lack of vitamin C makes sperm clump together, a problem called agglutinization that is readily apparent when sperm are examined under a microscope. "You can see them all stuck together, head to head, tail to tail, head to tail," Dr. Dawson says. The stickiness keeps the sperm from wriggling their way to an egg.

Adding enough vitamin C to a man's diet can correct the problem, Dr. Dawson has found.

In one study, a group of 30 men, all with sperm agglutinization problems and all unsuccessfully trying to get their wives pregnant, were divided into three groups. Two groups got vitamin C, either 200 or 1,000 milligrams a day. The third group got a placebo (blank pill). At the end of 60 days, every one of the men taking vitamin C had impregnated their wives; none of the placebo group reported a pregnancy.

In another study, researchers found that men who cut back on vitamin C from 250 to 10 or 20 milligrams a day had 2½ times the amount of genetic damage to sperm. When the men increased their intake of vitamin C to 60 to 250 milligrams a day, the genetic damaged dropped.

"We know now that if your dietary intake of vitamin C gets below about 60 milligrams a day, you get into trouble," says researcher Bruce Ames, Ph.D., of the Division of Biochemistry and Molecular Biology at the University of California, Berkeley. "And smokers, who have lots of damage-causing oxidants in their bodies, may have genetic damage even at higher intakes." In fact, smokers may need two to three times as much vitamin C, up to about 180 milligrams a day, "just to keep even with nonsmokers," Dr. Ames says.

To be safe, Dr. Ames recommends eating two fruits and three vegetables a day. "That gives you not just the vitamin C you need, but also folate and lots of other protective nutrients," Dr. Ames says. "It will benefit you and your children yet to be born."

Find your most fertile weight. Doctors who specialize in infertility have known for ages that women who are too thin or too thick have more trouble than usual getting pregnant.

"That's because body fat plays an important role in estrogen levels in the body," says reproductive endocrinologist G. William Bates, M.D., professor of obstetrics and gynecology at the Medical University of South Carolina College of Medicine in Charleston.

Body fat stores estrogen and can convert other hormones into estrogen, Dr. Bates says. Thin women may have too little estrogen, and overweight women too much, for a successful pregnancy, he says.

Dr. Bates has found that women who reach their normal body weight, either by dieting or gaining weight, increase their chances of becoming pregnant.

"We've seen women who were trying to conceive for years, and they gain some weight, and they conceive," he says. "We expect pregnancy within six months of attaining normal body weight."

Thin women need to gain an average of 8½ pounds to become fertile; overweight women don't need to become svelte, but they do need to lose enough weight to allow their periods to normalize. "The target weight for most obese women is 140 to 160 pounds," Dr. Bates says.

Women gaining weight are encouraged to temporarily load up on high-fat, high-calorie goodies like cheesecake, pastries and ice cream. This regimen puts pounds on fast; once the weight is gained, the women go back to healthy foods. Those losing weight are steered toward a moderate weight-loss and exercise program that allows them to shed a pound a week.

"I'm amazed how often body fat causes infertility problems," Dr. Bates says. "As many as 15 percent of couples may have an overweight or underweight problem. And I am amazed at how often it is overlooked."

MOTHER-TO-BE

Eating for two? A successful pregnancy can also benefit from good nutrition, from the moment of conception to the day of delivery—and even beyond if you are breastfeeding. A balanced diet helps prevent certain complications of pregnancy. And it may also guard against low birth weight and infant mortality.

A healthy diet provides the raw materials your body needs to produce a baby, which weighs an average of seven pounds. It also supplies the building blocks for the extras that go along with pregnancy. Increased blood and fluid volume, the placenta, amniotic fluid and bigger breasts, not to mention those "fat stores" the body stashes away during pregnancy for future breastfeeding, add up to 25 to 35 pounds of new tissue, all manufactured during pregnancy.

That comes to an average of about 300 extra calories a day, or a total of about 81,000 calories over the course of a pregnancy, says Elyse Sosin, R.D., supervisor of clinical nutrition at Mount Sinai Medical Center in New York City.

Those calories need to be chosen carefully. Pregnant women need extras of just about everything, including vitamin A, thiamine, riboflavin, folate, vitamin B_{12}, calcium, phosphorus, magnesium and iron.

But dietary surveys indicate that pregnant women tend to come up short, consistently getting well below the RDA for eight nutrients—vitamins B_6, D and E, folate, iron, zinc, calcium and magnesium. "If it's severe enough, any one of these deficiencies can pose dangers for both mother and fetus," says John Repke, M.D., associate professor of obstetrics, gynecology and reproductive biology at Harvard Medical School.

Many obstetricians *do* recommend prenatal supplements. If your doctor hasn't, you may want to bring the topic up at your next visit.

PREVENTING BIRTH DEFECTS

Good nutrition is important right from the start . . . even *before* the start! Why? Because certain serious defects that have been linked with poor diet are present by the fourth week of pregnancy. That's about the time most women first realize they're pregnant, Sosin says.

Neural tube defects, for instance, have been strongly linked with a deficiency of folate, a B-complex vitamin. Neural tube defects can be deadly—they result in spina bifida (failure of the spinal column to close) or anencephaly (failure of the brain to develop).

In a large study, researchers found that adding four milligrams of folate to pregnant women's diets cut by 72 percent their risk of having a baby with neural tube defects. These women were considered at high risk, because they'd already had one baby with this defect.

Ask your doctor about folate—before you become pregnant. The Centers for Disease Control recommend that women who've had one baby with neural tube defects start taking four milligrams of folate daily starting *at least six weeks prior to attempting to become pregnant.* All other women of childbearing age are advised to take 0.4 milligrams (400 micrograms) of folate daily.

AVOIDING ANEMIA

It's hard enough hauling around that extra baggage. If you're anemic as well, your pregnancy can be a time of bone-weary, tail-dragging fatigue.

Iron requirements double during pregnancy, from 15 to 30 milligrams daily. The National Academy of Science recommends a daily 30 milligram iron supplement, beginning in the fourth month, because it's so hard for a pregnant woman to get all the iron she needs through diet. Most prenatal vitamins contain at least some iron.

Ask your doctor about iron supplements. Some obstetricians recommend iron supplements from the start of a pregnancy, based on a woman's iron status. Others, though, wait until iron stores begin to dip. "During the 16th through 24th week, a woman's hemoglobin is at the lowest point ever during her pregnancy, and that's often why iron supplementation is started at this point or a little before," Sosin says.

KEEPING A LID ON BLOOD PRESSURE

Pregnancy-induced high blood pressure, with its accompanying bloating and protein breakdown, can be risky to both mother and baby. Some doctors believe this condition is caused by poor nutrition. Many, though, claim the cause is unknown. Some studies do suggest that pregnancy-induced hypertension is linked with an imbalance of minerals—too little calcium, magnesium or potassium and too much salt. The link currently is strongest for calcium.

Bone-building calcium demands shoot up to 1,200 milligrams a day for a pregnant woman, the amount found in about a quart of milk. Most studies show women coming up short on calcium. "We found poor pregnant women got about 65 percent of their RDA," Dr. Repke says.

In one study by Dr. Repke and others at Johns Hopkins Hospital in Baltimore, women who were given two grams of calcium a day had lower blood pressure and a lower incidence of pregnancy-induced high blood pressure, than women not receiving calcium supplements. They also were less likely to have premature or low-birthweight babies. "We felt calcium supplementation provided some protection from this disorder," Dr. Repke says.

Ask your doctor about calcium supplements. Most pregnant women need to add calcium-rich foods to their diet or take calcium supplements, Dr. Repke says. The average prenatal vitamin contains only about 20 percent of the RDA. The National Academy of Science recommends calcium

CRAVINGS: FOODS PREGNANT WOMEN CAN'T RESIST

For one expectant mom, it was chicken liver pâté; for another, M&Ms—plain, not peanut; a third couldn't get enough ice cream—but it had to be strawberry, and only one brand would do.

Food cravings are common during pregnancy. Studies show that as many as 75 percent of women find certain foods irresistible. The cravings often begin in the first few months of pregnancy, when levels of appetite-stimulating hormones are highest, and for many, continue until childbirth.

What foods do women desire most? That varies from study to study, but milk, ice cream, salty foods and snacks, sweets, chocolate and fruit seem to top most lists, says researcher Judith Brown, Ph.D., at the University of Minnesota's School of Public Health.

Apparently these hankerings can be fairly intense. In one study, women indicated they'd be willing to steal the food items they craved.

Pregnant women also tend to develop aversions to some foods: colas, coffee, alcohol, fried foods and meat seem most likely to cause turned-up noses.

One theory proposes that women are gravitating naturally toward foods that contain nutrients they need: pregnant women who crave salty foods, for instance, really

supplements for pregnant women who consume only one serving of calcium-rich food a day.

Make sure you're getting enough of other minerals. Several preliminary studies suggest that pragnancy-induced hypertension may also be influenced by levels of magnesium and zinc. "Right now, though, most doctors believe evidence supporting those links is weak," Dr. Repke says. Intravenous magnesium sulfate is given to stop pregnancy-induced hymay need more salt. That theory is shaky, though, since women don't always pick the food richest in a particular nutrient. "If a woman craves chocolate because she needs more magnesium, why doesn't she crave a better source of it, like green vegetables?" Dr. Brown asks.

As for aversions, some researchers think the distaste (often to the point of nausea) some women develop for some foods may be their bodies' reaction to substances that are potentially harmful to their babies. A distaste for alcohol and coffee, for example, often occurs early in pregnancy. Alcohol's harmful effects on an unborn baby are well known. In moderation, though, caffeine seems to do no harm. So the aversion theory, too, remains to be proven.

What should a pregnant woman do about cravings? "If it's for a healthy food, like milk or fruit, indulge and don't think yourself strange," Dr. Brown says. "If it's for a food that's giving you mostly empty calories, like chocolate or ice cream, try to limit portions." If you are having a hard time avoiding unhealthy foods or find yourself craving nonfood items, such as ice, clay or laundry starch (strange as it seems), it may pay to have a nutritional analysis done, she says. And make sure you discuss it with your health-care provider. Some researchers believe these nonfood cravings are the result of nutritional deficiencies, especially iron deficiency, which is common in pregnant women who are not taking iron supplements.

pertension (also called preeclampsia) from progressing to eclampsia, a full-scale medical emergency that may include seizures.

Avoid salt-laden foods. Pregnant women do need extra salt, so a severely salt-restricted diet is less likely to be used these days to control pregnancy-induced hypertension. Still, doctors do nix very salty foods like pickles, potato chips and pepperoni.

GOOD NUTRITION FOR BREASTFEEDING MOMS

You don't necessarily have to eat right to have health-giving breast milk, but you *do* need a balanced diet if you don't want to rob your body of nutruents while you're breastfeeding.

"A woman's body will see to it that most of the nutrients needed in the milk get in the milk, even if it means robbing minerals, fat or protein from other parts of the body to do so," says Judith B. Roepke, R.D., Ph.D., associate provost, dean of continuing education and professor of home economics at Ball State University in Muncie, Indiana, and a member of the La Leche League International professional advisory council.

If you're not getting enough calcium (1,200 milligrams a day) to meet your breastfeeding needs, your body will borrow it from your bones. The price you pay may be osteoporosis later in life. You don't necessarily have to drink milk to make milk, Dr. Roepke says, "but it is true that milk is an easily absorbed source of calcium."

Breast milk uses up to 0.5 to 1 milligram of iron a day, Dr. Roepke adds. Over a month that adds up to less than the amount lost during menstruation. However, many doctors recommend that breastfeeding mothers continue to

FOOD TAMERS FOR PMS

Could what you eat ease or exacerbate the irritability, bloating, breast tenderness and fatigue some women have in the week or so prior to menstruation? Could certain nutrients, such as vitamin B_6, influence a woman's production of hormones promoting premenstrual syndrome (PMS)? No one knows for sure, but there's some evidence to indicate that good nutrition may ease this rough spot in a woman's monthly cycle.

take an iron supplement to build up their iron stores after pregnancy.

Breastfeeding is also an energy-intensive activity. You'll need 500 extra calories a day, 200 more than you did while you were pregnant, to keep up with the calorie needs of breastfeeding. This will slowly use up the eight or so pounds of fat your body stored during pregnancy just for this use. "Women who breastfeed generally lose a pound or two a month, so that by the time the baby is four to six months old, they are back to their prepregnancy weight," Dr. Roepke says.

Breastfeeding also requires extra fluid. "But the only rule of thumb is: Drink to satisfy your thirst," says Betty L. Crase, La Leche League International's director of scientific information. "Women who force themselves to drink large amounts of milk or water can overload their bodies, which can be just as detrimental to milk production as dehydration."

According to the American Academy of Pediatrics, a good breastfeeding daily menu includes 5 servings of milk or milk products and 4 two- to three-ounce servings of protein foods such as meat, chicken or fish. The U.S. Department of Agriculture also recommends at least 3 to 5 servings of fruits and vegetables and 6 to 11 servings of breads, cereals, rice and pasta.

Along with countless theories about the causes of PMS have come many remedies, from hormones to psychotherapy. Special diets, and sometimes nutritional supplements, have been popular treatments for PMS for years, even though studies that would conclusively support such measures are few and far between.

Vitamin B$_6$, vitamin E, evening primrose oil and a certain "PMS formula" multivitamin/mineral supplement all seem to show some benefits, according to studies and clinical experience. Eliminating caffeine and alcohol and cutting back on sugar have also been shown to help in some studies, says Susan M. Lark, M.D., author of *The Premenstrual Syndrome Self-Help Book* and director of the PMS and Menopause Self-Help Center, in Los Altos, California.

Based on research studies and her own experiences, Dr. Lark has designed a PMS diet that she says many women find offers across-the-board symptom relief.

"It emphasizes the same kind of healthy eating habits recommended to most people these days," she says.

The PMS diet cuts out what several studies have suggested are PMS-aggravating foods: coffee, refined sugar, chocolate, alcohol, salty and fatty fried foods and anything that qualifies as "junk food" (few nutrients, lots of calories and/or fat). It emphasizes whole-grain complex carbohydrates, including whole-grain cereals, breads, crackers, pancakes, waffles and pasta; legumes, such as lentils and kidney beans; lean meat, especially chicken and fish; raw seeds and nuts; vegetables, especially root vegetables and leafy greens; fresh fruits; and cold-pressed oils such as sesame, olive, corn and safflower oil.

"By reducing simple sugars and caffeine and increasing fiber and complex carbohydrates, this diet helps to stabilize blood sugar, which may play a role in PMS," Dr. Lark says. "It also provides nutrients thought to be important in the management of PMS—B-complex, vitamin E, various minerals and certain types of vegetable oils."

SAILING THROUGH MENOPAUSE

Today, many symptoms of menopause, especially hot flashes and vaginal dryness and thinning, are treated with hormone replacement therapy. But some doctors recommend dietary changes and vitamin/mineral supplements, both for their patients taking hormone replacement therapy and for those who can't or won't take hormones.

What's a menopause diet like? "It's a basic, healthy diet," says Dr. Lark, in her book *The Menopause Self-Help Book*.

The menu is packed with whole grains, vegetables and fruits, leaves plenty of room for fish, allows small portions of meats and poultry, emphasizes vegetable oils over saturated fats, and edges out sugar, high-fat foods, caffeine and alcohol.

Dr. Lark also recommends a range of vitamin and mineral supplements, including calcium and magnesium, which help prevent osteoporosis and may help relieve fatigue, nervousness and irritability; vitamin E, which in some older studies seemed to help reduce the frequency and severity of hot flashes; and bioflavonoids (found in the membranes of citrus fruits), which older studies show also help to reduce hot flashes.

"For women with fibroid tumors, endometriosis or some other condition that prevents them from taking estrogen when they reach menopause, I find that vitamin E and other nutrients are the answer to their problem," Dr. Lark says.

CHAPTER 26

Nutritional Healing

An A-to-Z Guide

"Take two zucchini and call me in the morning." Imagine your doctor scribbling out such a prescription. You might think he's blown a fuse from filling out endless medical insurance forms.

But studies show that dietary changes can sometimes be as effective as drugs in the treatment of certain illnesses—without potentially harmful side effects.

High blood pressure, gout, indigestion and headaches are just a few examples of the health problems that may be completely controlled in some cases with a few judicious dietary adjustments. Even when a health problem requires medical care, proper nourishment often adds a healing advantage. And when it comes to preventing diseases such as cancer and heart disease, studies clearly show that dietary factors—plenty of fruits and vegetables, for instance, and fewer fatty foods—can help provide protection.

In this chapter you'll read about a number of disorders that respond to dietary changes, along with key research findings that detail exactly how to eat for maximum benefits.

In some cases, as we've indicated, good nutrition is considered secondary to proper medical care. In other cases, such as cancer, dietary changes play a purely preventive role; they are not considered part of treatment.

ACNE

Just about anyone who's made it through adolescence is familiar with the bumps and embarrassment of acne. These blemishes occur when skin pores clog up and become infected, usually just before a big event. Hormones, stress and genetics are involved.

While medications—benzoyl peroxide products, topical or oral antibiotics and vitamin A—derived drugs (Retin-A, Accutane)—are the cornerstones of medical treatment, poor diet has long been thought to play a part. And although its role more recently has been downplayed, it hasn't been totally dismissed.

Several studies done during the 1970s and 1980s showed that people eating what's considered a typical Western diet (high in fat and salt and low in fiber) were more likely to have acne than people eating the traditional diets of their region. One study showed that Eskimos who changed to a Western diet developed a number of new diseases, including acne. Another found less acne among blacks in Kenya eating a traditional low-fat, high-fiber diet than among blacks in the United States.

If diet does aggravate acne, no one knows for sure what components are to blame. The usual list of suspects includes chocolates, shellfish, iodized salt, cheese, fatty foods and colas. But studies have failed to show that restricting these foods clears up acne, and most dermatologists now simply advise their patients to eat a well-balanced diet and eliminate only those foods that consistently cause flare-ups. Those foods vary from person to person.

Other nutritional recommendations for acne include:

Get more zinc. Two studies showed that people with acne had lower zinc levels than people without acne. In four studies, supplemental zinc led to fewer breakouts.

Get enough vitamins A, E and B$_6$, folate, selenium and chromium. All have been found to reduce acne breakouts in some studies.

ALCOHOLISM

Problem drinkers (people who have three or more alcoholic drinks a day) also tend to eat poorly. So their bodies have to endure a double insult—from overindulgence and malnourishment. The combination can be deadly.

The usual treatment for alcoholics trying to stop drinking is to substitute tranquilizers for alcohol, then slowly reduce the dose over time. These drugs ease symptoms of withdrawal. In some cases, nutritional therapy may be included to counteract alcohol's toxic effects and to restore severely depleted nutrients. Some addiction experts believe good nutrition can reduce cravings for alcohol, making it easier to stay on the wagon. Their recommendations:

Take a good multivitamin/mineral supplement. Thiamine, folate, magnesium, potassium and calcium are just some of the nutrients alcoholics often lack. Most doctors give supplements until a person is stable and eating well.

Add extras of some vitamins to reduce alcohol's harmful effects. Vitamins C and E, zinc and selenium may help protect the liver; thiamine may help prevent nerve damage; and vitamin E may protect the heart. Discuss dosages with your doctor.

Upgrade your diet. Make sure you're getting enough protein, fruits and vegetables and whole grains. Research is limited, but several animal studies suggest alcohol craving is stronger when it's compounded by poor diet. And one study shows that alcoholics getting nutritional support (individual nutritional counseling and a menu designed by a dietitian) are more likely to abstain than those getting traditional therapy.

ALLERGIES

Does your immune system get all worked up over nothing? Allergies are an overreaction by the immune system to substances normally considered harmless. People with allergies are usually advised to avoid whatever is causing their symptoms, to take drugs that suppress symptoms or to get desensitizing shots.

Diet usually isn't addressed in allergy treatment unless a person reacts to a particular food or food additive, such as sulfites. But some doctors believe certain nutrients may aid the sneeze-prone by tempering allergic response. Their suggestions:

Add vitamin C. Studies show that people with low vitamin C levels have higher-than-normal blood levels of histamine, a biochemical that produces allergic symptoms. In one study, adding extra vitamin C to allergy sufferers' diets resulted in reduced histamine levels.

And vitamin E. In another study, this nutrient dampened histamine-related allergic response.

Try flavonoids. These compounds, found in the membranes of citrus fruits, and in other fruits, vegetables, nuts and seeds, also seem to inhibit some allergic responses. "Data indicate that a number of flavonoids inhibit *in vitro* [test tube] allergic reactions, and may have an influence on many immunologic actions," says Elliott Middleton, Ph.D., of the State University of New York at Buffalo School of Medicine and Biomedical Sciences. Flavonoids are not considered to be vitamins. One widely marketed flavonoid is Quercetin.

ANGINA

Nobody likes getting shortchanged, and when it's your heart running low on oxygen, the result is downright painful.

Angina pectoris is chest pain that occurs when blood flow to the heart is impaired, so heart muscles don't get enough oxygen. Angina usually occurs during physical activity, which increases oxygen needs. Rest or nitroglycerin (which opens arteries, improving blood flow) both relieve angina. Dietary changes can help keep blood vessels clear of fatty deposits and make them less likely to go into spasms. Recommendations include:

Eat low fat. The same lean menu that prevents heart disease can help ease symptoms of angina by preventing further buildup of artery-choking fat deposits. (And a very low fat diet may *shrink* deposits.) A low-fat diet also makes blood cells less likely to clump together or to adhere to blood vessel walls.

Take vitamin E. In one study, low levels of vitamin E were associated with more than double the risk of angina. Although no clinical trials have been done to show vitamin E helps prevent angina, there's good reason to think it might. It has been proven to reduce symptoms of intermittent claudication, a kind of "angina of the leg."

Add magnesium. In several studies, magnesium given intravenously was effective in stopping *variant angina,* spasms in the coronary arteries that are not related to a permanent blockage. It's not the drug of choice in hospitals but magnesium seems to work by relieving the spasms that occur with this type of angina. However, at normal dosage levels it does not seem to help people with *stable effort angina,* which is caused by a permanent blockage. Ongoing research shows that getting adequate magnesium in the diet can be helpful in preventing complications from heart disease.

ANOREXIA NERVOSA

If you think you can't be too thin or too rich, you're only half right. People with anorexia nervosa are obsessed with the fear of becoming overweight. They may eat so little they need to be hospitalized.

Most people who develop anorexia nervosa are women between the ages of 12 and 18. The condition is classified as a psychiatric disorder. It is treated with psychotherapy and a structured eating program. Nutritional recommendations include:

Eat right with a professionally designed diet. Nutrition therapy includes a carefully balanced diet that offers enough calories to first regain weight, and then maintain normal body weight. Monitoring the minerals that control heart rate and blood pressure—potassium, calcium, magnesium and sodium—is particularly important. Imbalances can cause serious problems.

Get adequate zinc in your diet. Some researchers believe correcting a zinc deficiency can help break the cycle of chronic anorexia.

Studies show that women with anorexia nervosa are more likely than normal to be low in zinc. That's important because a zinc deficiency can produce symptoms similar to anorexia nervosa—lack of appetite, depression, changes in taste and smell, cessation of menstrual periods.

"A woman who goes on a weight-loss diet low in zinc may slowly become zinc deficient," explains Laurie Humphries, M.D., associate professor of psychiatry at the University of Kentucky Medical Center in Lexington. "That may lead her into a vicious sycle. She eats less, becomes even more zinc deficient and finally loses her appetite altogether."

Studies also show that women with anorexia nervosa tend to become *more* zinc deficient during refeeding if they are getting only the RDA of zinc. (That's because extra zinc is needed to metabolize the extra calories.)

"Even if an anorexic woman is not clearly zinc deficient when she begins treatment, she can become zinc deficient within 30 days of refeeding unless she gets adequate supplemental zinc," Dr. Humphries says. "Even if they regain weight, women who remain zinc deficient may go back to their old eating habits."

ANXIETY

Anxiety is considered a psychological state—a mix of fear and anger—but it has a definite physical dimension. Along with clammy hands comes rapid heartbeat and fast, shallow breathing, the result of adrenaline pouring into your system.

Traditional treatment includes psychological counseling and anti-anxiety drugs such as tranquilizers. Nutritional recommendations involve avoiding foods that may heighten the physical aspects of anxiety. They include:

Sidestep symptom producers. Anxiety-provoking food components may vary from person to person, but they often include caffeine, alcohol and sugar. Caffeine is a known stimulant. Alcohol is often considered a mild tranquilizer, but when it's abused, withdrawal symptoms can include anxiety. And sugar and other refined carbohydrates can lead to a quick rise, then a big drop in blood sugar. It's the drop that generates anxiety in some people.

Rule out nutritional deficiencies. Some studies suggest that B-vitamin deficiencies can cause anxiety-related symptoms. And some researchers contend that calcium and magnesium deficiencies can cause jumpiness and frayed nerves. But experts in this area say that more research is needed.

ASTHMA

Air may be one of the best things in life that's free, but perhaps you're having trouble getting your fair share. Coughing, wheezing and shortness of breath are the trademarks of asthma.

Anti-inflammatory and other inhalant spray drugs that relax bronchial passages, allergy shots and avoidance of environmental triggers are the usual medical treatments for asthma.

Nutritional therapy is based on eliminating the foods and food additives (such as sulfites) that may cause attacks, and adding nutrients some doctors believe make the lungs less reactive. Recommendations include:

Add vitamins C and E. Some doctors recommend these nutrients as a way to protect the lungs from damaging air pollution and to help tame "twitchy" bronchial muscles.

Havva cuppa java. (Better make that two.) A study suggests drinking coffee regularly may reduce the number of attacks you have. Although not a substitute for medication, a couple of cups of strong coffee might have a short-acting beneficial effect on asthma, adds one allergist. Caffeine and the popular asthma drug theophylline are almost identical, although the latter is much more powerful.

BLADDER INFECTIONS

Burning pain when urinating and the unpleasant sensation of having to go, go, go, even when you've just gone are familiar signs to some people. They could mean a bladder infection is brewing.

Most bladder infections happen when *E. coli* bacteria normally found in the colon make their way into the bladder and multiply, infecting the lining and causing pain and, sometimes, bleeding.

Most bladder infections are easily treated with antibiotics. To help prevent chronic bladder infections, some doctors suggest dietary changes in addition to drug treatment.

Drink plenty of fluids. Urinating frequently helps flush bacteria out of the bladder and stops them from multiplying. Drink enough water and other fluids to make your urine clear; if it's a deep yellow color, you aren't drinking enough, experts say.

Try a cranberry chaser. Although it controversial and not scientifically proven, many stand by the claim that cranberry juice can help get rid of a bladder infection. The theory: It contains substantial vitamin C, which acidifies the urine and inhibits bacterial growth.

Toss down some vitamin C. Doses of 1,000 milligrams a day are sometimes recommended to deter chronic infections.

CANCER, BREAST

Breast cancer shares top billing with lung cancer as the leading cause of cancer deaths among women. Despite that, premenopausal breast cancer is considered to respond well to medical treatment, especially when the tumor is detected early. Breast cancer appears to have some links with diet, and many experts believe women can cut their risk with changes in eating habits. Their recommendations:

Eat a low-fat diet. Some researchers suggest you try to keep fat intake at 20 to 25 percent of total calories. High-fat diets have been implicated as a cause of breast cancer; in animal studies, the connection is particularly strong.

Fill up on fiber. Preliminary studies suggest that fiber (cereal fiber in particular) reduces blood levels of estrogen, even in the face of a high-fat diet. Too-high blood levels of this hormone seem to promote the development of breast cancer. Aim for 30 grams of fiber a day.

Include vitamins C, E and A, beta-carotene and selenium. In animal studies low intakes of each of these nutrients has been associated with an increased risk of breast cancer.

CANCER, CERVICAL

Thanks to the Pap smear that detects cell changes *before* they become cancerous, the death rate for cervical cancer is at its lowest ever. And healthy eating may pare your risk of developing cervical cancer. Studies indicate cervical cancer is less common in women who get adequate amounts of certain nutrients. Recommendations include:

Fill up on folate. Researchers have found that the risk of cervical cancer climbs sharply in women whose diets are low in this B-complex vitamin found in green leafy vegetables. They speculate that sufficient amounts of folate protect genetic material in cervical cells from virus-induced damage.

Color away risk. In some studies, women who filled up on carotenoid-rich red, yellow and green fruits and vegetables had a reduced risk of cervical cancer.

Add vitamins C and E. Deficiencies of either vitamin have been associated with a higher risk of invasive cervical cancer. Citrus fruits are your best dietary source of vitamin C; for E, it's nuts and vegetable oils.

CANCER, COLON

Of all the types of cancer thought to have dietary links, colon cancer stands out as one of the most obvious. Researchers speculate that most cases of colon cancer are linked with diet. Their findings point to these dietary changes.

Eat low fat and high fiber. Fat itself isn't carcinogenic. But it sets off a chain reaction that enhances the development of tumors. Some researchers suggest cutting fat back to 20 to 25 percent of calories. Fiber may help prevent colon cancer a number of ways—decreasing bowel transit time, diluting toxins and carcinogens, lowering blood levels of hormones and binding with cancer-promoting secondary bile acids. Experts suggest increasing fiber intake to about 30 grams a day (double what most people get.)

Drink your milk. A calcium-rich diet has been tentatively linked with reduced risk of colon cancer.

Add vitamins A and D. Both promote the normal development of cells in the colon.

Disarm toxins with vitamins E and C. Both help protect the colon by neutralizing cancer-promoting nitrosamines (chemicals produced during the digestion of nitrates, which are found in preserved meats and some other foods).

CANCER, LUNG

Cancer occurs when a cell mutates and starts multiplying out of control, eventually crowding out or taking over vital organs, causing them to fail. In lung cancer, delicate lung tissue turns into a fibrous tangle that can no longer absorb oxygen. By the time signs of cancer (bloody sputum, persistent cough, shortness of breath) are present, the disease is usually advanced. Treatment involves surgery and chemotherapy. Prevention includes avoiding cigarette smoke and asbestos, both well-known lung cancer promoters. Prevention may also be linked to diet.

Treat your lungs to a salad. Researchers don't know for sure yet if certain nutrients can protect people at high risk for lung cancer. They're studying that right now. But they *do* know that lung cancer rates are lower in people who eat several servings a day of foods high in carotenoids, including beta-carotene, found in green leafy vegetables such as kale and spinach, and in yellow, orange and red fruits and vegetables such as carrots and cantaloupe.

Add vitamins A, E and C and selenium. These nutrients may also cut your risk for lung cancer, although they don't seem to offer as much protection as carotenoids.

CANKER SORES

One good thing about canker sores: They're *inside* your mouth, not on your lips where everyone can see them. These small, painful ulcers are common, but doctors can't seem to figure out what triggers them. Injury to the mouth, stress and certain foods may play a role in triggering these lesions, but an altered immune response appears to be the most plausible explanation. Topical antibiotics can rid the sore of the accumulated bacteria that can prolong healing. Astringents, antiseptics or a baking soda rinse may also help in reducing pain.

Nutritional recommendations include:

Check for dietary shortcomings. Iron, vitamin B_{12} and folate deficiencies have been linked to canker sores in some people, according to a study from Scotland. Supplementation for six months improved symptoms in most of the people studied. However, these findings could not be duplicated in several other studies.

Ferret out food sensitivities. They may be associated with canker sores. In one study, about 18 percent of people with canker sores traced their occurrence to eating specific foods. Citrus, chocolate and nuts are the most common offenders.

CARDIAC ARRHYTHMIA

In a love song a wild heartbeat may signal romance, but in real life it signals trouble. Cardiac arrhythmia means your heart is beating out of sync, making this vital pump much less efficient at moving blood throughout your body.

Arrhythmia can be caused by many things, including damage to heart muscles caused by heart attack, reactions to heart drugs and an imbalance of heartbeat-regulating minerals known as electrolytes (sodium, calcium, magnesium and potassium).

Cardiac arrhythmias are usually treated by correcting an electrolyte imbalance or by using drugs that help stabilize heart rhythm. Sometimes doctors remove tissue in the heart that is causing the erratic electrical impulses, or implant a pacemaker or other device capable of delivering an electrical impulse to the heart. Nutritional measures include:

Make sure a doctor checks your electrolyte balance. A potassium deficiency is the most commonly diagnosed electrolyte problem. Intravenous or oral potassium supplements (available only by prescription) may correct the problem. Intravenous magnesium sulfate can sometimes correct serious arrhythmias when potassium alone will not work. That's one reason some researchers believe a magnesium deficiency can contribute to heart arrhythmia. A calcium deficiency, or too much calcium can also cause arrhythmia.

Cut back on coffee. Too much caffeine seems to set some hearts aflutter, especially if abnormalities already exist.

Be on the lookout for food instigators. Foods or food additives are a rare cause of heart irregularities in some people.

CARPAL TUNNEL SYNDROME

The carpal tunnel is a sheath of bones and tendons in your wrist that normally protects a major nerve to your hand, the median nerve. If this tunnel collapses and begins to squeeze the nerve, you have carpal tunnel syndrome.

Numbness, pain, weakness and a pins-and-needles sensation in the thumb, index finger and middle finger are your first clues. If untreated, the pain can radiate to the elbow, upper arm and even the shoulder. Eventually, the nerve can be permanently damaged.

Carpal tunnel syndrome seems to go hand in hand with jobs that require repetitious manual motions. Meat cutters, data processors, cashiers and assembly-line workers are especially vulnerable.

Splints that keep the wrist straight, physical therapy, cortisone injections and surgery that cuts ligaments to free the nerve from any underlying adhesions are all standard medical treatments. A few doctors have only one nutritional recommendation.

Take vitamin B$_6$, with medical supervision. The vitamin is thought to help preserve the integrity of synovian, the thick, slippery sheath that surrounds the bones and tendons in the wrist.

Fairly large doses of B are used (100 to 300 milligrams daily). Since large doses may *cause* sensory nerve problems, it's important to have your treatment monitored by a doctor. Improvement from B$_6$ supplementation is said to start within a few weeks, with a complete cure in 8 to 12 weeks for 85 percent of patients.

CATARACTS

Cataracts occur when proteins in the lens of the eye lose their crystal-clear properties, becoming opaque and hard to see through.

Smoking, years of exposure to sunlight, damage to the eyes or an accumulation of sugar in the lens (usually associated with diabetes) can all contribute to cataract development.

Several dietary strategies seem to help shield eyes from the damage that causes cataracts. Recommendations include:

Become a fruit and vegetable fan. In one study, people who ate more than 3½ servings per day of fruits and vegetables had only one-sixth the risk of developing cataracts as people who ate fewer than 3½ servings a day.

Take C and see. Another study found that people taking supplements of vitamin C had a 70 percent reduction in their risk of developing cataracts, compared to the general population.

Make "E" stand for eyes. Research in animals has demonstrated that vitamin E is able to prevent cataract formation to some degree. In one study, people taking 400 I.U. of vitamin E a day reduced their risk for cataracts by more than 50 percent.

CELIAC DISEASE

Bread may be the staff of life for most of us, but for people with celiac disease, it means trouble.

People with this disorder are sensitive to gluten, a sticky protein found in wheat, rye, barley and oats. When they eat gluten, the lining of their intestine is damaged. They develop bloating, cramping and diarrhea and can become malnourished because they have trouble absorbing nutrients. Celiac disease often becomes apparent as soon as cereal is introduced into an infant's diet. Sometimes, though, the first signs of the disorder appear in adulthood.

Steer clear of gluten. A diet that completely eliminates gluten is standard treatment for celiac disease. That means no food that contains wheat, rye, barley or oats. Symptoms usually improve within days or weeks.

Do a temporary bypass around dairy foods. Some people with celiac disease develop lactose (milk sugar) intolerance as well, so these foods may be restricted initially, and slowly added back as the bowel recovers. (Some people will continue to have problems digesting dairy products, and may need to permanently limit their intake.)

Replace missing nutrients. Celiac disease often causes malabsorption, which can create vitamin and mineral deficiencies even in people who are eating well. (The only way to minimize malabsorption is to keep the disease under control with a gluten-free diet.) Using blood tests, your doctor can determine if you are developing nutritional deficiencies. Anemia, especially, may be a tip-off that you need to get more iron, B_{12} or folate.

COMMON COLD

The symptoms—head congestion, sneezing, coughing, runny nose and eyes—begin a few days after your nose is invaded by a virus. You probably know the signs of a common cold all too well, even if you go years between bouts.

Antibiotics are considered inappropriate treatment for a cold. Most doctors suggest you simply let it run its course, or use over-the-counter drugs to ease symptoms. Nutritional suggestions range from symptom-soothing soups to virus-fighting vitamins. They include:

Opt for oranges. Some doctors dispute its effectiveness, but there's no doubt vitamin C remains a popular remedy for colds, perhaps with good reason. One study found that men taking large doses of vitamin C (2,000 milligrams a day) had half the symptoms of men taking look-alike sugar pills. Vitamin C is known to boost immune system response.

Suck on zinc. In one study, cold-infected volunteers who sucked on zinc gluconate lozenges every two hours had less nasal secretion than those using sugar pills. Like vitamin C, zinc is important for boosting immunity.

Go Italian. Dine on garlic, a tasty bulb with proven virus-taming talents.

Turn up the heat. Season foods with chili peppers, curry or cumin, spices with head-clearing, mucus-thinning effects.

Load up on liquids. Plenty of fluids, especially hot soups and herbal teas, may help clear your head by thinning mucus and opening airways.

CONSTIPATION

In medical-ese, constipation is "the infrequent and difficult passage of stool." What's considered infrequent? Less than three times a week. What's considered difficult? Well, if you keep a copy of *War and Peace* by the toilet, and are finding time to read it, you may have a problem.

Drugs, iron supplements, dehydration, poor diet and laxative abuse can all block you up. Knowing what's causing your constipation is important: You may need medical treatment.

If poor diet is contributing to your problem, however, it's time to revamp your habits.

Eat more fiber. Slowly increase your intake of whole-grain breads and cereals, prunes, figs, raisins, corn and other sources of insoluble fiber, giving yourself time to adapt, until you're regular. Also eat foods high in soluble fibers—beans, oat bran, barley, peas, carrots, apples and citrus fruits. Insoluble fibers add lots of *bulk,* moving things along faster. *Soluble* fibers dissolve in water to form a gel that helps keep stools soft.

Drink lots of liquids. Experts suggest one to two quarts a day. That's especially important because fiber needs to absorb fluid before it can have its bulking effect on the stool.

Once you start such dietary measures, always answer nature's call without delay. Even with a high-fiber diet, stools kept "on hold" in the colon become dry and hard.

CROHN'S DISEASE

Crohn's disease is a chronic inflammation that can occur anywhere in the intestine. Most often, it attacks the lower bowel. Diarrhea, cramping, fatigue, loss of appetite and weight loss may all be symptoms. Typically, Crohn's disease starts at around age 25, with attacks every few months. If the disease continues without treatment, the bowel gradually deteriorates.

Most people do get better if they eat no solid food at all, so that treatment is sometimes suggested. They go on an elemental diet, fed through a naso-gastric tube, that puts all the nutrients they need, already broken down, into the intestine. Anti-inflammatory drugs are another treatment option. Dietary recommendations include.:

Throw out the junk. Some studies suggest diets low in sugar and refined carbohydrates help people with Crohn's disease. One study, by researchers in Sweden, found that people who ate fast foods at least twice a week were 3½ times more likely to develop Crohn's disease than people who ate these foods less frequently. It also found that people who ate more than 55 grams of sugar per day (the equivalent of about 13 teaspoons) were 2½ times more likely to develop Crohn's disease.

But most U.S. doctors don't think a low-sugar diet would help much. "Unlike celiac disease, Crohn's is not a classic allergy condition. There's no standard diet that's proven to work," says Theodore Bayless, M.D., director of the Meyerhoff Digestive Disease Center at Johns Hopkins Medical Institutions in Baltimore. Dr. Bayless works with patients individually to eliminate symptom-aggravating foods such as milk, and makes sure they eat nutritious meals with adequate protein and calories.

DEPRESSION

It's normal to be sad sometimes. It's part of being human. What's called clinical depression, though, goes beyond sad. Its symptoms include troubled sleep, fatigue, tearfulness, weight loss or gain, and the lost capacity to experience pleasure. Clinical depression is *not* something you can talk yourself out of, or shake off with a smile.

These days, depression is usually treated with drugs that treat brain chemistry imbalances as well as by psychotherapy.

Many nutritional deficiences have depression as a symptom, but doctors treating depression do not usually test for nutritional deficiencies because normally there's no reason to. Some doctors, however, *do* consider nutritional deficiencies as a possible factor in depression. Their recommendations include:

Ask your doctor if it's appropriate to test for nutritional deficiencies. Especially if you also have fatigue, muscle weakness or irritability. Depression has been associated with deficiencies in folate, vitamin B_{12}, vitamin C, iron, magnesium and potassium.

Cut out caffeine, sugar and refined carbohydrates. Studies suggest avoiding these foods can improve mood in some depressed people.

DIABETES

Diabetes occurs when the body produces too little insulin (called insulin-dependent diabetes) or when it becomes resistant to insulin (called non-insulin-dependent diabetes).

Insulin is needed to break down glucose for energy. When insulin isn't available, this sugar builds up in the bloodstream and organs, causing damage to blood vessels, eyes and kidneys.

Nutritional recommendations for diabetes are designed to maintain normal blood sugar level and to reduce the risk of cardiovascular disease, which is higher-than-normal in those with diabetes. They include:

Reduce to the lean side of normal. Since 85 percent of diabetics are overweight at the time of diagnosis, weight loss is an important part of treatment. They can often keep their blood sugar levels in line with a weight-reducing diet.

Say "no thanks" to dessert. Although restrictions on carbohydrates have been eased, keeping sugar intake to a minimum is still recommended for most people with diabetes. That means you may even need to limit fruit intake.

Put some balance in your diet. Balanced meals with a mix of protein, high-fiber complex carbohydrates and fat are recommended.

Ward off damage with vitamins. There's evidence that vitamin C can help prevent blood vessel damage in those with diabetes. And some studies suggest that B-complex vitamins can help prevent diabetic nerve damage.

Monitor your minerals. Chromium deficiency may be at fault in the development of non-insulin-dependent diabetes. Chromium must be present for the body to move glucose out of the blood and into cells; chromium is also needed for cells to metabolize glucose. In one study, supplementation with 200 micrograms chromium daily brought both high and low blood sugar back toward normal.

Potassium deficiency (associated with the use of some diuretics) is a well-known cause of insulin resistance. In many cases, insulin resistance occurs even though the body is producing plenty of insulin, but it's not being properly utilized by the body's cells.

DIVERTICULOSIS

Diverticulosis occurs when pouches form in the walls of the colon, likely as a result of constipation. Trying to pass hard, dry stools creates so much pressure on the colon walls that they develop permanent pockets. These pockets or pouches can become inflamed or infected. That condition is called diverticulitis.

Large, soft stools help prevent diverticulosis, and tame inflammation in people who already have the disorder. Dietary recommendations include:

Bulk up on fiber. Include both soluble fiber sources (like oat bran, barley, apples, citrus fruits and prunes) and insoluble fiber sources (such as wheat bran, corn bran and vegetables).

Avoid fiber, though, during an acute attack of diverticulitis. In fact, your doctor may want you to avoid solid foods altogether for a few days.

Wash it all down with lots of fluids. Fiber absorbs fluid, so to keep things moving smoothly, it's important to drink plenty of water. Try for eight big glasses a day.

Steer clear of seeds, such as poppy or sesame, and popcorn. Some doctors suspect that small, hard particles such as these can become lodged in the pouches, causing inflammation.

EPILEPSY

If you have been diagnosed with epilepsy, consider yourself lucky to have been born during this day and age. Exorcism will not be considered one of your treatment options.

In epileptics an electrical misfiring of cells in the brain can cause a variety of seizures—from convulsions to vacant staring. More than 50 percent of all cases are considered idiopathic—that is, doctors don't know the cause. Antiseizure drugs are standard treatment for most forms of this disorder.

Most cases of epilepsy are *not* treated with dietary changes. But some are, quite successfully. Dietary recommendations include:

Ask your doctor to check for nutritional deficiencies. Low levels of calcium, magnesium and vitamin B_6 may make some people more seizure-prone. And certain epilepsy medications make nutritional deficiencies more likely.

Make sure you get enough folate. Antiseizure drugs can deplete the body of this important B vitamin. Check with your doctor if you are taking drugs. Folate deficiencies have been associated with serious birth defects.

Check out vitamin E. In a study by researchers at the University of Toronto in Ontario, children with epilepsy whose seizures could not be controlled by medication were given 400 I.U. of vitamin E daily over a period of three months, along with their regular medication. The frequency of seizures was reduced by more than 60 percent in 10 of the 12 children. Six of them had a 90 to 100 percent reduction in seizures.

Vitamin E may protect brain cell membranes from the damaging effects of oxygen or toxic chemicals, making the cells less prone to seizures, researchers say. And it may work in adults as well. (Adults weren't included in this study since they are much less likely than children to have severe epilepsy.)

FATIGUE

Feel like your get-up-and-go got up and went? Join the crowd. Twenty-five percent of all the people in the United States say their tails are dragging. Because there are so many possible causes, the real reason for your fatigue may be hard to pinpoint.

Many nutritional deficiencies have tiredness as a symptom. In some people, multiple deficiencies work together to cause fatigue, so a complete dietary overhaul is in order. Aging, dieting, pregnancy, heavy menstrual periods, absorption problems and, of course, poor eating habits can all set the stage for weariness.

Have your doctor check your iron status. Especially if you are a menstruating woman, iron deficiency is a common and easy-to-diagnose problem.

Beef up your vitamin B intake. Deficiencies of folate, B_6, pantothenate and B_{12} are all associated with fatigue and sometimes also with depression and nerve problems.

Make sure you're getting enough magnesium. This mineral is essential for biochemical reactions that allow the body to burn carbohydrates. In one study, people with chronic fatigue syndrome had low quantities of magnesium in their red blood cells. Receiving magnesium injections to boost their intake improved symptoms in 12 of 15; those with the least energy improved most.

FIBROCYSTIC BREASTS

Breast lumps that ebb and swell with the menstrual cycle are not unusual. They can be the size of peas, grapes or even golf balls. And they can hurt! This condition used to be called fibrocystic breast disease. But since it's so common, the "disease" label has been dropped.

Studies that looked at diet's role in triggering fibrocystic breasts have had mixed results. Still, some doctors suggest their patients try making dietary changes. Among their suggestions:

Avoid coffee, tea, chocolate and cola. These foods contain compounds called methylxanthines. In several studies, women who completely eliminated these foods from their diets had a significant reduction in symptoms.

Eat a low-fat, high-fiber diet with a calorie count that maintains your ideal weight. This kind of diet helps to reduce body levels of estrogen, a known breast-tissue stimulant that is stored in body fat. It may reduce your risk of breast cancer. And some doctors say it can help relieve breast pain. (Some women say avoiding fat-rich dairy products is especially helpful.)

Take vitamin E. Several studies have shown that vitamin E seems to ease monthly breast pain and swelling perhaps by reducing levels of certain biochemicals implicated in the disease. In one study, improvement was found in 15 of 17 women with fibrocystic breast condition who took 600 I.U. of vitamin E daily for two months.

GALLSTONES

One good thing about gallstones: They develop in an organ you can afford to lose.

The gallbladder is a pear-shaped sac tucked beneath the liver. It holds bile, an important digestive fluid formed by the liver. When food reaches the small intestine, the gallbladder squirts bile through a duct into the intestine. The bile breaks food down into particles small enough to be absorbed.

Bile carries large amounts of cholesterol, which helps digest fats and other foods. Gallstones form when the excess cholesterol in bile "precipitates." Instead of remaining fluid, the cholesterol forms tiny, waxy spheres that slowly become larger and larger, until they are the size of stones. Gallstones may happen because of obesity, diet or a genetic tendency. Not eating for long periods of time also tends to concentrate cholesterol in bile.

Gallstones may be symptomless; if they lodge in a duct, however, the pain will be memorable. These days, stones can be dissolved with drugs or removed by surgery. More frequently, the entire gallbladder is removed.

Dietary measures to sidestep gallstones include:

Stay lean and trim. The more overweight you are, the greater your chances of getting gallstones. Researchers at Harvard University found that women who were slightly overweight had a 70 percent greater risk than ideal-weight women of developing gallstones. And those who were very obese had a 600 percent greater risk.

If you're losing weight, do so gradually. Overweight people who lose weight rapidly on a very restricted diet may be at special risk of forming gallstones, according to a study from Cedars-Mt. Sinai Hospital in Los Angeles.

Up your fiber intake. Fiber, especially water-soluble fiber, escorts cholesterol-laden bile from the body and may also lower your risk for gallstones.

Be a grazer. Small, frequent meals may pare your risk for gallstones by regularly emptying the gallbladder of bile, researchers have found. In one study people who regularly went about 14 hours without eating were more likely to develop gallstones.

GOUT

You're in good company if you have gout—Michelangelo, Leonardo da Vinci and Henry VIII all had this disease.

A form of arthritis, a gout attack starts when crystals of uric acid form in the fluid surrounding joints. (Gravity puts the big toe first in line for an attack, but other joints may follow.) The sharp crystals cause painful swelling.

Dietary therapy is designed to reduce body levels of uric acid. That can best be achieved by losing weight. It's also advisable to avoid foods containing purine, an amino acid that breaks down in the body to form uric acid.

Steer clear of purine-containing foods. Anchovies, asparagus, consommé, gravies, organ meats (kidney, liver, heart, sweetbreads), herring, mincemeat, mushrooms, mussels and sardines are all high in purines. Beans, cauliflower, fish (other than those mentioned above), nonorgan meats and poultry are moderately high sources.

Go easy on alcohol. Beer, especially, is high in purines. Moderate beer drinking causes increases in uric acid levels, which may contribute to gout, British researchers have found.

Try cherries. This popular home remedy for gout has been around for a while, and some people claim it does work. Unfortunately, no research has been done on cherries or any of this tasty fruit's components to prove this one way or another. One study indicated that vitamin C improved uric acid clearance from the kidneys, but there are better sources of vitamin C than cherries.

HEADACHE

A headache is a *symptom,* not a disease in itself. Most can be traced to stress-related muscle tension or migraine problems. Some headaches, though, may be linked with food sensitivities, dehydration or caffeine withdrawal.

Toss out your trouble foods. Red wine, caffeine, chocolate, aged cheeses, eggs and milk are all known headache causers for some people. So are foods containing additives like monosodium glutamate (MSG, a flavor enhancer that may be found in many processed foods), nitrates and nitrites (found in preserved meats like hot dogs, salami and bacon), tartrazine (yellow dye #5) and yeast (found in wine and raised baked goods).

Bathe your brain. If the thobbing in your head comes after too much fun and sun or too much alcohol, it is probably due, in part, to dehydration. After a night on the town or a day on the beach, a big glass of water before bed may help avert "morning after" symptoms.

Beware of withdrawal symptoms. Not getting your normal fix of caffeine may cause a headache. If you're trying to cut back or stop drinking coffee, cola or tea, do so gradually to avoid head-pounding symptoms.

HEARTBURN

Considering the strange assortment of foods we toss down, it's no wonder our stomachs sometimes rebel. A bout of heartburn occurs when hydrochloric acid escapes from the stomach into the esophagus, the tube between the stomach and mouth. That produces smoldering pain behind the breastbone and an acrid taste in the mouth. If the condition becomes chronic, the acid can actually erode the esophagus. Changing how you eat is an important part of treatment.

Know when to stop. Stuffing yourself silly is the main cause of occasional heartburn. Your stomach becomes so distended that its contents are pushed back up the esophagus. So eat smaller, more frequent meals. When you're eating out, ask for a doggie bag.

Avoid flame-fanning foods. South-of-the-border dishes are the prime trigger of heartburn, a poll reports, followed by Italian cuisine. In addition to spicy foods, some people have problems with acidic foods like tomatoes, orange or grape-fruit juice and red peppers. Others find that grease-laden burgers and French fries, chocolate, alcoholic beverages or peppermint fan their flames. These foods relax the ring of muscles around the lower esophagus that normally keep stomach acid in its place.

HIGH BLOOD PRESSURE

High blood pressure is a serious problem that requires a doctor's attention. Often pressure-lowering drugs are prescribed. But dietary changes are a proven way to prevent or reduce high blood pressure in many people. Among the most important:

Shake the salt habit. This is often recommended as the first line of defense for high blood pressure, with good reason. The sodium in salt makes the body retain water, and too much fluid retention causes blood pressure to rise. Studies show that Americans get up to 20 times as much salt as they need—the equivalent of 2 teaspoons a day, when ⅛ teaspoon would suffice.

Make sure you're getting enough potassium, calcium and magnesium. These minerals along with sodium, help to regulate the amount of fluid retained in your body. A well-balanced diet generally provides proper amounts of all four minerals and is necessary for normal blood pressure. But studies show that, all too often, potassium, calcium and magnesium come up short. Adding these minerals back by a change in diet away from high-salt foods to more fresh vegetables, grains and fruits often leads to a drop in blood pressure.

Shed pounds. Obese people are three times as likely to have high blood pressure as people of normal weight. In some cases, even losing just half that excess weight normalizes blood pressure.

Add fiber. Some studies show that adding fiber to the diet helps reduce blood pressure.

Eat low fat. Steering away from fatty foods may lower blood pressure directly, and it helps prevent heart disease, a cause of high blood pressure.

Do it all. Studies show a combined approach works best— a low-salt, low-fat, high fiber, high-potassium, high-calcium, high-magnesium diet. That translates into lots of fruits and vegetables, whole grains, lean meats and low-fat dairy foods.

HYPERACTIVITY

Most of us wouldn't mind having a bit more pep, but people (usually children) who are hyperactive have more energy than they can handle.

Hyperactivity (also called attention deficient hyperactivity disorder) includes many symptoms: fidgeting, excitability, impulsiveness, poor sleep habits, short attention span, compulsive aggression, and memory, reasoning and reading problems.

No one knows for sure what causes hyperactive behavior. Some people believe that, in those vulnerable to hyperactivity, certain compounds found naturally in foods or added to foods play an important activating role.

The Feingold diet, developed by the late Benjamin Fein-

. gold, M.D., is a dietary program that eliminates foods containing these compounds. Many pediatricians and food industry spokesmen contend there's little evidence to support the Feingold diet's recommendations. But a National Institutes of Health Consensus Panel Report stated that there were enough individual instances of improvement to warrant a trial of the Feingold diet for one to two months, "after thorough and appropriate evaluation of the child and family—including consideration of other possible therapies." Here's what's involved:

Avoid certain food additives. Avoid *all* food colorings, *all* artificial flavors and three preservatives (BHA, BHT and TBHQ). And avoid medicines containing artificial colors or flavors.

Forgo foods containing salicylates. These naturally occurring substances are found in almonds, apples (also cider and cider vinegar), apricots, all berries, cherries, cloves, coffee, cucumbers and pickles, currants, grapes and raisins (also wine and wine vinegar), nectarines, oranges, peaches, peppers (bell and chili), plums and prunes, tangerines, tea, tomatoes and oil of wintergreen. Aspirin also contains salicylates.

INFERTILITY

About one of every six couples has trouble conceiving. They have tried, without success, for a year or more, to produce a baby. There are lots of reasons for infertility. But when it's not associated with something obvious, infertility may sometimes be traced to poor nutrition.

Check your vitamin C intake. If you're a man, make sure you're getting at least the RDA of 60 milligrams of vitamin C daily. (Smokers should aim for more than 100 milligrams.) Vitamin C helps prevent sperm from sticking together, which keeps them from wriggling toward an egg. It also protects them from genetic damage that can cause birth defects.

Get enough zinc. In adult men, zinc deficiencies lead to reduced levels of testosterone, the main male hormone. And low testosterone levels reduce sperm production. Improving zinc status can normalize testosterone levels, but it may take months.

If you're a woman, maintain your normal weight. Being too thin, or seriously overweight, upsets female hormones and may cause infertility, researchers have found. Gaining or losing weight may be all it takes to become pregnant.

INFLUENZA

It's almost impossible to avoid meeting up with at least a few of the viruses that cause the flu. But whether or not you get laid low is determined in part by your immune system's ability to fight back. And that depends on good nutrition.

Bone up on the Bs. B_6 and other B-complex vitamins play a vital role in immune function. They help produce the cells and chemicals that allow your body to gear up for an attack.

Zero in on zinc. This mineral is important for the proper functioning of the thymus, a gland that produces immune cells. People deficient in zinc have a number of immune system weaknesses that make them much more prone to infection.

Add vitamin E. This antioxidant shields immune cells from the oxidative reactions that are part of the battle against viral infections.

Stock up on vitamin C. Like vitamin E, vitamin C protects frontline infection fighters. Some immune cells have up to 150 times the amount of vitamin C found in other cells. Vitamin C is used up quickly during infections and is not stored in the body, so it's important to get a fresh supply every day.

Toss down some carrots. Beta-carotene, a pigment found in carrots, sweet potatoes, cantaloupe and other orange-yellow vegetables and fruits, seems to have potent immune-stimulating powers. One study found that about 30 milligrams a day of beta-carotene (about four carrots' worth) produced significant increases in natural killer cells and T-helper cells—two types of immune cells.

IRRITABLE BOWEL SYNDROME

Some people are fussy; they want things to be *just so,* and when they're not, they grumble and have trouble adjusting. Well, some innards react like that, too. A day full of rude people or the wrong foods produces pain, cramps, gas and diarrhea.

This condition, known as irritable bowel syndrome, does not stem from a *physical* problem. There's no inflammation or ulceration of the intestines, for instance. But there is a *functional* problem. Instead of moving food along with co-ordinated waves of muscle contraction, the bowels go into spasms.

Dietary changes are usually the first course of treatment for irritable bowel. Often, careful eating is all that's needed to relieve symptoms.

Find out if you're lactose intolerant. Lots of people with irritable bowel syndrome are really lactose intolerant. They have a hard time digesting lactose, the sugar found in dairy products. A breath hydrogen test is the surest way to determine if you have this problem.

Fence off the worst offenders. Besides dairy foods, these other foods top the list of culprits: alcoholic beverages, fatty foods, beans, cabbage, onions, spicy or acidic foods, coffee and other caffeinated beverages and foods containing sorbitol or fructose (mostly fruits). Try avoiding these items for a week or so to see if your symptoms ease up.

Take the high-fiber route. A high-fiber diet can soothe spastic intestines. Just make sure you chase the fiber with a big glass of water. (Note: You may need to avoid some high-fiber foods, such as beans, which contain a hard-to-digest starch that can cause gas.)

Opt for acidophilus. Some people with irritable bowel find yogurt or acidophilus tablets helpful. Both contain bacteria that tend to normalize bowel function.

KIDNEY STONES

The majority of kidney stones form as a result of excess calcium in the urine. Tha calcium combines with other substances, oxalates or phosphates, to form crystals. The resulting stones cause pain in the middle back that radiates around the abdomen toward the genitals.

Some people simply inherit the tendency to form kidney stones, but eating habits also play a role. Dietary measures cannot remove already-formed stones. But they may cut your chances for a recurrence.

Float 'em. Kidney stones can start to form during a single incident of dehydration. So don't let yourself get too dry; drink at least eight glasses of fluid a day.

Factor in fiber. Fiber helps to reduce the amount of calcium in your urine, a major risk factor for calcium oxalate stones, the most common kind.

Save a steer. Vegetarians have a 50 to 60 percent decreased risk of kidney stones compared to meat eaters. Animal protein increases calcium excretion.

Avoid oxalates. Limit these oxalate-containing foods: beans, cocoa, instant coffee, parsley, rhubarb, spinach and tea.

Make sure that you are getting enough magnesium and vitamin B$_6$. Deficiencies have been associated with an increased tendency for stone formation.

Shake the salt habit. Salt increases calcium excretion in urine.

Don't be too sweet. Sugar also increases urinary calcium concentration.

Cut back on caffeine. Caffeine increases urinary excretion of several minerals, including calcium.

Lupus

Most of the time a raring-to-go immune system is just fine. It keeps your body from becoming "home sweet home" to an array of opportunistic microbes.

With lupus, though, as with other autoimmune diseases, the immune system becomes overzealous. It begins to attack the organs and joints of the body, causing inflammation and tissue damage. One form of the disease, systemic lupus erythematosus, can be fatal. Another form, discoid lupus erythematosus, can cause disfiguring skin problems. Both types flare up, then go into remission. The drugs used to treat lupus often have their own serious effects.

In animal studies, low-fat, low-calorie diets help stop flareups. "But these are basically starvation diets that no doctor would recommend to a patient," says Daniel Wallace, M.D., an inflammatory disease expert at the University of California, Los Angeles, UCLA School of Medicine.

Put fish on the menu. Lupus is an inflammatory disease, and several studies indicate that the omega-3 fatty acids found in fatty fish such as salmon, mackerel and sardines can help reduce inflammation. Only a few studies so far have looked at fish oil and lupus. But all showed a beneficial effect. Dr. Wallace suggests his patients eat at least two fatty fish meals a week.

Avoid alfalfa. You can thank the monkeys at the Washington Zoo for this tip. Turns out that they all came down with lupuslike symptoms after eating a diet consisting mostly of alfalfa sprouts. These sprouts contain an immune-system stimulating chemical—enough, apparently, to trigger symptoms in lupus-prone individuals.

Macular Degeneration

Age spots on your skin are easy to see. But age spots of a different sort can appear on the retina at the back of your eye.

They're called *drusen,* and they're only visible to a doctor examining your eye. These yellow spots indicate that the cells in the middle of the retina—the macula—are dying, making your central vision fuzzy.

Simply getting old is the biggest risk factor for macular degeneration. The risk increases, though, if you're light-eyed and fair-skinned. And exposure to sunlight may also play a role.

Dietary suggestions for macular degeneration are meant to keep retinal cells healthy and ward off sunlight-related damage.

Make sure you're getting enough zinc. In one study, a group of healthy older people taking zinc supplements had significantly less loss of vision due to macular degeneration than a group taking blank pills. Zinc supplements should only be taken with medical supervision. Large doses interfere with other minerals such as copper.

Protect your retinas with vitamins C and E, beta-carotene and selenium. Results from studies using these nutrients show a significant retardation of vision loss in people with macular degeneration. Damage seems to be cut by about one-third.

MITRAL VALVE PROLAPSE

Normally, the valves that regulate the flow of blood through the heart close neatly, snapping shut with the sounds—*lub-dub*—that we recognize as a heartbeat.

With mitral valve prolapse, though, an additional click is added to the heartbeat, as the valve strains against the pressure of blood, almost like a parachute being snapped in the wind. If the valve lets some blood leak backward into the chamber of the heart from which it's just come, you have a heart murmur.

Mitral valve prolapse usually produces no symptoms. In some people, though, it's associated with chest pain, fatigue, heart palpitations, muscle cramps, episodes of low blood pressure and anxiety. Most doctors treat their patients with beta-blockers, drugs that help regulate heart rate. Some, however, prescribe magnesium, a mineral vitally important for proper functioning of the heart muscle.

Ask your doctor to check your red blood cell magnesium levels. Several studies have found that a high percentage of people with mitral valce prolapse have lower than normal magnesium levels.

In one study by researchers at the University of Alabama School of Medicine, people with mitral valve prolapse and low magnesium levels showed a marked improvement in symptoms after taking supplemental magnesium. Muscle cramps decreased by 90 percent, and chest pain was cut by 47 percent. Palpitations were also markedly diminished.

MOTION SICKNESS

There's no doubt that stomachs prefer terra firma. Send them spinning, bouncing or bobbing for too long and they're likely to get plenty upset.

Even though the symptoms settle in the stomach, motion sickness doesn't start there. It starts in your head, when your brain gets confused between motion your inner ears sense and motion your eyes see. The result is an unpleasant mix of dizziness, sweating, nausea and anxiety.

Some people are more sensitive than others, but a bumpy ride in the back of a pickup truck, a spin on the twirly-whirl or boating in choppy surf can eventually turn most stomachs sour. Drugs to prevent motion sickness are available in pill and patch forms, but there are also self-care cures.

Go gingerly. Pleasant, spicy ginger has proven antinausea effects. Some experts suggest taking two capsules (450 milligrams each) of powdered gingerroot at least ten minutes before movement begins, and more as needed. (The effects do not last very long.)

Travel on half a tank. Stomachs stay calmer if they have a bit of food in them, experts day. An empty stomach creates worse motion sickness symptoms. Try munching on soda crackers, a piece of bread or a hard pretzel.

Stick with quease-free foods. Foods that make you mildly queasy when you're standing still can bring on a case of the roaring heaves when they're combined with motion sickness, experts say. So save those foods for the times when your stomach has nothing else to contend with.

Save the martinis for port. Too much alcohol can disrupt the balance mechanism in your inner ear, setting your head spinning. That's enough in itself to make you sick, and it's likely to turn the tide against you when you're battling motion sickness. Sip ginger ale or a cola instead. Both have stomach-settling potential.

MUSCLE CRAMPS

They can grab you just about anywhere, but muscle cramps are most likely to go for your calves or feet, two body parts that do much of the work when you walk, and so are more likely to suffer abuse. These painful, prolonged contractions can be caused by various things: overuse, dehydration, muscle injuries or tightness, mineral imbalances and poor circulation.

To prevent muscle cramps, warm up with light exercise, such as easy walking, followed by stretching, before beginning a vigorous workout. Soothe cramped muscles with stretching and massage.

Nutritional recommendations to prevent muscle cramps are designed to maintain normal body levels of fluid and minerals, two factors vital to properly functioning muscles. They include:

Drink up. Drink a cup or more of water before you begin an exercise routine, and ½ cup every half-hour or so, whether you're thirsty or not. Drink more if it's hot and you're sweating a lot. Dehydration is a common cause of exercise-related cramps. Diuretics (drugs often used to control high blood pressure) can cause dehydration.

Make sure you're getting enough calcium, magnesium and potassium. These minerals are involved in muscle contraction and relaxation; too little, or too much, of any one can make muscles weak, trembly or quick to cramp. Calcium supplements have been shown to relieve leg cramps during pregnancy. Sodium is important, too. If you're on a low-sodium diet and have persistent muscle cramps, talk with your doctor.

Try vitamin E. A few studies suggest that supplemental vitamin E improves symptoms of intermittent claudication, a leg-cramping condition caused by poor blood flow. It seems to enhance the body's oxygen delivery system. Oxygen is important to hard-working muscles.

NAIL PROBLEMS

If you're using your fingernails as screwdrivers or staple removers, or nibbling on them for an afternoon snack, you already know why they're so beat up. If you have brittle or disfigured nails for no apparent reason, though, it's possible you may need a nutritional boost. Like skin and hair, fingernails can be an indicator of general nutritional status.

Ask your doctor about bliotin. Veterinarians give this B vitamin to horses with problem hooves, and it works wonders. So Swiss researchers decided to try it out on people with brittle and splitting fingernails. After three to four months of daily treatment, their nail flexibility was boosted significantly. Good sources of this nutrient include cauliflower, lentils, milk and peanut butter.

Check for other nutritional deficiencies. Horizontal furrows across a nail or spoon-shaped nails may indicate low iron status.

OBESITY

Those of us whose battle of the bulge has turned into the longest stand-off in history know at least one basic rule: To lose weight, we need to consume fewer calories than we burn up as energy. Sounds simple, but when it comes down to rationing out the Melba toast, most of us are soon ready to shout "Surrender!" We're *hungry*.

So what's the trick to successful weight loss? Here's what experts suggest.

Take aim at fat, not calories. Limit your intake of fats such as butter, mayonnaise, marbled meats, oils and most baked goods so that you aren't getting more than about 25 to 30 percent of calories from fat. Fats are the most concentrated source of calories; it's also easier for our bodies to make fat from fat, than from protein or carbohydrates.

Satisfy your hunger with fiber. High-fiber foods like oatmeal, carrots and beans fill you up, not out. Some doctors recommend raw vegetables with a meal or as a snack.

Don't go too low. Diets that offer fewer than 1,200 calories a day for women, or 1,400 for men, can backfire because they provide too few calories. Metabolism (calorie burning) slows down. It's much better to eat a few more calories and make exercise a regular part of your day. That way you build mucle mass and shed fat.

OSTEOARTHRITIS

Do your knees snap, crackle and pop when you kneel? It could be that your joints are developing some painful rough spots. Smooth, rubbery cartilage is wearing away; what's regrowing may be rough and hard. Doctors call the problem osteoarthritis, and it's considered an inevitable consequence of aging. By age 70, almost everyone has it.

Nutritional recommendations for osteoarthritis are meant to help repair cartilage and keep underlying bone strong.

Drop a load. Being overweight is a well-established risk factor for osteoarthritis of the knees. One theory is that obesity puts the squeeze on weight-bearing joints. Some patients who lose weight have less pain.

Eat an orange; better yet, eat two. Vitamin C is important for the formation of collagen, a fibrous material that's used to make both bone and cartilage. In animal studies, adequate vitamin C slowed the development of osteoarthritis. Some doctors advise their older patients with arthritis to take about 1,000 milligrams of vitamin C a day.

Check your calcium. Calcium helps maintain the underlying structure of the joint—the bones. Many people with osteoarthritis also have osteoporosis, and say that extra calcium helps ease their bone pain.

OSTEOPOROSIS

Imagine bones as weak and fragile as a termite-infested log. That's what can happen with osteoporosis. Instead of being strong and dense, the bones become porous, light and frail. The least blow, sometimes even the weight of your own body, can cause them to snap.

Postmenopausal women are at highest risk for osteoporosis. Nutritional recommendations are meant to enhance the bone-preserving effects of estrogen replacement therapy, which slows bone loss.

Bone up on calcium. Get at least the RDA of calcium during the premenopausal years. That's 800 milligrams daily for women aged 19 to 50. Studies indicate most women fall far short. After menopause, some doctors recommend 1,000 to 1,500 milligrams daily.

Make sure you're getting adequate vitamin D. This nutrient is essential for calcium absorption and utilization. Two cups of milk provide the RDA of 200 I.U. of vitamin D. Sunlight also allows the body to produce vitamin D.

Add other minerals. Manganese, magnesium, zinc, copper, boron and other nutrients also play a role in the formation of bone. The best way to get these nutrients? Eat a varied diet of wholesome foods, including nuts and seeds; leafy greens; sea vegetables such as nori, laver and kombu; fruits; whole grains; beans; shellfish and lean red meat.

Limit coffee to two cups a day. Studies show that caffeine increases urinary and fecal calcium loss.

PARKINSON'S DISEASE

Imagine being trapped in a body that balks at the simplest tasks. That's what can happen with Parkinson's disease. Brain cells that produce an important chemical messenger slowly die; the result is slowness and reduced movement, rigid muscles, trembling and balance problems.

Parkinson's disease may be caused by a combination of factors: exposure to toxins or viruses, genetic vulnerability, even aging. Only recently has nutrition been thought to play a possible role. Researchers suspect some nutrients may help delay or prevent the brain cell death that causes symptoms.

Add antioxidants. A preliminary study suggests that large amounts of antioxidant nutrients—vitamin E and C—slow the progression of Parkinson's disease, delaying by 2½ to 3 years the time when a symptom-reducing drug, L-dopa, is required.

If you're taking L-dopa, watch daytime protein. High-protein meals may interfere with your body's ability to use L-dopa. One dietary program saves high-protein foods (meats, fish, eggs, legumes, dairy products) for your evening meal, eaten shortly before bedtime. That way, amino acid levels peak while you're asleep, blocking L-dopa when it matters least.

PERIODONTAL DISEASE

Periodontal means "around a tooth" and it refers to any disorder of the gums or other supporting structures of the teeth.

In periodontal disease, sticky deposits of bacteria, mucus and food particles, called plaque, accumulate on teeth. Plaque causes the gums to become infected and swollen, forming pockets between teeth that trap even more plaque. The infection can eventually cause teeth to loosen as it eats away the bone in the jaw. Gum disease is usually treated with professional cleaning, antibiotics to treat infection, and sometimes, surgery to remove infected gum tissue and reshape the bone.

Nutritional treatment to control gum disease includes avoiding foods that promote plaque formation, and adding foods that help fight infection and rebuild gum and bone tissue.

Avoid dental enemy number one. That's sugar. When you eat it, you set the stage for plaque-forming bacteria to take over your mouth. If you do eat sugary foods, eat them as part of a meal, not as snacks. And brush afterward.

Eat an orange. Even a borderline deficiency of vitamin C increases your chances of developing bleeding, infected gums. And if you're vitamin C deficient, studies show that increasing your intake may help reduce gum inflammation.

Say Mo-o-o-o-o-o-o. . . . Teeth need calcium to stay anchored in the jawbone. Calcium deficiency is associated with bone loss around the tooth. In addition to making teeth wobble, that makes room around the gumline for bacteria to move right in.

Balance your act with other nutrients. Folate, vitamins A and E, zinc and magnesium are also important for healthy teeth, gums and jawbone.

PREMENSTRUAL SYNDROME

Premenstrual syndrome (PMS) includes an array of physical and psychological changes, including bloating, breast tenderness, headache, fatigue, anxiety, depression and food cravings. These symptoms are associated with hormonal shifts in a woman's body, but just why one woman suffers so much while another breezes through this time of month is a mystery.

Studies show mixed results when it comes to any particular dietary regimen, but many women say they feel better following a special nutritional program. Most emphasize well-balanced, low-fat, high-fiber meals, along with nutritional supplements.

Dietary recommendations include:

Axe PMS-aggravating foods. Certain foods seem to aggravate PMS symptoms. Coffee, sugar, chocolate, alcohol and salty and fatty fried foods stand out as the main culprits in some studies; you may need to do some experimenting to determine which, if any, affect you.

Eat all-around healthy foods. One very popular PMS eating program, designed by Susan M. Lark, M.D., author of *The Premenstrual Syndrome Self-Help Book,* fulfills all the requirements of a healthy diet. It offers whole-grain cereals, breads, crackers, pancakes and waffles and pasta; legumes, such as lentils and kidney beans; lean meat, especially chicken and fish; raw seeds and nuts; vegetables, especially root vegetables and leafy greens; fresh fruits and oils such as sesame, olive, corn and safflower. A diet featuring these foods, followed conscientiously—not just before your period—may help alleviate some of the symptoms of PMS.

Ask your doctor about supplemental nutrients. Vitamins B_6 and E, calcium and certain PMS formula multivitamin/mineral supplements all seem to show some benefits, according to studies and clinical experience.

PROSTATE ENLARGEMENT

Enlargement of this walnut-size gland, located just below the bladder, is the most common prostate problem. The growth, called benign prostatic hyperplasia, occurs in more than 80 percent of men older than age 60. If you have an enlarged prostate, you may need to get up to urinate at night or

have trouble completely emptying your bladder. You may develop bladder infections, or, with prolonged urinary obstruction, kidney problems. The enlargement is thought to be due
to hormonal changes that occur as a man ages.

Any prostate problem deserves a doctor's diagnosis and
monitoring. That's because prostate cancer is one of the most
common cancers among men and the second leading cause of
cancer deaths.

Most doctors treat benign prostate enlargement with drugs
that shrink the gland or surgery that removes excess tissue
blocking the urinary passageway. However, a few doctors
may suggest a trial of nutritional therapy first.

Ask your doctor about zinc. Some doctors suggest their
patients with benign prostatic hyperplasia take zinc sulfate.
(Zinc gluconate, the more common form of zinc supplements,
apparently does not reach the same level of absorption in the
prostate.) There's some clinical evidence (but no studies with
a control group of men not taking zinc) that indicates zinc may
be helpful for benign enlargement. But zinc apparently does
not help the firm, nodular variety of prostate enlargement. (A
urologist can easily feel the difference between the two types.)

One urologist who prescribes zinc sulfate for his patients
with benign prostatic hyperplasia recommends a preparation
that also contains vitamin C, magnesium and B vitamins. He
says these nutrients seem to help the body absorb and use the
zinc more efficiently.

PSORIASIS

The dry, silvery scales that sometimes characterize psoriasis most commonly appear in spots on the scalp, elbows and
knees, back or buttocks. In more severe cases, the scales may
cover the entire body.

One out of three cases of psoriasis is thought to be inher-
ited. Scaling occurs because the cells that produce skin, called

epidermal cells, have cranked up production. Instead of taking 28 to 30 days to produce a new layer of skin, they take only 6 to 8 days. The result: a birthday suit with plenty of quantity but little quality.

Tar ointments, cortisone creams and ultraviolet therapy are the usual treatments.

Psoriasis generally is *not* considered to be caused by poor nutrition. Nevertheless, nutritional intervention has offered relief in some cases.

Ask your doctor about fish oil ... In some studies, omega-3 fatty acids found in fish oil improved symptoms of people with psoriasis. (In one study, it also improved symptoms of psoriatic arthritis, a related condition.) The fish oil worked best when used in addition to other treatments; by itself, improvement was only modest.

... And about new synthetic vitamin treatments. In several studies, either topical or oral forms of vitamins A and D have reduced scaling in people with psoriasis. Since these experimental drugs can have serious side effects, their use requires medical supervision. Over-the-counter versions of vitamins A and D are not considered to help psoriasis and can be harmful in large amounts.

RAYNAUD'S SYNDROME

It's normal for blood vessels in your hands and feet to constrict somewhat when they are exposed to cold, or when you're under stress. Most of us don't even notice it. With Raynaud's syndrome, though, the response is exaggerated. Blood flow is severely restricted and sometimes stops completely. The condition can cause discomfort, numbness, even pain.

In severe cases, hands change color—from white, as blood leaves, to blue, as venous blood pools, to deep red, at the end of the attack as freshly oxygenated blood rushes in. The whole process can last from less than one minute to as long as several hours.

Most cases of Raynaud's are mild and have no known cause. They are usually treated simply by taking care to keep hands warm. More serious cases may be caused by a connective tissue disorder or repeated physical stress, especially vibration. These cases may be treated with drugs that help maintain normal blood flow.

Mild cases, with no known cause, may respond to a dietary addition: fish oil.

Take a mackerel to lunch. The omega-3 fatty acids concentrated in fatty fish seem to help keep blood vessels open in some people with Raynaud's syndrome.

In one study, symptoms stopped altogether in 5 of 11 people taking fish-oil capsules daily for 12 weeks. The other 6 extended the time they could keep their hands submerged in cold water from 31 to 46 minutes (an increase of 50 percent) before blood flow to their fingers shut down. In a comparison group of 9 other people with Raynaud's taking olive oil, only 1 showed any improvement.

RESTLESS LEGS SYNDROME

You're not camping out under the stars, but you feel like a whole forest of creepy crawlers is attacking your legs. Unfortunately, even the strongest insect repellents won't help. The strange, crawling sensation is a neurological condition called restless legs, so named because the odd feelings (people describe them as "like writhing worms" or "crawling with ants") make the urge to move your legs irresistible.

People with restless legs syndrome notice these sensations most often when they're at rest—often in bed. Walking seems to ease symptoms.

Although restless legs is considered a malfunction of the nerves in the legs, dotors find no apparent neurological abnormalities or other evidence of disease. The disorder is most likely to develop in people with higher-than-normal blood levels of uric acid, including people on kidney dialysis and those with diabetes. Pregnant women sometimes develop restless legs; the condition usually disappears after delivery.

Some cases of restless legs respond to a variety of muscle-relaxing or antiseizure drugs; others, to nutritional therapy.

Make sure you're getting enough iron. Restless legs syndrome has long been associated with iron-deficiency anemia. Menstruating women and older people who are taking drugs for rheumatoid arthritis may have low iron status.

Check your folate intake. Restless legs, sometimes includes symptoms of pain or numbness. Studies suggest that folate may help these symptoms.

Junk the java. Doctors report that some patients who stop drinking caffeinated beverages get relief.

RHEUMATOID ARTHRITIS

For decades, some people with rheumatoid arthritis have contended that eating certain foods made their joint pain and swelling worse, and that avoiding those foods eased their symptoms. Some doctors listened, but most pooh-poohed the idea. More recently, there has been enough hard evidence to help sort fact from fiction and provide some nutritional guidance when it comes to arthritis relief. Even the Arthritis Foundation, a longtime holdout against the notion of a diet-arthritis link, now says, "There are some scientific reasons to think that diet might affect certain kinds of arthritis in some patients."

Dietary changes seem to work best used along with such standard treatments as exercise, heat or cold and medications.

Dietary strategies seem to help rheumatoid arthritis in some patients by reducing joint tenderness. Avoiding bad flare-ups is important; it may spare your joints from additional damage.

Talk to your doctor about fish oil. Several studies have shown that the omega-3 fatty acids found in highest concentrations in fatty fish like salmon, mackerel and sardines help reduce tenderness, possibly by reducing inflammation. Some doctors suggest eating fatty fish a few times a week.

Rule out food flare-ups. Some people with arthritis have increased joint pain soon after they eat particular foods. (That's one reason short-term fasting or vegetarian diets seem to help some people.) Since just about any food—or component of food—can be implicated, it's important to work with a doctor who can help you pinpoint your symptom-producing foods, if any.

Make sure you're eating extra well. Nutritional deficiencies might exacerbate rheumatoid arthritis in some people: Studies from researchers around the world suggest that copper, selenium, zinc, vitamins C and E and pantothenate may all play a role in this disorder.

STROKE

The results of a stroke can be devastating. Because it's your brain that's injured, you may lose the ability to move parts of your body. You may also lose the capacity to see, feel or speak. Imagine not being able to converse with people you've known all your life, or being unable to say the words "I love you."

A stroke is usually caused by a blood clot that disrupts blood flow to parts of the brain, allowing brain cells to die, or by a hemorrhage that destroys brain tissue. Some people have a mini-stroke, which does little damage but is a serious warning that a full-blown stroke may be coming. It is possible to reduce your risks of a major stroke by reducing blood pressure, not smoking, lowering high cholesterol, losing weight, if necessary, and improving your eating habits.

Cut the fat. Eighty-four percent of strokes are caused by a blockage of the blood supply to the brain, either from a blood clot or fatty plaque that obstructs the cerebral arteries. This obstruction causes a kind of a "heart attack of the head." Reducing blood cholesterol by cutting back on dietary fat can reduce your risk of this kind of stroke.

Toss your salt shaker. High blood pressure can dramatically increase your risk of stroke, especially hemmorhagic strokes. For many people, a high-salt diet sends blood pressure creeping upward.

Eat an extra serving of fruit or vegetables each day. In one study, one additional serving of fresh fruit or vegetables a day was associated with a 40 percent reduction in the risk of a fatal stroke. It is believed that the high levels of potassium in fruits and vegetables are responsible. This mineral plays a vital role in the regulation of blood pressure.

Lay off the hard stuff. Several studies have shown that drinkers, and especially heavy drinkers and binge drinkers, are more likely to have the kind of stroke caused by hemmorhaging within the brain.

TASTE IMPAIRMENT

Some people might think it would be just dandy if they couldn't taste foods. Then they wouldn't be lured into overindulgence by their mouthwatering response to flame-broiled burgers or fresh-baked brownies.

The fact is, though, that people who can't taste—or who have a distorted sense of taste—often lose their appetite altogether and become malnourished. Plus, they make terrible cooks!

Nasal viruses and exposure to toxic chemicals are common causes of taste (and smell) disorders. They may cause a temporary problem, but sometimes the effects are permanent.

One nutrient—zinc—has been associated with taste and smell disorders.

Ask your doctor to test for zinc deficiency. Zinc deficiency is a possible cause of taste and smell impairment. Zinc-depleting drugs, poor eating habits, alcoholism, kidney disease or the stress of surgery or severe burns can all set the stage for zinc deficiency. Even if your blood zinc level is normal, your doctor might detect a deficiency with a 24-hour urinary zinc excretion test.

If they're going to work at all, zinc supplements should improve symptoms within weeks. In studies, 440 milligrams of zinc sulfate (equivalent to 176 milligrams of elemental zinc) or 15 to 25 milligrams of zinc acetate or gluconate were effective. Some doctors recommend their patients continue to take supplements for a few weeks after their symptoms improve, then cut back to RDA levels—15 milligrams for men, 12 milligrams for women.

TINNITUS

Experts estimate that 40 to 50 million Americans experience the internal jangle of hums, roars, buzzes, clicks, or, of course, ringing, that characterizes tinnitus.

For most, the sounds are barely noticeable annoyances that last from a few minutes to a few days. For others, though, the noise becomes increasingly loud and persistent, to the point where it disrupts their lives and sends them on the search for treatment. Ringing ears can be caused by loud noises, drugs, allergies or health problems. In some cases, symptoms can be relieved with a small electronic device, known as a masker, which is usually combined with a hearing aid. The masker produces a competitive but pleasant sound that for some people masks the tinnitus.

Most dietary recommendations for tinnitus are designed to address some of the whole-body ailments that can contribute to the problem: high blood pressure, high cholesterol or diabetes. A few recommendations, however, address tinnitus directly.

Avoid caffeine and alcohol. In people who already have tinnitus, over-indulging in these foods can make symptoms worse. Red wine, in particular, can turn up the volume for some people. (Nicotine, although not a food, does the same thing. So do aspirin-containing drugs.)

Hold the MSG. In some people, this common food additive causes ears to buzz.

ULCERATIVE COLITIS

This serious inflammatory bowel disease strikes the colon, causing the intestinal wall to break down. Bloody diarrhea, mucus, pain and fever signal a flare-up. Treated promptly with anti-inflammatory drugs, symptoms usually subside.

Dietary treatment for ulcerative colitis involves avoiding foods that aggravate symptoms, and filling up on those that help.

Go fish. In one study by researchers at the University of California at Davis, daily doses of inflammation-fighting fish oil soothed the symptoms of ulcerative colitis. Eleven men who took 4.2 grams of fish oil a day for three months had a 56 percent decline in the severity of the disease, while another group taking a placebo (harmless blank pill) had only a 4 percent decline. Eight of the men taking fish oil were able to reduce or eliminate their medication. There were no side effects from the fish oil.

Pinpoint trouble foods. Foods aren't thought to cause ulcerative colitis, but once you have developed the disorder, certain foods seem to make symptoms worse. One study found that people with ulcerative colitis had developed a sensitivity to cow's milk. In another, 10 of 13 ulcerative colitis patients on a dairy-free diet remained symptom-free, compared to 5 of 13 people on a control diet that contained dairy products. Fatty foods also seem to cause problems for lots of people. Raw fruits and vegetables, along with other high-fiber foods such as popcorn and bran, are often restricted, too.

Ask your doctor about pectin. Doctors often restrict solid food during a flare-up. In one study, people with ulcerative colitis fed a liquid diet containing pectin (a soluble fiber found in fruits and used to thicken jellies) fared better than those fed the usual liquid diet.

ULCERS

Doctors used to think gastric ulcers were caused by too much stomach acid or a combination of acid and stress. Treatments were designed to decrease or neutralize stomach acid, one way or another. Bland diets were often recommended.

Now, though, it's thought that the development of gastric ulcers is more complex. Researchers believe bacteria *(Helicobacter pylori)* that lodge in the stomach and upper intestine are probably involved in the development of some, if not most, cases of ulcers. The bacteria, thought to secrete chemicals that attack the lining of the stomach or intestine and make it vulnerable to acid erosion, can be found in more than 50 percent of people age 60 or older. Although most people who have the bacteria *do not* develop ulcers, those who do are much less likely to have a recurrence if the bacteria is eradicated with a combination of drugs.

Dietary recommendations are designed to help minimize symptoms while an ulcer is healing and to provide the materials a body needs to heal properly. They include:

Aim for optimal nourishment. Vitamins A and C, zinc and other nutrients are essential for wound-healing. In one study, large amounts of vitamin A helped ulcers heal faster. In another, extra vitamin A reduced formation of ulcers in people with severe burns, injuries or postoperative complications. And in another, zinc supplements resulted in faster healing and reduced pain. In an animal study, vitamin E reduced the occurrence of stress ulcers. Several studies suggest vitamin C helps ulcers heal faster.

Eat full-size meals at regular intervals. "Snacking stimulates stomach acid production but doesn't provide enough food to buffer the additional acid," explains William Ruderman, M.D., chairman of the Department of Gastroenterology at the Cleveland Clinic in Fort Lauderdale, Florida. "I tell my snackers to become meal eaters."

Eat whatever you want, but avoid foods that have given you an upset stomach in the past. Coffee and strong tea stimulate gastric acid secretion, irritating an already fussy stomach. Spicy hot foods have pretty much gotten a bum rap—they don't *cause* ulcers. But if they upset your stomach, stick with tamer fare.

Don't count on milk to soothe your stomach. Initially, it may neutralize acid and you may feel better. But milk actually stimulates acid release: Thirty minutes or more after drinking milk, your acid level goes up. Rely on antacids instead.

Vaginal Yeast Infections

The main sign of a vaginal yeast infection is an itch that won't quit in a place that's never scratched in polite company.

Yeast is normally found in the vagina, but with a yeast infection, it grows out of control. Antibiotics, birth control pills, even semen can upset the vagina's slightly acidic balance and allow yeast to flourish. The yeast can be killed with over-the-counter creams designed just for this purpose. The creams are very effective, with few side effects.

Nutritional therapy is not meant to cure an existing infection. But it can help reduce the number of infections a woman gets. It's aimed at edging the yeast out with beneficial bacteria and restoring the vagina's normal acid balance, which helps keep the yeast population in check.

Eat a cup of live-culture yogurt every day. Yogurt is a popular home remedy for vaginal infections—women eat it or apply it topically. A study confirms that eating yogurt really does work, and even helps women with chronic, drug-resistant vaginal yeast infections. In the study, women who ate one cup a day of yogurt containing live *Lactobacillus acidophilus* (a beneficial type of bacteria that colonizes the vagina and colon) had a clear-cut reduction in symptoms of itching, burning and discharge. During a six-month yogurt-eating period, the average number of infections in the group fell from 2.5 per woman to less than 1.

PART 4

USING FOODS WISELY

CHAPTER 27

Basic Strategies

Pick an Eating Plan You Can Live With

In *The Wizard of Oz,* Dorothy asks Toto the way to the Emerald City. The Scarecrow, hanging nearby, points in *both* directions.

Americans, when it comes to their diets, are a lot like Scarecrow. We want to be healthy *and* feast on pizza, lose weight *and* grab some ice cream. In other words, we not only worry about our cake, we eat it, too.

A Gallup poll perfectly illustrates our yes/no relationship with nutrition. According to the poll:

- Nearly three in four Americans worry about nutrition.
- More than half of all adults say they have significantly changed their eating habits in recent years.
- More than half of grocery shoppers say they read the labels on new foods most or all of the time.

Are we on the road to nutritional health? Not quite. When the people polled were asked to plan a "perfect" meal, nutrition wasn't necessarily the first thing on their minds. Like their parents before them, they craved steak and potatoes, followed by cheesecake or ice cream for dessert.

There's quite a difference between what we think we should eat and what we actually eat, says Marion Nestle, Ph.D., professor and chairperson of the Department of Nutrition, Food and Hotel Management at New York University in New York City.

"The general attitudes toward dietary change in this country reflect a one-third, one-third, one-third trend," adds C. Wayne Callaway, M.D., associate clinical professor at the George Washington University Medical Center in Washington, D.C. According to Dr. Callaway, one-third of people learn about nutrition and make changes in their diet. Another third know they should change their habits, but don't. The last group, unconvinced of the merits of dietary reform, are best described as the still-alive club: "I ate hamburgers and fries yesterday and I'm still alive."

MAKING NUTRITION WORK FOR YOU

Whichever group you belong to, launching a healthy-eating lifestyle can be a confusing process. "There are so many guidelines out there, it's easy for people to throw up their hands and shout, 'I give up,' " says Jeannette Miller, R.D., a nutrition consultant and newspaper columnist in Carbondale, Illinois. "But if they pick just one sensible set of guidelines that they can follow and live with, they'll have a much easier time of it."

In a bit, we'll discuss some of the specific guidelines that can help you plan a nutritious, eminently enjoyable diet. But first let's look at some general rules that can help make your path (whichever one you finally choose) as easy as possible.

Be creative. "There are many ways to eat an adequate diet," says Paul R. Thomas, R.D., Ed.D., project director of the Food and Nutrition Board of the National Academy of Sciences in Washington, D.C., "Make sure you eat a wide variety of grain products, fruits and vegetables. Flexibility is the key." If you usually eat spaghetti, for example, try some spinach fetuccine, instead. Instead of a three-bean salad, make it four or five types of beans.

Expand your horizons. There's no reason for a nutritionally sound meal to be a culinary snooze. Let your imagination fly. Have you ever tasted low-fat cheese with a tart green apple? Try topping your grapefruit half with thinly sliced kiwi. Or sprinkle warm spinach leaves with lemon and hard-boiled egg whites for an unusually tasty breakfast treat.

Take one step at a time. "Never expect your family to make a lot of big changes all at once," Miller advises. "For example, don't give skim milk to someone who is used to drinking whole milk. Give them 2 percent milk for a few weeks, then 1 percent milk and eventually, skim. If you walk away from something gradually, you won't miss it."

Banish temptation. Even staunchly sensible eaters occasionally are tempted by cookies, ice cream and the many other "diet traps" that will sabotage the best of intentions. Protect yourself by stocking the pantry with foods you know you should eat—not those you can't resist. "If good food is in the house, that's what you'll eat," Miller says.

Watch the big picture. The best-laid schemes, said poet Robert Burns, often go awry. That's especially true for dietary improvement plans. Nearly everyone occasionally indulges in a sugary snack or "forgets" and has two helpings of steak. "People should think about their food intake over time and not just focus on single food items," says Dr. Callaway. "You need to look at your food intake the way you look at your checkbook—it's something you have to balance over weeks, months, years and a lifetime."

Now that you understand the basics, it's time to take a look at some of the different plans nutritionists recommend for healthy eating. Each approach has its own strengths and weaknesses. Which you ultimately pick is entirely up to you. Let's begin this discussion by looking at the grand-daddy of nutritional guidelines, the Basic Four.

SETTING YOUR PRIORITIES

Of all the hundreds of dietary habits you can possibly adopt, which ones are the most powerful for preventing disease and promoting optimum health? Should you put a lot of energy into reducing the amount of cholesterol in your diet? Or is it more important to avoid alcoholic beverages? Where exactly is the biggest health payoff?

The question was posed to more than 300 top nutrition experts in a poll conducted by Medical Consensus Surveys, a research arm of *Prevention* magazine. These black belts in nutrition were asked to rate 44 nutritional actions (all purported to benefit health) as follows: extremely important, very important, important, not important but may help or probably worthless.

The nutritionists' responses were then compiled and statistically weighted to create a list of dietary "top priorities" for preserving and boosting your health.

Priority/ Ranking	Action
Very High Priority	
79	Control calorie intake to control your weight
76	Reduce all dietary fats
75	Control fat intake to control your weight
High Priority	
71	Increase physical activity to enable greater nutrient intake
71	Enjoy your food
70	Balance your diet among the four food groups
69	Ensure adequate intake of vitamins and minerals to meet the RDAs
65	Replace saturated fats with monos and polys
65	If not pregnant or trying to conceive, limit your alcohol intake to one or two drinks per day

High Priority	**Action**
63	Replace whole-milk products with low-fat and nonfat dairy products
63	Avoid raw eggs, raw meat and raw seafood
62	Increase total fiber to at least 20 grams per day
62	Eat more complex carbohydrates, such as grains, rice, beans, potatoes, bread and pasta
61	Eat more fish in place of meat
59	Ensure adequate intake of soluble fiber
57	Avoid very low calorie diets
56	Cut meat portions to three to four ounces
55	Reduce dietary cholesterol
54	Ensure adequate intake of insoluble fiber
54	Eat at least five fruit and vegetables per day
54	Eat breakfast
51	Reduce sodium intake
Moderate Priority	
49	Increase intake of cruciferous vegetables, such as broccoli, cauliflower, kale and others
49	Avoid eating large meals and snacking excessively in the evening when activity levels tend to be low
48	Switch from butter to margarine
48	Restrict intake of tropical oils
47	Drink six to eight 8-ounce glasses of water (or decaffeinated, low-calorie and low-fat fluids) every day
47	Avoid nitrates and nitrites (smoked and cured foods)
44	Reduce trans-fatty acids (e.g., stick margarine, hydrogenated vegetable shortening)
43	Reduce sugar intake
41	Eat three square meals a day with a minimum of snacking in between

continued

Moderate Priority	**Action**
41	Eat only when you're hungry (regardless of whether it's mealtime or not) and only to satiety
40	Limit your daily caffeine consumption to the amount in four cups of coffee
38	Peel or wash fruit before eating to avoid pesticides
37	Increase beta-carotene intake
37	Switch from stick margarine to soft (tub) and liquid margarine
35	Have a regular nutritional assessment
30	Eliminate alcohol from your diet
29	Restrict your intake of phosphorus
Low Priority	
24	Increase intake of vitamin E beyond the RDA without exceeding safe limits
23	Increase intake of vitamin C beyond the RDA without exceeding safe limits
16	Make breakfast the biggest meal of the day
14	Avoid irradiated foods
13	Avoid overgrilled (i.e., charred) or blackened foods

NOTE: The numbers in the left column represent the relative importance of each positive action, based on a scale of 0 (not important) to 100 (extremely important).

FOUR GROUPS, THOUSANDS OF CHOICES

In 1956 the U.S. Department of Agriculture divided the wide world of foods into four groups: grains, meats, dairy products and fruits and vegetables. For Americans to have a balanced diet, experts said, they need only eat several daily servings from each of the groups. They called this plan the Basic Four Food Groups.

Imagine a cube or circle divided into four equal sections. The dairy group typically is represented by a wedge of cheese or a milk bottle. In the meat compartment goes a pork chop or a chicken and an egg. A carrot and peach may represent the fruit and vegetable group, while a loaf of bread typifies the grain group.

The Basic Four is to nutrition what the three Rs—reading, writing and 'rithmetic—are to education: A strong foundation to support a lifetime of good habits. "There was an understanding early on that what one ate had a strong influence on one's health," says Dr. Thomas.

PUTTING THE PLAN TO WORK

Now that you understand the Basic Four, you can begin "building" nutritious meals from each of the four groups. Keep in mind the minimum recommended number of servings: two dairy products; two servings of meat, fish, poultry or eggs; four helpings of fruits and vegetables; and four servings of bread, flour or whole-grain cereals.

To get your daily allotment of grains, for example, you could eat a bowl of cereal, two slices of whole-wheat toast, a serving of rice and a zesty bowl of tabbouleh during the course of your day. The fruit and vegetable category offers even more variety: apples, oranges, melons, berries, peas, beans and spinach are among the foods that you can choose from. There's just as much variety in the meat and dairy groups. You could eat different foods seven days a week and always have a square meal!

Indeed, eating different foods can be a nutritional boon, Dr. Thomas says. "The greater the variety of foods you eat, the better you'll do." By contrast, the more limited the variety, "the greater the risk of not getting enough nutrients."

SQUARE MEALS OR WISHFUL THINKING?

Mmmmm. I'll have the 16-ounce steak, onion rings and chocolate cake with vanilla ice cream, please. Meat? Check. Vegetable? Yep. Grain? Check. Dairy? Check. Okay—now I have all four of the Basic Four Food Groups. Must be a good, square meal, right?

Hardly. But with wishful thinking, "virtually any food can be made to fit into one of the food groups," says Paul R. Thomas, R.D., Ed.D., project director of the Food and Nutrition Board of the National Academy of Sciences in Washington, D.C.

Take the meal above. Technically it meets the requirements for the Basic Four plan. But the meal is so heavy on protein and fat, and so light on healthful grains and vegetables, it's probably worse then following no plan at all.

When you begin "building" meals based on the Basic Four, try to be realistic, Dr. Thomas advises. The idea isn't to fool yourself but to lay down a healthy foundation of grains, vegetables and fruits with smaller amounts of dairy products and meat or meat alternatives such as legumes. Once you have a firm base, then you can treat yourself to the occasional potato chip or strawberry sundae. What's the category? Just call them the *fun* food group!

SERIOUS OMISSIONS

Although the Basic Four provides an easy-to-follow framework for healthy eating, some nutritionists worry it's a bit too simple. Yes, by following the guidelines you're unlikely to become malnourished. But what about eating too much? When it comes to dietary *excess,* Dr. Nestle says, the Basic Four is basically silent.

Foods that are high in calories, fat, salt or sugar and low in nutrients may appear in any of the four groups, and no distinction is made between them and more healthful options.

For example, cheesecake might be found in the dairy category, although few people would suggest it's the nutritional equal of yogurt. Similarly, a slice of sponge cake might appear in the grain category, although it's scarcely a rival for seven-grain bread.

The same problem occurs with "related" foods that have vastly different nutritional values. For example, both broccoli and iceberg lettuce occupy the vegetable niche, yet broccoli contains a great deal more fiber, vitamins A and C and other nutrients, says Dr. Nestle. In short, it's a superior food, although you wouldn't know this if your only information came from the Basic Four.

Despite these "crimes of omission," doctors agree the Basic Four is a useful guide on the road to good nutrition. For more detailed guidelines, look at the plan below.

THE NATIONAL DIETARY GUIDELINES

In many parts of the world, people are more likely to get too little food than too much. In this country, the opposite is true. Dietary excesses are a leading cause of obesity, diabetes, heart disease, high blood pressure and many other serious diseases.

To check our tendency to overindulge, experts have formulated the *Dietary Guidelines for Americans*. The guidelines aren't meant to replace the Basic Four. What they do is encourage people to concentrate on healthy foods, says Dr. Callaway.

"Rather than come at it from a restrictive point of view and tell people what they shouldn't eat, the Dietary Guidelines emphasize the positive: the delicious foods people can add to their diets," he says.

SEVEN STEPS TO HEALTH

The guidelines are simple: Eat more fruits, vegetables and grains, and limit your consumption of sugar, fats, alcohol and salt. Specifically, experts say:

1. Enjoy nature's bounty. There are more than 40 nutrients that are essential to good health. The best way to get enough of these nutrients is to regularly eat many foods, says Dr. Nestle. So experiment. Try new foods in new combinations. Instead of eggs for breakfast, have a grapefruit. Follow your noon sandwich with an apple or pear. Have turkey breast instead of pot roast. Add several vegetables to the dinner menu, and follow up with fruit for dessert. The more healthful foods you try, she says, the less likely you are to come up short—or overweight.

2. Be a lean machine. Study after study has shown that diets high in fat contribute to everything from diabetes and cancer to high blood pressure and heart disease. If you do eat meat, stick to lean cuts such as flank steak or chicken breast (without the skin). A low-fat diet is the best short-cut to keeping your cholesterol low, your arteries clear and your weight down.

3. Plan to eat more plant foods. On the nutritional road to good health, the plant kingdom should be your first stop. Most fruits, vegetables and cereal grains are low in fat, high in fiber and positively packed with important vitamins and minerals.

The guidelines call for three servings of vegetables, two servings of fruit and six servings of grains every day. This may sound like a mountain of food, but it's all in a normal day's dining. For example, a single slice of whole-grain bread takes care of one of your grain servings. A bowl of oatmeal and a small biscuit take care of two more. Add to this a grapefruit, an apple and several servings of salad or cooked vegetables, and you've fulfilled one part of the guidelines. The others are just as easy.

4. Sack the sugar. It's unfortunate, but many of the foods we love the best—cookies, candy bars and ice cream, to name just a few—don't love us back. The arithmetic is simple: Processed sugar, whether packed into peanut butter fudge or stirred into coffee, adds up to empty calories. To satisfy your sweet tooth *and* protect your waistline, get your sugars the natural way—from grapes, watermelon and other fruits.

5. Go lightly on salt. In small amounts, sodium and chloride—the main ingredients in table salt—are essential nutrients for good health. Taken in excess, however, they can cause high blood pressure and a host of other problems.

Salt is tough to avoid. Even if you shun the shaker on your table, it's found in everything from canned soups to store-bought bread. That's why you *must* read the labels, experts say. Whenever possible, buy foods that have little or no added salt. In the kitchen, don't add salt while you're cooking. In time you'll lose your "salt tooth," and your health will be the winner.

6. Maintain a healthy weight. Doctors agree that obesity is one of the leading causes of disease and early death. If you've tried to lose weight and can't, see your doctor. When you succeed, the benefits will last a lifetime.

7. Drink only in moderation. There simply are no great benefits to be had from drinking alcohol, and there are plenty of risks. If you do drink, doctors say, do so in moderation— no more than one to two drinks a day. And remember: The calories in alcohol are "empty." As the drinks go down, your weight may go up.

THE FOOD GUIDE PYRAMID

Here's still another approach to healthy eating. Designed by the U.S. Department of Agriculture, the Food Guide Pyramid displays the types of foods you should eat each day: grains, vegetables, fruits, meats and dairy products. (Fats, oils and sweets are included but are optional.) The Pyramid also lists the recommended number of servings for each group.

Did you just hear an echo from the Basic Four Food Groups? The plans are similar. However, the Food Guide Pyramid doesn't treat the food groups equally. (You'll remember this was a complaint leveled against the Basic Four.)

Instead, it recommends eating more of some types of foods and less of others. Let's take a look.

Like the Egyptian landmark, the Food Guide Pyramid is a triangle planted wide-end down. The inside is divided into four tiers, with the broadest at the bottom and the smallest at the top. The size of each tier corresponds to the amounts of food you should eat. For example:

Begin with grains. Rice, pastas, breads and cereals occupy the Pyramid's largest tier, and with good reason: They represent the *foundation* for your diet. These foods give you a firm base of complex carbohydrates, B vitamins, protein and fiber. The plan calls for 6 to 11 servings a day.

Then add fruits and vegetables. These form the second tier of the Pyramid. Fruits (two to four servings daily) and vegetables (three to five servings) will help you meet your daily requirements for fiber, vitamins C and A and many other important nutrients.

Add some protein. The third tier of the Pyramid includes red meat, poultry, fish, dry beans, eggs, cheese, milk and yogurt. Nutritionists say you should eat two to three daily servings of the meat, bean and egg group, and the same number of servings of dairy products. Together, these groups will give you an abundance of protein, B vitamins, calcium and other minerals.

Watch out for fats. Unlike the Basic Four, the Pyramid doesn't ignore fats, oils and sweets. Instead, they're perched on the Pyramid's pinnacle—along with a warning to use them sparingly.

Too Many Choices?

As with the Basic Four and the Dietary Guidelines, the Food Guide Pyramid offers a complete, easy-to-understand guide for a lifetime of healthy eating. So long as you properly apportion your diet among the four tiers, you can eat pretty much everything you want—within your caloric limits, of course! "The actual foods you choose are a matter of personal preference," says Dr. Thomas. In other words, the Pyramid emphasizes groups—you pick the foods.

For beginners, however, the Food Guide Pyramid can seem daunting. They may wonder, "Must we stuff ourselves with up to *11* servings of breads, cereals and grains? Is there enough time in the day to eat as many as *9* helpings of fruits and vegetables? Won't we burst?"

The servings quickly add up, Dr. Thomas says. "Just a sandwich can give you a third of the minimum six servings of grain products," he explains. In fact, if you drink juice in the morning, add dried fruit to your cereal, snack on fruits and vegetables and add carrots and potatoes to your casserole, you're well on your way.

THE NEW FOUR FOOD GROUPS

Doctors have known for a long time that people who base their diets on high-fiber, low-fat foods tend to be healthier than those who fill up on pizza, hamburgers and shakes. Large studies such as the Framingham Heart Study, the China Health Study and work by Dean Ornish, M.D., all have shown that diets based on plant foods can help cut the risk of cancer, diabetes, heart disease and high blood pressure. That's why experts nearly are unanimous in recommending that people eat fewer meats and more grains, fruits and vegetables.

The New Four Food Groups plan takes this approach a step further. Designed by the Physicians Committee for Responsible Medicine, it recommends that people build their diets from whole grains, legumes, vegetables and fruits. No meat. No sweets. No dairy products.

"The New Four Food Groups do not mean you should *never* eat meat or dairy products," explains Neal Barnard, M.D., president of the physicians committee. "What we are saying is that they should be considered options, not essentials."

PYRAMID POWER

Let's compare your diet to the Food Guide Pyramid. First count the servings you eat every day from each of the different groups. Then compare them to the daily servings recommended below. This will help you decide which foods you need more of, which you may cut back on and which are just right.

Food Group	Servings per Day	Serving Size Examples
Bread, cereals, pasta, other grain products	6-11 (include several whole-grain products every day)	1 slice of bread bun ½ hamburger bun or English muffin 1 small roll, biscuit or muffin 4 small or 2 large crackers ½ cup cooked cereal, pasta, rice or other whole grain, such as barley or buckwheat 1 ounce ready-to-eat cereal
Fruits	2-4	1 med. apple, orange or banana ½ grapefruit 1 melon wedge 6 ounces fruit juice ½ cup berries ½ cup cooked or canned fruit

Food Group	Servings per Day	Serving Size Examples
		¼ cup dried fruit, such as raisins, apricots or prunes
Vegetables (dark green or yellow vegetables, potatoes, dry beans and peas or other legumes)	3-5	½ cup cooked vegetables
		½ cup chopped, raw vegetables
		1 cup raw, leafy vegetables, such as spinach or lettuce
Meat, poultry, fish and alternates (eggs, dry beans and peas, nuts and seeds)	2-3	Servings should total 5 to 7 ounces of cooked lean meat, poultry or fish per day
		1 egg, ½ cup cooked beans or 2 tablespoons peanut butter count as 1 ounce of meat
Milk, cheese or yogurt	2 (3 for pregnant women)	1 cup milk or yogurt
		1½ ounces natural cheese
		2 ounces processed cheese
Fats, oils, sweets and alcohol	—	Avoid too many fats and sweets. If you drink alcoholic beverages, do so in moderation.

WEED OUT TEMPTATION

So you're ready to begin cutting fat, adding fiber and otherwise improving your diet. Where to begin?

For starters, nutritionists say, take a look at the foods in your larder. Are white bread and salted crackers really the best choices for one of your food groups? Do you have to buy hamburger, or would lean flank steak do as well? The next time you go shopping, nutritionists say, begin replacing inferior foods with their more nutritious counterparts. For example:

Low Fiber	High Fiber
White bread	7-grain bread
White rice	Brown rice
Spaghetti	Whole-wheat pasta
Instant pilaf mix	Lentils and chick-peas
Corn flakes	Corn bran cereal
Fruit juice	Oranges and apples
Watermelon	Fresh berries

High Sodium	Low Sodium
Canned beans	Dry beans
Canned vegetables	Frozen or fresh veggies
Mix-n-eat oatmeal	Regular oatmeal
Cold cuts	Fresh cuts of meat and poultry
American cheese	Low-salt Swiss cheese
Soy sauce	Lemon juice

High Fat	Low Fat
Ice cream	Low-fat frozen yogurt
Whole milk	Skim or 1 percent milk
Cheddar cheese	Skim-milk cheese
Corned beef	Lean roast beef
Spareribs	Skinless chicken breast
Sardines	Tuna packed in water

These are just a few examples to help you begin your nutritional make-over. Before long, stocking your pantry with low-fat, low-sodium and high-fiber foods will be second nature.

WE HAVE A LONG WAY TO GO

Though Americans have become increasingly savvy about nutrition, we still have room for improvement, says Marion Nestle, Ph.D., of New York University in New York City. Polls have shown:

• About 36 to 38 percent of Americans' calories come from fat. That's down slightly from the 1960s, although it is well above the recommended 30 percent or less.

• We still eat a lot of steak, hamburger and pot roast, despite warnings about the health risks of eating too much red meat.

• Only 33 percent of Americans ate the recommended minimum of five servings of fruits and vegetables on the day they were surveyed. In fact, 7 percent said they ate *no* fruits or vegetables.

It doesn't have to be this way. According to Paul R. Thomas, R.D., Ed.D., of the National Academy of Sciences in Washington, D.C., people can make healthful changes in their diets without going crazy. "Making relatively minor changes in the diet—for example, decreasing the size of the meat portion and including a fruit or vegetable in each of your meals—can lead to substantial changes toward healthier diets," he says.

People should have five servings a day of breads, pastas, rice, corn or other grains, Dr. Barnard says. Three servings a day each of beans, vegetables and fruits completes the requirements.

Because the plan represents quite a departure from the traditional American diet (hot dogs and hamburgers come to mind), it may be a challenge for people who aren't seriously motivated, Dr. Thomas says. And if they don't plan carefully, they may put themselves at nutritional risk. Those who suc-ceed in making plant foods the center of their dietary circles, however, may be well rewarded—with lower cholesterol, healthier arteries and perhaps slimmer waistlines, too.

FIVE A DAY FOR HEALTH

The Five-a-Day Plan, which is being promoted by the Na-tional Cancer Institute, focuses on the disease-fighting power of fruits and vegetables, says Elizabeth Pivonka, R.D., Ph.D., director of nutrition and sciences for the Produce for Better Health Foundation in Newark, Delaware. "It's a completely positive message—we're not telling anyone what *not* to eat," she says.

The idea is simply to eat a minimum of five servings of vegetables and fruits daily as part of a low-fat, high-fiber diet.

"The Five-a-Day program is something that everybody should feel really comfortable about supporting," says Dr. Nestle. "Eating five fruits and vegetables every day would make a big difference in the American diet." Adds Dr. Pivonka, "The plan is easy to remember, easy to follow, and it's tasty." It's also an easy way to plump healthy amounts of fiber and vitamins A and C into your daily diet.

Don't be lulled into a false sense of security, though, by adding a few extra vegetables and fruits to your diet and doing little else. You can't *really* keep the doctor away with an apple a day—not if every day you eat three eggs for breakfast, fast food for lunch and greasy pizza for supper.

Still, some people aren't prepared to change their entire diet, Dr. Pivonka says. For them, adding a few oranges, green salads, broccoli and other fruits and vegetables might make a big difference.

CHAPTER 28

Cooking Light

Techniques and Tips

Your shelves may bow under packages of dry beans and pasta, but the benefits they bestow can be overwhelmed in dishes that ooze butter or cheese.

Your refrigerator bins overflow with fresh vegetables, which, in turn, overflow with vitamins, but their nutrients can be nullified by boiling them away.

Your freezer is packed with poultry and fish, but their low-fat goodness will be lost if you coat them with batter and deep-fry them.

Cooking methods that obliterate foods' nutritious goodness are sheer folly when your priority is to give your diet a healthful lift. The not-so-healthful techniques that scarcely deserve a good-bye wave as you usher them out of your kitchen include boiling vegetables into green-gray mush, deep-frying and extra oily sautéing, butter-based baking, marinating and basting with fat and salty sauces, and adding fat- and salt-drenched gravies and toppings to otherwise healthful dishes. Good riddance.

Clear your culinary thinking of those poor preparation choices and you're left with a rich array of cooking methods that lend such flavor and variety you'll never miss your old ways. The good news is that you can begin today to take control of your healthful eating strategy by adopting cooking methods like these.

HOW LONG SHOULD YOU STEAM?

Steaming vegetables is an imprecise art, because of the great ranges of sizes and densities. You can use this table, though, to gauge the time at which you should begin checking the food for doneness.

Time (min.)	Vegetable
3	Asparagus
	Broccoli rabe, whole leaves
	Greens, beet, kale, etc.
	Peas, shelled
	Snow pea pods
5	Beans, green or wax
	Beans, lima
	Corn, off the cob
	Snap pea pods
7	Broccoli, medium stalks
	Corn on the cob
	Potato chunks
	Summer squash chunks
8	Cabbage, quarter heads
10	Brussels sprouts
	Carrot chunks
	Fennel, quarter heads
	Parsnip chunks
12	Cauliflower florets
	Turnips, quartered
15	Eggplant slices, peeled
18	Potatoes, whole, medium
20	Winter squash chunks
30	Artichokes, whole

STEAMING

It's hard to resist the fresh flavor of steamed vegetables cooked to perfection, splashed with lemon juice, sprinkled with basil, dill or any fresh herb and presented without a hint of added fat. Although vitamin-robbing boiling water is the cooking agent in this method, foods never actually touch it, so more of the vitamins in fresh and frozen vegetables are yours to keep, as long as steaming time is short, says Susan Witz, R.D., Director of Nutrition at Heartland Health and Fitness Retreat and Spa in Gilman, Illinois.

Put a lid on it. For the best steaming results, bring about an inch of water to a boil in a pot with a tight-fitting lid. Place vegetables in a steaming basket that fits into the pot without getting dunked, and cover. To conserve color and vitamins, steam vegetables until they are tender, but no longer. Steaming is an excellent, no-fat-added, quick way to cook broccoli, summer squash, asparagus, carrots and spinach. It is also a better choice than boiling for longer-cooking vegetables such as potatoes, turnips and parsnips.

"Some people might think steamed vegetables are going to be tasteless; they want a sauce on everything," says Nancy Leicht, former sous chef at Heartland. "But steaming lets us get down to the essence of eating fresh foods. It's a matter of learning that we don't need all those rich calories to enjoy them."

POACHING

"A lot of people feel they don't have time to cook," Leicht points out. Yet you can quickly prepare healthful and elegant foods by starting with fresh, high-quality ingredients that don't need a lot of time-hungry cooking methods or embellishments, she says. Poaching is a quick, gentle, no-fat-added method that rivals the results of much more elaborate techniques.

Depend on these liquid assets. Poach foods by briefly simmering them in a shallow pool of whatever liquid you choose: water, broth, fruit or vegetable juice. No-fuss poaching works especially well for delicate fillets of fish, such as sole, that cook in minutes, and for fragile fruits, such as ripe, skinned pears. The water, broth or juice in which the food is cooked can then be seasoned and reduced—boiled down to a fraction of its original volume—to intensify its flavor, then poured over the food for a light, refreshing sauce.

STIR-FRYING

Stir-frying vegetables, meats and fish with little or no added fat is one of the fastest ways to put a remarkably healthful meal on the table. "The basic idea behind stir-fry cooking is to cook at high heat for a short amount of time, which retains vitamins and keeps food intact so it doesn't become limp or lose its appeal," says Leicht.

Bring on the vegetables . . . any vegetables. You can cook colorful, delicious and nourishing vegetable masterpieces in minutes by stir-frying. Almost any combination of vegetables—oriental cabbages, carrots, onions, peppers, snow peas, squash, broccoli, asparagus, you name it—can be whipped up in a hot wok or large sauté pan.

"The key to easy stir-frying is cutting the foods up into similar sizes beforehand so that it all cooks evenly and is ready at the same time," says Leicht. Vegetables are done when they take on an intense color but have not lost their crispness. "Carrots or other hard vegetables should be cooked for a few minutes before most of the other foods go in, and you can throw pea pods in at the last moment to prevent them from being overcooked," she suggests.

A dab of cooking oil guarantees a stick-free dish, but for the ultimate low-fat vegetable stir-fry, try tossing your vegetables with a few tablespoons of water, wine, broth or fruit juice, says Joanne D'Agostino, R.N., author and low-fat-cooking consultant based in Easton, Pennsylvania. Stir-frying without oil is a no-stick snap as long as your wok or sauté pan is large enough to keep the food sizzling hot and moving rapidly. "I really find that vegetables taste better without the oil, and they stay crisper," says D'Agostino. Go easy on salt in your vegetable stir-fry by splashing on a reduced-sodium soy sauce, if you like. Or, skip the salt altogether by adding a dash of ginger juice. Finally, your amazingly healthful and colorful creation is ready for a bed of rice, barley or pasta. Or add a side dish of cooked, dried beans instead of meat for a vegetarian stir-fry feast.

Add lean meat, poultry or fish and wok away from fat. "In traditional Chinese and Asian cusine, meat is used as a flavoring ingredient or as a supplement or condiment rather than a main ingredient," says Martin Yan, chef, food consultant and public television cooking show host. A little bit of marinated meat, poultry or firm-fleshed fish can go a long way when it is stir-fried with lots of crisp vegetables. "You don't need a lot of oil, whatever you stir-fry," says Yan.

For stir-fried combination dishes, cook the meat or fish first until it is almost done, before adding vegetables, which need only a quick toss in a hot wok. "You don't want to worry about thinly sliced peppers being overcooked while the chicken or shrimp is still raw in the center, for example," says Leicht. "Another way to hasten the cooking of chicken, shrimp and scallops in a stir-fry is to marinate them in an acid, such as lemon or lime juice, with some herbs. The marinade adds flavor and also actually firms up the flesh so that when you put it in the wok it will cook faster because it's already on its way."

For an exciting change of pace, add diced apples, orange segments or pineapple chunks to your next stir-fry.

GRILLING AND BROILING

Almost any food would do well to jump *out* of the frying pan and into the fire—or at least *close* to the fire—from a grill

GETTING INTO HOT WATER

Despite the reputation that boiling has as a vitamin robber, there are a few types of foods on your healthy-eating menu that just have to be cooked in hot water. Pasta, grains and dry beans.

Pasta. To take full advantage of the low-fat, high-carbohydrate, low-sodium nature of pasta, unlearn the urge to cook it in salted water with a layer of anti-stick oil floating in it. Cook dry or fresh pasta in rapidly boiling, plain water. Use enough water for the pasta to swim freely when you gently stir it once or twice during cooking to avoid sticking.

"Any pasta dish can also be made with the colorful pastas that are available, although there is so little spinach, tomato or other vegetable added to them for color that they're not significantly more nutritious than plain, white pasta," says Susan Witz, R.D., of Heartland Health and Fitness Retreat and Spa in Gilman, Illinois. "Whole-wheat pasta does have a little more fiber and protein, though, and there are various types of high-gluten, high-protein pastas that do provide more of that nutrient."

Grains. If boiling a batch of white rice is your idea of grain cooking, be prepared to widen your horizons. "Two of the most popular healthy grains are bulgur and millet, and they're both very easy to prepare," says vegetarian cookbook author Mollie Katzen, of Berkeley, California. Bulgur is chopped, or cracked, pre-steamed, whole-wheat grains. "To cook bulgur, put some in a bowl, pour in up to twice as much boiling water, cover and wait 15 or 20 minutes for the grains to absorb the moisture," says Katzen. The result is a pleasantly chewy, nourishing grain dish that can be used instead of rice as a bed for stir-fried vegetables. Or serve it cold, mixed with parsley, tomato, garlic, olive oil, mint and lemon juice, as tabbouleh, a healthful Middle Eastern salad.

Millet is another quick-cooking, nutritious whole grain that is ideal for pan toasting, a low-fat method that gives grains a nutty flavor and keeps them from turning mushy when simmered as a base for fluffy pilaf. Toast the pale yellow spheres of millet over low to moderate heat in a large, heavy pan, stirring frequently until the grains turn tawny. Add boiling water or fat-free stock to the grains, and whatever seasonings and vegetables you like, such as diced onions, peppers and carrots. Cover the pan tightly and simmer until all the water is absorbed. Fluff it with a fork and your perfect pilaf is served. "You can do this with just about any grain or combination of grains to add flavor and interest to them," says Katzen, "but the amounts of water and cooking times will vary."

Most other whole grains—long- or short-grain brown rice, whole-oat groats, wild rice, barley and cracked corn grits also turn out very well when you simply measure the grain, add it to the correct amount of boiling water or broth in a heavy saucepan, cover it tightly and simmer it very gently for the called-for amount of time. No peeking or stirring while it cooks or the grain may turn out underdone or sticky. To add flavor to the grains without adding salt, fat or calories, try adding lemon pepper, Italian seasonings or curry powder to the water. To cut most grains' cooking times in half, simmer them in a pressure cooker, instead.

Beans. Because they, too, must be reconstituted, many of the cooking methods for dry beans and lentils are similar to those for grains. They can also be simmered in slow cookers or crock pots or speed cooked (relatively speaking) after overnight soaking. Follow the directions on dry bean packages for the best results. Cooking with canned or precooked, dehydrated beans are instant ways to add these high-fiber, low-fat little wonders to your healthy diet.

or broiler. Grilling and broiling have similar advantages: Foods cook over or under direct, high heat, and neither method calls for adding fats. Any fats that do cook out of foods fall into the grill or are drained away into a pan beneath the broiling rack. The idea is to keep fat levels down as much as possible, so barbecued ribs and other fat-laden items are out. To keep grilled or broiled foods moist and flavorful, marinate or baste them with citrus fruit juice, defatted broth or fat-free sauces.

Keep it simple. Poultry, lean cuts of meat and firm-fleshed fish are naturals on a grill or under a broiler. "Grilling, by its nature, is a healthy style of cooking because it produces a lot of flavor on its own, and it doesn't call for a lot of accompaniments," says Chris Schlesinger, chef and co-owner of the East Coast Grill in Cambridge, Massachusetts. "For example, you can grill a piece of plain fish or beef and that's all you need; no herb butter, no cream sauce," he explains.

Or, perhaps you like to show off your flair for dressing up foods. There are plenty of ways to do so without reaching for fatty or salty barbecue sauces. "Top grilled meat or fish with fruit relishes, salsas or chutneys instead," Schlesinger suggests. "And you can add lime juice, ginger, garlic and other spices to fish, rather than loading it down with rich sauces."

Take special care with fish. Firm fish, such as swordfish and tuna can stand up to just about any cooking style, but more tender types of fish need a bit more care in their handling, says Leicht. "When you grill or broil fish such as salmon or trout, the heat of the grill and the amount of cooking time are the most important factors to consider. The coals should be medium hot. That means they're not flaming anymore and are powdery on the surface," she says. "When you put a small piece of fish on a grill that is so hot, it won't take very long at all to cook, so watch it closely.

"The appearance and feel of the fish are important indicators of doneness. When a dense fish, like salmon, is approaching the overdone point, a white residue appears on the surface and tells you it is definitely time to get the fish away from the fire. More delicate fish, like sole, turn from a translucent state to a pure white state and take on a firmness when they are done," she explains.

If you have been shy about grilling fish because of its delicate nature, try cooking fish steaks, rather than fillets. They're a bit easier to handle. Also, fish does have a tendency to stick to grills, and could be hard to turn or remove, says Leicht. "To prevent that, brush or spray a little bit of canola oil on the grill or on the fish itself and there won't be any problem," she suggests.

Try meatless kabobs. You need not put your grill away if you rarely eat meat. Most vegetables can easily and quickly be broiled or grilled. Leave small veggies—such as cherry tomatoes, mushrooms, small onions and pea pods—whole and grill them in a mesh rack, or skewer them on shish-kabob spears. Large vegetables, such as summer squash and potatoes, can be sliced diagonally to give them a large surface area for resting on the grill. Marinate or baste vegetables with lime or orange juice or with low-fat salad dressing to keep them moist while they cook.

For a special, fruity treat, try grilled or broiled sliced apples, bananas, pineapple, oranges, peaches, or pears. Season them with ginger, cinnamon or lemon or lime juice. Wrap fruit in foil for grilling or broil it directly. Or thread chunks of fruit onto skewers and enjoy grilled or broiled fruit kabobs.

BAKING AND ROASTING

Baking and roasting might conjure images of belt-busting holiday feasts, but your oven is also a great place to prepare lots of everyday foods in a healthful way.

Curtail fat without fuss. Most meats and poultry can go directly from the refrigerator into the oven, without much fuss, after a quick rinse and dry-off with paper towels, and certainly without adding fats, oils or salt. Place meats and poultry on a rack in an ovenproof pan to melt away and drain off much of the fat you cannot trim off. Once the food is put in the oven at the recommended temperature, it is basically on "automatic pilot," thriving on minimum attention until your oven timer goes off.

Make it moist with marinade. For added flavor interest, and to help meat and fish stay moist, baste them with broth, fruit juice or a low-fat marinade. Marinating can be a flavor and moisture boon to low-fat foods that could otherwise become dry or tough when you bake or roast them. "Marinating can be especially healthful if you limit the oil. Use just a scant amount of olive oil in marinades or eliminate it altogether. Concentrate more on herb-lemon or herb-vinegar blends for marinating. There are virtually no calories in these, but there is a lot of flavor," says Leicht.

Be quick with fish. "Slow roasting is one method that does not usually lend itself well to fish. It's better to bake fish quickly, at relatively high heat, so that it doesn't become tough," says Leicht. "The more delicate a fish is in flavor and texture, the more you must guard against taking away from that delicacy. You can bake delicate fillets of sole or flounder, if you do it carefully. Denser fish, like salmon or tuna, can be baked, too, but they also stand up to cooking by just about any method," she explains.

"Overcooking by just a few minutes can make fish dry, and you can't reverse overdoneness," Leicht says. To prevent that, check the fish frequently when it is approaching the time limit called for in recipes.

Don't stop with just potatoes. "Roasting and baking are slow-cooking methods that can be used for dense vegetables, such as potatoes and sweet potatoes, winter squash, onions and garlic," says Leicht. Baking vegetables can be as simple as washing them, pricking the skins to prevent steam buildup, which can cause vegetables to explode, and placing them on a baking sheet in a hot oven. Vegetables are done when they can easily be pierced to the center with a fork.

Moisture-lending vegetables, such as zucchini and pumpkin, are quite at home in flavorful, baked quick breads and muffins, too, says D'Agostino. They give baked products a moist texture that can make people forget egg-enriched or butter-burdened cakes.

Bake some sweet treats. Various fruits, such as apples, bananas and pears, can be baked whole for simple, warm desserts. Add a sprinkle of cinnamon or nutmeg for a spicy flavor boost without added calories.

Baked goods that include fruit for flavor, sweetness and moisture can be the crowning glory of low-fat cooking. Apples, bananas, pears, peaches and other sweet, moist fruits can be used in breads, quick breads, cookies and muffins to replace eggs and fats and to add fiber and nutrients. Fresh or frozen berries as well as raisins, chopped figs or other dried fruits are sweet, fiber-rich delights when you add them to fruit tarts, cobblers, pies and crisps. The concentrated sweetness of very ripe berries and dried fruits can replace some of the sugar in many dessert recipes.

Fiber-up with flour power. Baking breads, quick breads, cakes, muffins, waffles and cookies using whole-grain flours is a good way to add fiber to your diet. You can do it in an extra healthful way by cutting in half (or better) the amount of butter, margarine or oil called for in recipes that contain fruit, vegetables or other moistening ingredients, such as nonfat yogurt, says D'Agostino.

You can also give your baked goods a fiber lift by adding wheat germ or bran to your recipes, replacing an equal amount of flour. The secret to working with bran, says Linny Largent-Mayer, executive chef at the Los Olivos Grand Hotel near Santa Barbara, California, is to soak it in hot water for at least 10 minutes to soften it. This will make your fiber-rich baked goods much lighter and moister.

A LITTLE OF THIS, INSTEAD OF THAT

When you begin cooking in more healthful ways, usually you need not deprive yourself by giving up your favorite dishes. In many cases, you can substitute healthful ingredients for less healthful ones and come up with a dish that satisfies both your hunger for the foods you like and your desire to eat in the most healthy way possible.

"The first thing you can do to any recipe is find the source of fat in it, and reduce it. Cut it in half, or just eliminate it, in most cases," says Joanne D'Agostino, R.N., a low-fat-cooking consultant in Easton, Pennsylvania. "When a recipe calls for butter or shortening, use a whipped, diet, polyunsaturated margarine and use a third to a half less," she suggests. "Or, if a recipe calls for oil, as many muffin recipes do, substitute half as much corn syrup or honey in place of the oil and decrease the amount of sugar."

"In most cases, you can substitute turkey for red meat in recipes without making any other changes," says D'Agostino. Use ground, skinless turkey in meat loaf, chili or spaghetti sauce. And, turkey breast cutlets can be marinated and poached or used in low-fat, stir-fried dishes, for example.

The representatives of Project LEAN (Low-fat Eating

BRAISING

Braising, like baking, takes place in an oven. It is a slow, moist cooking method in which foods simmer in a covered pan in a moderately hot oven. Braising is a good way to tenderize dense vegetables, such as whole potatoes, quartered rutabagas, whole onions and large carrots as well as some of the leanest cuts of meat, such as fat-trimmed flank cuts, which can be tough.

for America Now), based in Chicago, and other cooking experts, suggest these additional fat-busting, salt-reducing substitutions.

If the Recipe Calls for . . .	**Substitute**
Milk	Skim or 1% milk
Light cream	Equal portions 1% milk and evaporated skim milk
Baking chocolate (1 oz.)	3 tablespoons cocoa plus 1 tablespoon vegetable oil
Sour cream	Blend 1 cup low-fat (1%) cottage cheese with 1 tablespoon skim milk and 2 tablespoons lemon juice
Eggs	Two egg whites for one whole egg
Salt	Lemon or lime juice
	Fresh herbs
	Spicy salt substitutes
	Low-sodium hot sauce
High-fat sauces	Fat-free mayonnaise mixed with nonfat yogurt
	Fruit or vegetable salsas
	Chutney
	Reduced stocks or fruit juice

Sear first, simmer later. Braising is especially healthful as long as meats are well trimmed and no fats are added to the pan. Prepare meat for braising by first searing it in a hot, heavy pan on top of the stove. Cook off as much fat as possible and drain it off. Searing browns and seals the surface so the meat stays moist. Then, place the meat, along with whatever vegetables and seasonings are called for in your recipe in a covered, oven-safe dish or roasting pan. Add enough liquid to cover about a third of the food, and cook it according to your recipe's instructions. The result is a medley of flavors that meld and blend like the voices in a barbershop quartet.

MICROWAVING

Microwaving is probably the next best thing to eating foods raw. Vitamins are conserved especially in vegetables, because cooking times are short and little or no water is needed. Also, added fat is not necessary.

Let your veggies ride the waves. "Vegetables in the microwave are marvelously healthful because they cook in one-fourth the time needed for other methods and require only two tablespoons of added water per quart of fresh vegetables," says Joan Toole, certified home economist, cookware designer, author and microwave-cooking instructor in Wilmington, Delaware.

Toole offers a few more rules of thumb for making microwaved vegetables as healthful and appealing as possible: Cut vegetables into uniform slices, always cover and vent them and cook on high power for six to seven minutes per pound, depending on the liquid content of the food. Low-moisture veggies like carrots take longer. To cook vegetables with different densities or sizes, such as peas and carrots, start the carrots a few minutes before adding the peas.

Because microwave energy heats liquid first, drain the liquid from canned vegetables before heating them in the microwave. For the same reason soups and very saucy dishes with chunks of vegetables or meats will not cook evenly unless you carefully follow the directions in a good microwave cookbook.

Stuffed, baked potatoes in ten minutes? It's possible in a microwave, says Toole. "First, pierce a potato all the way through, bake it on high power for about five minutes, then wrap it in a paper towel and let it finish cooking on the counter while you prepare low-fat cheese sauce (see page 563) and broccoli: Roll chopped broccoli in a damp, white, paper towel and put it on a paper plate. Into the oven it goes for two minutes. Split and fluff the potato with a fork, stuff it with broccoli and pour the cheese sauce over it," Toole says. "It's fun, delicious and fast."

Don't strain over grains. The time-cutting wonder of microwave cooking will not hasten grain cooking. "Rice and other grains have to be reconstituted, which takes almost as much time in a microwave oven as on the stove," says Toole. "They do come out beautifully, though, because they are not likely to stick to the cooking vessel," she explains, "and you *can* shave down the cooking time a little by starting them in very hot water."

Oatmeal and other whole-grain cereals, such as rolled barley, Wheatena and buckwheat kasha or mixed-grain Kashi, on the other hand, can be microwave-cooked right in a bowl, at 70 percent power, in about a third of the time it takes to cook them on a stove. It's quick, and there is no pot to scorch or scrub, which might encourage people to eat a hot breakfast when they might otherwise be inclined to skip it, says Toole.

Satisfy your sweet tooth. "Low-fat cakes, quick breads and muffins also can be quickly cooked in a microwave oven with good results, provided the recipe calls for fruit or low-fat yogurt. You don't really need lots of oil or egg yolks to get good results," says Toole.

"Fruits are just fabulous in the microwave, too," adds Toole. Four or five baked apples, cored and stuffed with raisins and cinnamon, take just eight minutes to cook on high power, in a covered, vented dish. To make quick, no-sugar-added apple, pear or peach sauce, just chop the fruit, add a little water and some cinnamon, if you like, and cook on high power, stirring every three or four minutes, Toole recommends. Fruit sauce can be added to baked goods as a no-fat ingredient for a tasty topping.

DAILY DAIRY DELIVERY—WITHOUT THE FAT

Low-fat milk, yogurt and cheeses have found their way into your fridge. Now here are many ways to help them find their way into your daily diet in place of the fattier products called for in many recipes. "In most recipes that call for milk and cheese, you can substitute low-fat or non-fat milk products with no changes to the recipe," says Melanie Polk, R.D., consulting nutritionist and author from North Potomac, Maryland.

"In some cases you won't get the same result, however," she warns. "Sometimes people need to use a little experimentation and creativity. For example, I've had lots of luck making lasagna with nonfat cheeses, but pizzas did not work out too well. My recommendation is to use the lowest-fat product that will give the results you find acceptable. Some products will work well in some dishes, but not in others."

Cheeses. "When you use a nonfat cheese, in many cases, you should use a lower cooking temperature or the cheese will get tough," says Polk. "Regular cheese is made of protein and fat, but if you take away the fat, all that's left is protein, which toughens when it's subjected to high heat." If possible, when you use nonfat cheese in a recipe, wait until near the end to add it.

Yogurt. "When you use yogurt—low-fat or otherwise—instead of sour cream in soups, dips or casseroles, add the yogurt at the end and stir it into hot foods gradually, or the yogurt will curdle," Polk warns.

Milk. "When using low-fat or skim milk in packaged puddings or custards, the finished product will be very similar to the versions made with whole milk. There's no reason to change your cooking method in that case," says Polk. What could be easier?

Make the most of meat, fish and fowl. "To microwave meat, fish and poultry, it's very important to begin with food that is the same temperature throughout," says Toole. "To cook fish in the microwave oven, place it in a microwave-safe dish and tuck under any thin tails of flesh on fillets so that the fish has a uniform thickness. As for meat, face the heavier pieces toward the outer edges of the oven, where the microwave energy is most powerful."

Say cheese. "Foods with cheese in them should be cooked in a microwave set at only 70 percent power. If you cook low-fat cheese at high power for too long, it will come out like rubber," says Toole. In most cases, however, grated, low-fat cheeses can be sprinkled on microwaved foods—such as a vegetable medley of red onions; green, red and yellow peppers; squash and broccoli—after cooking, during the standing time, and it will melt just fine.

Joan Toole's low-fat, microwaved cheese sauce: "Stir together ½ cup low-fat, imitation mayonnaise, ½ cup skim milk and ⅓ cup grated, low-fat cheese in a glass measuring cup covered loosely with plastic wrap, cook it at 70 percent power for 2½ minutes, stirring it every 60 seconds, and that's it. Pour some of it over your baked potato stuffed with broccoli (see page 561), stick the rest in the refrigerator, grab a beverage, and you can sit down to eat in about 10 minutes," Toole exclaims.

High Nutrition Recipes

MICROWAVE LASAGNA

This recipe takes a lot of the fuss out of preparing lasagna. You can brown the ground turkey (or lean beef, if you prefer) in the microwave. Then you assemble the dish without cooking the noodles first. This recipe was created by Anita Hirsch, a nutritionist at the Rodale Food Center.

8	ounces lean ground turkey	2	tablespoons minced fresh parsley
4	cups tomato sauce	½	teaspoon ground black pepper
½	cup water		
1½	cups nonfat ricotta cheese	9	lasagna noodles
¼	cup fat-free egg substitute	8	ounces nonfat mozzarella cheese, shredded
2	tablespoons minced fresh basil	¼	cup grated Parmesan cheese

Crumble the turkey into a large glass bowl. Microwave on high for 2 minutes. Break up the pieces and stir well. Microwave on high for 1 minute, or until the turkey is cooked through. Drain well. Stir in the tomato sauce and water.

In a medium bowl, mix the ricotta, egg, basil, parsley and pepper.

Spoon about 1 cup of the tomato mixture into the bottom of an 8" × 12" glass baking dish.

Top with 3 of the noodles. Spread with about ½ cup of the ricotta mixture. Sprinkle with some mozzarella and Parmesan. Top with about 1 cup of the tomato mixture. Repeat the layering procedure twice to use all the ingredients.

Cover with wax paper. Microwave on high for 4 minutes. Give the dish a quarter turn. (If your microwave isn't deep enough to hold the dish sideways, give it a half-turn.) Microwave on high for 4 more minutes.

Turn the dish again. Microwave on medium-low (30% power) for a total of 30 minutes; stop every 10 minutes to turn the dish.

Let stand 15 minutes before serving.

Serves 9
Per serving: *191 calories, 1.5 g. fat (7% of calories), 1.8 g. dietary fiber, 22 mg. cholesterol, 371 mg. sodium*

Mahi Mahi with Jamaican Tartar Sauce

Poaching is a very easy, low-fat way to cook fish. This recipe was developed by Tom Ney, director of the Rodale Food Center. You may substitute other types of firm fish, such as salmon, cod, snapper or sablefish.

⅓ cup finely chopped papaya	2 quarts water
⅓ cup nonfat mayonnaise	3 tablespoons white-white vinegar
¼ cup thinly sliced scallions	3 lemon slices
2 tablespoons finely chopped lime flesh	4 bay leaves
1 tablespoon minced fresh coriander	1 tablespoon pickling spices
½ teaspoon hot-pepper sauce	¼ teaspoon celery seeds
	1 pound mahi mahi fillet

In a small bowl, mix the papaya, mayonnaise, scallions, lime, coriander and hot-pepper sauce. Cover and refrigerate for at least 1 hour.

In a large frying pan, combine the water, vinegar, lemon slices, bay leaves, pickling spices and celery seeds. Bring to a boil, then reduce the heat to medium-low and simmer for 10 minutes.

Add the mahi mahi to the pan. If necessary, add more water to the pan to cover the fish. Simmer for 15 minutes, or until the fish is just cooked through.

Use 2 metal spatulas to remove the fish from the liquid without breaking it. If desired, remove some of the spices from the fish (but they're edible, except for the bay leaves). Serve with the papaya sauce.

Serves 4
Per serving: *120 calories, 0.8 g. fat (6% of calories), 0.2 g. dietary fiber, 83 mg. cholesterol, 355 mg. sodium*

SAVORY ROASTED ONIONS

Roasting gives onions a sweet, mellow flavor, making them a delicious side-dish vegetable for fish, poultry or meat.

4 large onions	2 teaspoons balsamic
¼ teaspoon olive oil	vinegar
¼ teaspoon dried savory	

Peel the onions and cut in half lengthwise. Coat with the oil and sprinkle with the savory. Place, cut side down, in a shallow baking dish. Bake at 350° for 50 minutes, or until tender. Sprinkle with the vinegar before serving.

Serves 4
Per serving: *66 calories, 0.5 g. fat (7% of calories), 2.6 g. dietary fiber, 0 mg. cholesterol, 5 mg sodium*

SCALLOP STIR-FRY

Stir-frying is a quick cooking method that retains the fresh flavors of foods. And it's very adaptable to whatever is in your pantry. In this recipe, you may replace the scallops with shrimp or strips of chicken breast. And you may use other vegetables, such as broccoli florets, mushrooms, onions, snow peas or peppers.

1 pound medium sea scallops	2 large carrots, thinly sliced on the diagonal
1 tablespoon cornstarch	1 celery stalk, thinly sliced on the diagonal
¾ cup orange juice	
2 tablespoons low-sodium soy sauce	½ cup sliced water chestnuts

1	tablespoon honey	2	teaspoons peanut or
1	tablespoon minced fresh		canola oil
	ginger	3	cups hot cooked rice
¼	teaspoon red-pepper		
	flakes		

Cut the scallops crosswise into rounds about ⅓" thick. Pat dry on paper towels and set aside.

In a small bowl, dissolve the cornstarch in the orange juice. Stir in the soy sauce, honey, ginger and red-pepper flakes. Set aside.

In a wok or large frying pan over medium-high heat, stir-fry the carrots, celery and chestnuts in 1 teaspoon of the oil for 5 minutes, or until crisp-tender. Remove with a slotted spoon and set aside.

Add the remaining 1 teaspoon oil to the pan. Add the scallops and stir-fry for 2 minutes, or until just cooked through. Return the vegetables to the pan. Pour in the orange sauce. Stir until thickened, about 2 minutes.

Serve over the rice.

Serves 4
Per serving: *359 calories, 4.6 g. fat (12% of calories), 4.3 g. dietary fiber, 37 mg. cholesterol, 515 mg. sodium*

CHAPTER 29

Restaurant Savvy

Dining Out Without Damage

If calories consumed were dollars spent, a not-so-unusual restaurant meal for two of chicken wings, New England clam chowder, tossed salad with blue cheese dressing, prime rib with sour cream and horseradish sauce, twice-baked potato stuffed with Cheddar cheese, buttered corn-on-the-cob, garlic bread, deep-dish apple pie à la mode and Irish coffee would cost almost enough to buy the restaurant owner a gold Rolex.

Lucky thing that's not the case. But a meal like this *can* cost you plenty in terms of your calorie, salt, fat and cholesterol budget. Dining out—whether breakfast with the boss, a fast-food jaunt with the kids, lunch in the company cafeteria or a romantic dinner—can be a nourishing adventure, though, when you take your healthy eating habits with you.

Before you leave the house and head for the neon signs that virtually cry out, "Eat here, eat here," there are two general guidelines to keep in mind about dining out without damage. They apply to all types of establishments, including diners, pizza parlors, sandwich shops, cafeterias, convenience stores, full-service restaurants, bar-and-grills, fast-food places and even other people's homes.

First, be on the lookout for meals that fulfill both your flavor *and* nutrition needs. They can be found almost anywhere, but it's easier to select a healthy and tasty balance of foods in eateries that offer a wide variety of dishes.

Next, strive for moderation in your eating habits, even though many restaurants make it all too easy to overindulge. You can hold the line on calories, salt, fat and sugar even when you're not doing the cooking. It's just a matter of making smart choices and sticking to them.

CHEFS WHO CARE ABOUT HEALTH

The healthy bandwagon is traveling at a dizzying pace as more and more people like you jump on. Restaurant owners and chefs are not only among the wagon-hopping crowd— they're often leading the band. "It's become the responsibility of restaurateurs to educate and show customers that there's a healthy way to eat without giving up the excitement of the restaurant experience," says Michael Franks, proprietor of several West Coast restaurants, including Chez Melange in Redondo Beach, California.

Franks is national chairman of the chefs' committee of Project LEAN, a group whose objective is to creatively reduce fat in the American diet. Innovative chefs around the country are finding substitutes for and cutting back on offending ingredients; devising menus that depend less on fatty meats and more on vegetables, grains and other heart-smart items; and borrowing pearls of healthful wisdom from the cuisines of other cultures. A peek into a few inspired chefs' kitchens will show you how they do it.

At Chez Melange, the game, in many cases, is substitution. Franks explains. "We try to replace high-fat items with low-fat items. Nonfat yogurt replaces sour cream. We also cook with reduced stocks in place of butter. Instead of rich sauces we use fresh, nonfat salsas. We often replace fatty meat, like hamburger, with a low-fat protein like ground turkey. We try to replace things while still giving customers what they're used to. And we do it by using products that are fresh and natural."

Are you afraid that by going to a health-oriented restaurant you might be faced with boring, tasteless dietetic foods? One taste of a typical Chez Melange lunch—peppered fresh tuna with Japanese salsa over oriental greens, with basmati rice and steamed vegetables—may quell your fears. This dish weighs in at just 240 calories, 25 milligrams of cholesterol and 4 grams of fat.

TEACHING THE RIGHT TECHNIQUES

Some chefs emphasize moderation, rather than eliminating certain ingredients altogether, explains Robert Briggs, a chef instructor at the Culinary Institute of America in Hyde Park, New York, where students attend classes in nutritional cooking as well as gourmet cooking. "We're teaching students who are going to be chefs to use ingredients they're already comfortable with, but to use less of them when they can. For example, we show them how they can do a lot with a lot less butter than usual. One way to drastically reduce the amount of melted butter we use is to put it in a spray bottle," Briggs explains. In many cases, just a spritz can boost flavor without significantly increasing calories from fat.

At the institute, student chefs are taught techniques for cutting fat in everything from salad dressings to desserts: "Normal salad dressing, for example, is about 75 to 95 percent fat," Briggs says. "But we can cut that by about two-thirds by using a small amount of very high quality fat—like avocado puree—that has a lot of flavor. Then we replace the fat we've taken out with juice, stock or water and thicken it lightly with cornstarch or arrowroot, so it's the same consistency as oily dressing. By adding vinegar or citrus juice and whatever seasoning we want to that basic recipe, we can make an infinite number of different dressings, and no one knows they're lower in fat."

The four basic sauces in traditional cooking—velouté, bechámel, brown and hollandaise—make up another fat-laden area that lends itself well to the institute's method. "The basic sauces can all be made low-fat by using evaporated skim milk instead of cream and by thickening them with a plain starch instead of roux or egg yolk. By adding flavorings like mustard, defatted chicken stock or fish stock, the possibiliteis are limitless," says Briggs.

Chefs at the institute who teach the health-wise classes have even developed a low-fat version of crème anglaise— the creamy basis for many rich desserts—from a mixture of ricotta cheese, nonfat yogurt and sugar, corn syrup or honey. By adding gelatin and meringue to the base, rather than real cream, it is transformed into low-fat Bavarian cream. In another metamorphosis it becomes a rich-tasting frozen delight.

Another way some chefs cater to their guests' health concerns is to offer low-fat options in addition to a "regular" menu. "We have a separate menu insert that lists all our reduced-fat items together with the amount of total fat, calories and percentage of calories from fat in each dish," says Richard Wright, senior chef at Hawk Prairie Inn in Olympia, Washington. For example, guests can order a 'typical' prime rib roast beef dinner or another beef dish featuring meat that was raised and processed to contain less fat.

A WORLD OF LOW-FAT CUISINES

Another way chefs are helping Americans change the way they eat is by borrowing ingredients and cooking techniques from the global community. "International cuisines are frequently built around rice or other grains, and they use more naturally low-fat foods, such as fish, lentils and beans," says Franks.

A CAFÉ THAT'S REALLY SPECIAL

Nutrition education for chefs is a trend for the 90s and beyond. The Culinary Institute of America, in Hyde Park, New York, teaches low-fat cooking and nutrition to its future chefs during a three-week course conducted at St. Andrew's Cafe, one of the school's four public restaurants. The healthy philosophy there calls for moderating calories, fats, sodium and cholesterol, while bolstering complex carbohydrates. "Meals at the café provide about 800 to 1,000 calories each, compared with a typical restaurant meal's calorie load of 2,000 to 2,200 calories," explains Catherine Powers, R.D., a nutritionist at the institute.

The menu reveals a roster of treats that sounds anything but depriving. How about an appetizer of warm smoked duck with pasta, radicchio and shallot vinaigrette, followed by Michigan white bean soup scented with rosemary and sage, en entrée of roast chicken stuffed with fresh herbs, served with garlic-potato ravioli, glazed root vegetables and a salad of baby mixed greens with champagne herb vinaigrette?

Leave room for dessert. There's saffron-poached pears with rice pudding and kiln-dried cherry sauce. Or perhaps you prefer the fresh-baked Hudson Valley pear strudel with amaretto glacé. If you haven't drooled all over this page, you may want to show it to your favorite chef as an example of the lavish, yet healthful heights to which restaurant fare can soar.

"In traditional Chinese and Asian cuisine, meat is not served on a daily or even monthly basis," explains Martin Yan, chef, food consultant, and host of the PBS-TV series "Yan Can Cook." "Meat, when it is available, is mainly used as a flavoring ingredient or as a supplement to a variety of vegetable dishes. It's more of a condiment than a main ingredient. A lot of dishes are made by combining several vegetables that are in season."

We're not talking about piles of flavorless, boiled string beans with canned pearl onions, either. Innovative American chefs are combining colorful, crisp veggies from here and abroad with Mediterranean whole grains, pastas and fruits. Beans and seeds dance to a Latin beat, or they're dressed in lemongrass from Thailand, curries from India, ginger from China and sauces from Indonesia and Vietnam. Marco Polo himself would have been thrilled to sample the flavors that are flying in from around the world and landing in American restaurants.

"International foods are usually only healthy if they're prepared and eaten the way they are in their country of origin, though," says Franks. "The trouble comes when foods become too Americanized." To bypass that snag, many restaurants with a healthy bent borrow cooking techniques and philosophies as well as ingredients from international kitchens.

"The healthiest techniques in Chinese and Asian cuisine, for example, are steaming and stir-frying, with occasional braising and stewing," says Yan. "Deep-frying is rarely used. Stir-frying uses a minimum amount of oil, and the wok is heated before the oil and food are added. When meat is stir-fried, the heat sears and seals in its juices. By steaming, the food cooks in its own juice and moisture and never touches water or oil, so the food retains its original flavor and character."

READY TO TRY SOMETHING NEW?

Finally, there are chefs who believe the best way to change the way you eat is to change the way you think about food. "Instead of taking a dish that's meant to be very rich and trying to turn it into a healthy dish, I say just forget that dish al-

THE BEST AND WORST AT ETHNIC EATERIES

Living in a melting pot like the United States means you can have a taste of different cultures without traveling very far. Some of the world's healthiest fare comes from afar, too. The listings below, arranged according to restaurant type, will help you choose wisely when you explore the world with your fork.

Chinese

Dig into: Steamed rice; boiled, steamed or stir-fried veggies with little oil; skinless poultry; fish and shellfish (in moderation); tofu (not fried).

Steer clear of: Fried rice, salty soups, too much soy sauce, MSG, fried noodles, crispy duck, egg dishes and soups, sweet-and-sour dishes (they're deep-fried first), pickled foods.

Mediterranean and Middle Eastern

Dig into: Pita bread; legumes like lentils, chick-peas and broad beans; hummus; roast eggplant (babaghanouj) and olive oil in moderate amounts; wheat or cracked-wheat foods like couscous and bulgur; yogurt or pima; grape leaves.

Steer clear of: Too many olives and anchovies and too much feta cheese (use just a little of these as flavorings), baklava and other phyllo-dough dishes (except tiny servings), fatty lamb dishes, fried eggplant.

Japanese

Dig into: Rice (except fried), fish, raw vegetables, tofu, miso soup, yakimono (broiled foods), sukiyaki (stir-fried meat dish).

Steer clear of: Too much soy sauce or peanut sauce, deep-fried tempura, teriyaki, too many pickled foods.

Indian

Dig into: Yogurt-based curry sauce, salads, chutneys, raita (yogurt with shredded vegetables), tandoori chicken and fish (request no butter-basting), seekh kabob with lean lamb only, dal (lentils), rice, breads like pulkas and nan.

Steer clear of: Ghee (clarified butter), deep-fried meats.

Italian

Dig into: Pasta with vegetables or marinara sauce, garlic, salads and antipasto without oily dressing or too many meats, crusty bread without butter or oil, steamed leafy vegetables like kale and broccoli raab, zucchini, fresh tomatoes and fresh (unsalted) mozzarella, broiled or grilled meat or fish dishes, Italian ices.

Steer clear of: Cream-, butter-, or oil-and-wine-based sauces; meatballs and sausage; veal scaloppine; Parmesan-style or cheese-stuffed dishes; fried eggplant; spumone or tortoni ice creams; cappuccino.

Mexican

Dig into: Whole beans and rice, salsas, grilled chicken or fish, corn or flour tortillas in moderation (most are made with oil), seviche (marinade-cooked fish), colorful soups and stews, salads, onions and peppers, sliced avocado garnishes, fruit and fruit ices.

Steer clear of: Ground beef and pork dishes, heavy cheese, sour cream and guacamole fillings and toppings, chimichangas, refried beans cooked with lard, deep-fried churros (doughnuts) and other sweet breads.

French

Dig into: Salads with dressings on the side, steamed mussels, crusty baguettes without butter, fresh fruit, steamed vegetables, some "nouvelle" dishes, bordelaise and other light wine sauces in moderation, crêpes with fruit or lightly sautéed seafood.

Steer clear of: Pâtés; duck or goose with skin; au gratin dishes; hollandaise, béchamel, béarnaise, and other cream, egg, butter and high-salt sauces; buttery omelettes, croissants and pastries.

together and go have something completely different," suggests Chris Schlesinger, chef and co-owner of the East Coast Grill in Cambridge, Massachusetts.

"Look to fundamental change, not to substitutes," Schlesinger continues. "Eat something different, like grilled shrimp in tomatilla pineapple salsa with rice and beans. Or try grilled squid with lo mein noodles and ginger, garlic and lime juice. Don't just stop eating certain things. Instead, introduce a wider variety of foods into your diet."

Wide variety is truly the spice of life in cities like New Orleans, a place famed for spice and excitement. Just ask Emeril Lagasse, formerly executive chef at Commander's Palace, now owner of Emeril's. He strives to bring Creole dishes into the health-conscious 90s. "To do this, we start with the best ingredients and work from scratch. That way, we can really control the quality of the food we serve our customers," says Lagasse, a chef who really keeps pace with what his customers want.

"There's a growing interest in vegetables and vegetarian dishes," Lagasse observes. American poll-takers, ever alert to changes in the nation's pulse, concur. About one-third of all adults surveyed in one study said they are likely to order vegetarian meals if available. At Emeril's, their search would not be in vain.

"We do a lot of things with vegetables. For example, we offer a creative vegetable dish that consists of about 14 to 16 seasonal vegetables that are grilled, roasted, baked or pureed. In fall, for example, there may be two or three different types of baby beets, roasted sweet corn, roasted garlic, puree of two or three root vegetables or squashes and more-typical vegetables like zucchini, yellow squash, onions and stewed tomatoes with garlic. The foundation of the plate is a vegetable pasta tossed with herbs," Lagasse says.

Your Table Is Waiting

Makes you want to hop a plane just to sample the healthy fare in one of these restaurants, doesn't it? Well, you may not have to. An enlightened chef or restaurateur—or one who's willing to learn—may be right around the corner. Here's what you need to do.

Call ahead. To find such a restaurateur, call ahead, not just to make reservations or ask about prices, but to learn how well the establishment can serve your health needs. Ask for a few examples from the regular menu. If nothing stands out, find out if the chef is willing to make simple changes—such as serving sauces on the side, poaching or broiling fish or meat, preparing meatless dishes or omitting salt or butter. In response, the manager or chef may suggest a particular time when custom-made orders will be easiest to fulfill. Sudden demands for unusual fare at seven o'clock on a hectic Saturday night may find a less than flexible chef and staff. If they know your needs in advance, though, you will most likely be well accommodated, so don't be an anonymous caller. And if you enjoy your customized meal, a little praise for the staff and recommending the restaurant to others afterward, will go a long way toward making you a welcome and honored guest.

Take responsibility. Finding a restaurant that offers a variety of foods from which you may order a healthy meal is at least half the battle. But few restaurants—outside of health spas—offer nothing but low-fat, low-sodium, high-fiber foods. No matter how varied the offerings, there is only one person who can control the real impact this dining experience will have on your body. You guessed it. That person is you. And the decisions you make about how much and what types of foods you will order begin before you even look at the menu.

Eat something in advance. Don't risk a gut-splitting pigout by starving yourself before you get to the restaurant.

Stifle an urge to overindulge by eating normally earlier in the day. Otherwise, you may not be as resistant to high-fat appetizers and hors d'oeuvres, salty munchies or gigantic portions. A snack of bread or fruit may be helpful if dinner or lunch will be served very late.

MENU WARNING SIGNALS

To help you sort through the appetizer, soup, entrée and dessert offerings on a typical restaurant menu, here are two lists. These contain some common buzzwords that may tip you off to foods that could tilt your fat and sodium scales in the wrong direction.

High-Fat Warning Words   *High-Sodium Warning Words*

High-Fat Warning Words	High-Sodium Warning Words
• Rich	• Smoked
• Creamy	• Pickled
• Au gratin	• Barbecued
• Cheesy	• Broth
• Fried, including "pan-fried"	• Bouillon
• Fritter	• Cocktail sauce
• Gravy	• Soy sauce
• Saucy	• Teriyaki
• Breaded	• Cured
• Crunchy	• Marinated
• Crispy	
• Scalloped or escalloped	
• Buttery	
• Flaky	
• Pastry	

Remember, these are just clues. If there is any doubt about how a food is actually prepared, ask your server.

ARE YOU READY TO ORDER?

Here are a few guidelines for making your way through a typical restaurant meal. We'll begin at the top, with a health-smart cocktail and the free tongue ticklers that often get to the table before you do.

Drinks. An elegant meal need not begin with a high-calorie, alcohol-based drink. To quench your thirst or give your hands something to do before your meal arrives, you may wish to order fresh-squeezed orange juice, a glass of ice and a bottle of sparkling water to mix your own fruit spritzer. Or try sparkling water with a dash of bitters. Many mixed drinks can also be prepared "virgin-style" (without alcohol) as well.

Finger foods. Delve right into the relish tray, if one is offered. It may contain crisp, raw snow peas, red peppers, cauliflower, baby corn, carrots, celery, radishes or other colorful tidbits. Be wary of most other free hors d'oeuvres, however. Popcorn, crackers with pâtés or spreads, and hot hors d'oeuvres are usually loaded with fat and salt. They will entice you to drink. In this case, restaurants are not concerned so much about your health as they are about their own bottom lines.

Appetizers. "Stay away from anything deep-fried," advises Dotty Griffith, cookbook author, food editor of the *Dallas Morning News* and participant in Project LEAN. That includes fried vegetables, cheese or fish appetizers. "And anytime you find a dish that's had a lot done to it—if it's breaded, fried, sautéed in butter, pureed or has a sauce or other ingredient on it—chances are, the stuff they add is made of fat, because fat carries flavor," says Griffith. Better selections are simple appetizers, like smoked fish, roasted fresh vegetables or fruit.

Soups. "Cream soups are another thing to watch out for," says Griffith. Where there's a choice, go with clear soups that are hearty with vegetables, grains or pasta.

Salads. "Salads are not really healthy selections if they're globbed up with a lot of cheese or high-fat dressing," Griffith warns. Instead, look for salads that are topped with fresh herbs or crunchy treats, such as baby corn, water chestnuts or snow peas. A salad like that doesn't need to be overdressed. "A dash of herb vinegar or lemon or lime juice goes a long way," says Griffith.

Entrées. When you are ready to order your main course, you may wish to glance back at the menu's earlier course offerings. Some restaurants offer separate pasta courses in appetizer sizes, which you could order as an entrée, instead. Regardless of the portion size, you will probably have your choice of sauces: There's always marinara sauce, which is healthiest because there's very little fat in it, says Joanne D'Agostino, R.N., cookbook author and Pennsylvania-based restaurant consultant. Alfredo sauce, made mostly from cream and cheese is probably out of the question. Meat sauces may not look fatty, but often the meat and all the fat that cooks out of it go directly into the sauce without draining. D'Agostino explains. "Seafood sauces are healthier because the amount of fat that leaves the fish and cooks into the sauce is minimal, and, chances are, there won't be a tremendous amount of oil added."

As for more traditional entrées, if you have a choice between deep-fried and poached seafood, or between a fatty steak and a grilled chicken breast, the healthy selections are obvious. But if the choices are not so clearly spelled out, you may need to use a more savvy approach.

"If the restaurant does not mark the menu in some way to indicate which items are low-fat and which are not, it becomes incumbent on customers to know what kinds of ingredients they need to avoid," says Wright. "Then they need to decide which items on the menu are going to be good for them and which aren't, and start asking if certain ingredients can be withheld." For example, many sautéed or broiled meat or seafood dishes incorporate a lot of fat in the cooking process, or receive a shower of butter just before leaving the kitchen. The customer must learn to ask if there is a lot of butter, oil or salt in a dish and, if so, whether the chef can hold those ingredients, Wright explains.

"You can take this advice into any restaurant," advises Yan. "If you go into an Italian restaurant and there's too much olive oil in your pasta dish, next time ask them to use less. But ask with courtesy," he cautions. "You want to develop a working relationship with the chef and the staff in the restaurant. Most restaurateurs will gladly accommodate your request. Besides, they want your business, especially if you are a longtime customer. If they are unwilling to cooperate, it is time to switch to another restaurant and develop a working relationship there. After all, it is your health that matters most."

Whatever entrée you decide upon, the next challenge is controlling the amount you eat. For meat or fish entrées, one way to gauge the generally recommended three- to four-ounce serving is to use the "palm method," says Sheri Shansby Boyden, R.D., a dietitian at the Mayo Medical Center in Rochester, Minnesota, who advises diabetic patients about healthy eating. "The average woman's palm, without fingers, is about the size of a correct portion," she explains. "So, when the food arrives, a woman can discreetly compare the portion of meat, fish or poultry to her palm and decide how much she should actually eat." Men may wish to envision a deck of cards as their size guide, instead, experts say.

Others advise simply deciding beforehand not to overeat and relying on willpower to avoid getting carried away. One technique to avoid overeating that works for many people is to chew more. "Relax, eat slowly, chew your food thoroughly and let dinner last a long time," D'Agostino advises. "Chewing and really tasting food brings a lot of satisfaction. And extending the amount of time it takes to eat helps to overcome the tendency to stuff ourselves because it gives the stomach a chance to tell the brain that it's had enough."

Side dishes. Now that you are adept at entrée selection, you're ready for this side-dish quiz: Which of the following side dishes are good selections for a vitamin/mineral/fiber boost without excess fat?

- Fresh-cut French-fried potatoes
- Herbed new potatoes
- Cheese-stuffed baked potato
- Sliced tomatoes with basil
- Creamy coleslaw
- Broccoli florets marinated in dill vinegar
- Asparagus spears with hollandaise sauce
- Garden-fresh peas with pearl onions

Answer: Every other one, beginning with the second selection, is a healthy choice. Enjoy.

Bonus question: Which of the less-healthy dishes above can be modified most easily and how should you relay your request to the cook?

Answer: It's the asparagus, and one good way to phrase your special request is: "I'd like the asparagus, please. But will you ask the chef to put the hollandaise on the side so that I can use just a taste of it? Thank you."

Congratulations! You've won a chance to read about dessert.

Desserts. "When you have a choice, lean toward fruit desserts," advises Briggs. "They will generally be healthier. And it doesn't just have to be a poached pear or baked apple. Today, there are many frozen fruit yogurts and sorbets. Beware, though, that some can be loaded with sugar, even though they may be lower in fat than ice cream. A phyllo dough basket filled with fruit and served with fruit sauce is another possibility," he suggests.

"Fruit cup from the appetizer menu, and low-fat frozen yogurt or sherbet can be combined to make a low-fat sundae," D'Agostino suggests. "Angel food cake with fresh fruit is another good choice. And, if I really can't find anything else on

HEARTS ON MY MENU

They're popping up on menus all over the country: Little red heart-shaped symbols that signal heart-healthy items. Who decides which foods will have heart? Many restaurants are joining forces with hospital-sponsored or independent dietitians to help customers find foods that promote good health.

"We sponsor area restaurants that use recipes that are lower in fat, cholesterol and sodium," explains Vickie L. Spillane, R.D., who reviews menus to determine how well they fit with the HEARTCHECK Program of Our Lady of Lourdes Medical Center in Camden, New Jersey. Some of the parameters for eligibility in this program and others like it include:

• Preparing foods with two teaspoons or less of a polyunsaturated or monounsaturated oil or margarine per serving.

• Using low-fat cooking methods, such as baking, broiling, roasting, grilling, poaching and steaming instead of frying.

• Preparing foods without adding salt or MSG.

• Preparing broth-based soups.

• Serving polyunsaturated margarine as an alternative to butter.

• Trimming all visible fat from meat and limiting portion size to six ounces.

• Providing skim or 1 percent milk as an alternative to whole milk.

Dining in restaurants sponsored by hospital-based programs like HEARTCHECK takes the guesswork out of healthy dining. What could be easier?

the menu, I'd order fruit pie, but skip the crust and just eat the filling."

Even chocolate cake is okay to order once in a while, especially if you ask for just one piece to share among several people. This kind of mini-indulgence has become the norm, rather than the exception, in many restaurants.

The healthy dining methods above cover a lot of territory, and many are useful whether the meal is breakfast, lunch or dinner. The two earlier meals of the day have some interesting challenges all their own, however.

RISE AND SHINE

Breakfast. It's often called the most important meal of the day, yet it's the meal most often skipped. It's also the meal least frequently eaten out, although more and more people are eating breakfast away from home these days.

Many traditional diner-style breakfast foods have no-no reputations: triple-egg omelettes oozing cheese; pancakes, french toast and waffles slathered with butter and syrup; bacon, sausage, ham, pork roll and scrapple; plus home fries, corned beef hash and hash brown potatoes sizzling in the grease left on the grill. A long, slippery list, but it's easily countered by yes-yes breakfast dishes with a host of saving graces.

Fresh berries over crispy, buckwheat waffles, steaming oatmeal with raisins and cinnamon; a lightly toasted bagel with strawberry jam; oven-browned garlic-and-parsley potatoes; sweet slices of cantaloupe and honeydew melon; even yolkless omelettes stuffed with sweet red peppers, mushrooms, onions and broccoli are great-eye-openers. And with someone else doing the cooking, a healthy breakfast away from home can really light up your morning, says Tracy Ritter, a chef and owner of Vitality Cuisine, a food consulting firm in San Diego.

Breakfast and brunch buffets are especially easy places to eat too much. Here's where Clean Plate Club members may face their biggest challenge. Heaps of greasy sausage and eggs, mountains of deep-fried French toast, tray upon tray of home fries and buckets of steaming grits with tubs of butter and thick gravy beckon with oversized serving spoons and beg to be eaten or . . . gulp . . . go to waste. It may take gargantuan willpower, but reject the challenge to use up a whole stack of fresh plates by yourself. Remember, there are lots of people in line behind you who will help empty the tureens of cheese sauce. You don't have to do it alone.

Breakfast and brunch buffets offer a wide selection of foods, and if your main objective is to "get your money's worth," you can certainly do it without sending your cholesterol count through the ceiling. Take a good look down the line at the array of offerings before you fill your plate with the items closest to you. It's okay to shuffle along with an empty plate until you reach the cereals, fruits, juices and breads. With so many delicious and healthy ways to start the day, making it through to lunch should be a snap.

THE LUNCH WHISTLE

If you are one of the lucky few who have a company dining room or cafeteria that has leaped onto the healthy bandwagon, you know the joys of bean, vegetable or pasta salads and low-fat hot entrées that look good, taste great and keep you going strong all afternoon. If not, take some tips from Terri Seewald Klein, R.D., a Havertown, Pennsylvania nutrition consultant specializing in helping businesses improve their employee food and fitness services.

"First of all, do some advance planning," Klein says. "Look over the week's menu before you even walk into the cafeteria, and have some decisions made before you're confronted with items that may tempt you.

"Look for hot entrées that are steamed, broiled or grilled. Anything in a cream sauce or deep-fried will be higher in fat.

IN THE FAST LANE

For occasions that find you in fast-food places, here's a
short guide to items with some of the lowest proportions
of fat.

Food	Calories	Fat (g.)	Percentage of Calories from Fat
Breakfast Foods			
Hardee's Three Pancakes (with syrup and margarine)	292	8	25
McDonald's Hotcakes (with margarine and syrup)	440	12	25
Roy Rogers Pancake Platter (with ham)	506	17	30
McDonald's Egg McMuffin	280	11	35
Burgers			
McDonald's McLean Deluxe	320	10	28
Wendy's Jr. Hamburger	270	9	30
Hardee's Hamburger	260	10	35
Roast Beef			
Roy Rogers Roast Beef Sandwich	317	10	28
Hardee's Regular Roast Beef	280	11	35
Chicken			
Chick-fil-A Chargrilled Chicken Deluxe Sandwich	266	5	17

Food	Calories	Fat (g.)	Percentage of Calories from Fat
Carl's Jr. Charbroiler BBQ Chicken Sandwich	310	6	17
Hardee's Grilled Chicken Sandwich	310	9	26
Long John Silver's Batter-Dipped Chicken Sandwich	410	16	35
Fish			
Long John Silver's Light Portion Fish (2 pieces, with lemon crumb, rice and small salad)	270	5	17
Long John Silver's Baked Fish (3 pieces, with lemon crumb, rice, green beans, coleslaw and roll)	570	12	19
Potatoes			
Roy Rogers' Plain Baked Potato	211	0.2	0.9
Wendy's Plain Baked Potato	300	<1	<3
Carl's Jr. Lite Potato	290	1	3
Arby's Plain Baked Potato	240	2	8
Mexican			
El Pollo Loco Pinto Beans	110	1	8
Taco Bell Bean Burrito (with red sauce)	458	14	28
El Pollo Loco Chicken (with corn tortillas and salsa)	530	20	34

If the vegetables are steamed and you have the option of ordering them without butter or with sauce on the side, that's preferable," says Klein.

Eating your vegetables this way is a good way to increase your fiber intake. The sandwich and salad bar is another good place to bulk up on high-fiber items. "Salad bars have really been a great addition to company cafeterias," says Klein. They are also important parts of many restaurants and supermarkets as well. Wherever you graze, the general guidelines are the same: Select items like beans, tomatoes, peppers, sprouts, cauliflower, broccoli and spinach. Spinach is a better choice than iceberg lettuce as a base for your salad because of the additional vitamins and minerals it contains. Things to watch out for are potato salad, coleslaw, egg salad: Anything prepared with lots of added fats. That includes croutons. Many croutons are prepared with additional fat. "Another word of caution about salad bars concerns dressings," Klein adds. "They can really add a lot of fat to the diet. Good alternatives are reduced-calorie or fat-free salad dressing, lemon juice or vinegar with a little bit of oil."

Next stop is the sandwich line. "When you have a choice in the sandwich line, select whole-grain breads," Klein advises. "And steer clear of high-fat cold cuts, like salami and bologna. More heart-healthy choices are lean meats like turkey or lean ham. But, anyone on a salt- or sodium-restricted diet has to watch out for many deli items, which are processed with salt," she warns. What is the health rating of other standard sandwich fillings? "Anything that's prepared with mayonnaise will add a lot of fat to the diet. Some cafeterias or sandwich shops give you the option of reduced-calorie mayonnaise as a spread. Or opt for mustard, catsup or vinegar with just a splash of oil."

If fast food is more your speed, check out a burger joint that also serves up baked potatoes (hold the sour cream, cheese and bacon, though). Or, seek out a place with salads or a salad bar and follow the guidelines above. Hold the fries and think twice about having fried chicken or fish unless you *at least* remove the skin and crust.

Nearly anywhere and anytime you choose to eat out, you have at least some healthy options, and they're increasing as rapidly as new restaurants are opening. With a bit of communication and cooperation between restaurant owners, chefs and customers, it is becoming ever easier for *every* meal to be healthy as well as satisfying.

CHAPTER 30

Natural Food Stores

Naturally Better?

You wouldn't know it from the cramped shelves and less-then-posh decor, but chances are, your neighborhood natural food store contains the foods of the future.

Many of the nutritionally superior foods gracing supermarket shelves today got their start in health food and natural food stores. Among them are granola, herbal teas, ice cream substitutes, pita bread, rice cakes, salsa, sports drinks, soy meat and dairy substitutes, wheat bran and yogurt. "Really just about any innovative product you can think of," says Jeffrey Bland, Ph.D., a clinical nutritionist in Gig Harbor, Washington, and a senior investigator for the American Association of Clinical Scientists.

And then there are the natural food store items that perpetuate the convenience-store-to-the-counterculture mystique: mysterious potions, wacky literature (One actual headline: "Your Astrology Diet") and dubious supplements that promise to boost energy, renew your sex drive and build muscle—simultaneously.

"You have to be careful," says Kim Galeaz-Gioe, R.D., a spokesperson for the American Dietetic Association. "Just because something is sold in a health food store doesn't automatically mean it's healthy."

In fact, the average natural food store carries several hundred items—from herbs to organic peanut butter—each with its own purported health merits.

But once past the questionable products, your taste buds and body are in for an adventure: A smorgasbord of healthy foods awaits that you can't find in most supermarkets . . . *yet*.

NOT JUST FOR HEALTH NUTS ANYMORE

Here, overprocessed foods loaded with additives and refined sugar are out and products made with whole, natural and often organically grown ingredients are in.

And who's buying? Diabetics avoiding added sugar. Wheat- and yeast-sensitive people trying to find bread that doesn't make them feel bad. People with lactose intolerance turning to soy milk. Moms who want to give their kids nutritious snacks. Aspiring body-builders searching for a competitive edge. Not just folks with ailments, but folks who want to eat healthier.

"It just makes sense. The closer you can get to consuming food in its natural state, the better," says Mark Messina, Ph.D., a nutritionist with the National Cancer Institute's Diet and Cancer Branch in Bethesda, Maryland.

Health foods stores are definitely a hit: Americans now spend over $4 billion a year at natural food stores, according to the National Nutritional Foods Association, the industry's leading trade group.

Growth in popularity of natural foods has also meant growth in the sizes of stores. Over the past decade, nearly 200 supermarket-size health food stores have sprouted across the country, including chains like Mrs. Gooch's Natural Market in California, Kathy's Ranch Market in Las Vegas and Salt Lake City, and Massachusetts-based Bread and Circus. The nation's largest: Unicorn Village Marketplace, a 28,000-square-foot behemoth that includes a restaurant and a gift store, located in the posh Aventura section of North Miami Beach.

In addition to offering an even wider selection than mom-and-pop-size health food markets, these superstores often stock private-label products, organically grown produce (fruit and vegetables grown without the use of synthetic fertilizers or pesticides) and beef and poultry from grain-fed animals that have not been treated with growth hormones.

HEALTHY HUNT: FINDING A STORE YOU LIKE

But big or little, there are certain basic requirements for *any* good natural food store, says Sandy Gooch, owner of Mrs. Gooch's, one of the country's leading natural foods retailers. "If the establishment doesn't have a wide selestion of supplements, whole grains, cereals, legumes, spring water, fresh juices, natural yogurts, tofu, soy milk, healthy snacks, organically grown produce, and in some cases, fresh-prepared foods, you're in the wrong place," she says.

What if you feel daunted by that dizzying array of new or unusual products? Just browse and read the fine print, says Janet Savage, an Oakland, California, nutritionist who leads groups—from seniors to school kids—on educational tours of natural food stores. "We have to take time to find out what's going into our bodies," Savage says.

And if you're on a tight budget, you may also have to take the time to check the prices. In most cases, you'll pay at least 10 percent more for an item than for its nearest counterpart in a traditional grocery store. Reasons vary: Fewer preservatives usually mean a shorter product shelf life; most of the products are made by small companies with higher costs; small retailers can't always buy in larger quantities to get price breaks. The obvious exception: Bulk bins that sometimes offer deep discounts on dried fruits, beans, nuts and other items, while allowing you to select just the right quantity. But health food advocates suggest any short-term added expense is worth it in the long run. "It comes down to how much you are willing to pay for an improved quality of life," says Martie Whittekin, president of the National Nutritional Foods Association.

But before you reach for your wallet, join us for an exploratory trip down the aisles.

BEANS: THE HIGH-FIBER CULTURAL EXPERIENCE

One of the biggest advantages of shopping at natural food stores is exposure to a wide variety of healthful ethnic foods. In addition to offering the usual dry beans like lentils, chickpeas, red kidney beans and black beans, many stores also stock a few types that may make you feel like a globe-trotter.

But beans offer more than just an inexpensive cultural dining experience. Says Dr. Messina: "Beans as a whole are high in fiber and low in fat. If you have a chance to try some different ones, it's going to add some healthful variety to your diet."

Among the most unusual:

Adzuki beans. Small, red, kidney-shaped beans that do not need soaking before preparation, adzukis are popular in Japan and often used in confections.

Anasazi beans. These small palomino-colored, kidney-shaped beans, popular in Mexico and the American Southwest, are sweeter and meatier than most and contain generous amounts of protein and iron.

Mung beans. Tender and slightly sweet, mung beans are popular in China and India. They're most often green but may be yellow or black. Primarily used for sprouting, mung beans do not have to be soaked before cooking.

Soybeans. Perhaps the world's most versatile bean—used for making oil, tofu, soy sauce, soy milk and other products—

the small round soybean is also great cooked for dinner. High in protein, soybeans, contain fiber, calcium, iron, zinc, magnesium, thiamine, riboflavin and niacin, plus high concentrations of compounds that demonstrate anti-cancer properties, according to researchers.

SEA VEGETABLES: PRODUCE FROM THE DEEP

Harvesting vegetables from the ocean may seem like a relatively new concept, but the Japanese have been doing it for centuries. Don't be concerned, however, if you don't take to sea vegetables like Jacques Cousteau: With their salty, fishy flavor, they're definitely not for everyone.

But if you enjoy the taste, natural food stores often stock a variety of dried sea vegetables. Here are some examples of what you might find.

Arame. A vegetable side dish that need only be rinsed and soaked for five minutes before cooking.

Dulse. A popular ingredient in stir-fries, sandwiches and soups.

Hijiki. A black, erect sea grass that can be added to soups and salads.

Kelp. Rich in iodine, it can be used in salads and as wrapping for other dishes.

Kombu. Can add flavor to beans or vegetables and simultaneously prevent the rice from sticking to the bottom of the pan during cooking.

Nori. Used to wrap sushi, comes in toasted strips which are a zesty complement to rice or vegetables.

BREADS: MAN DOES NOT LIVE BY WHITE ALONE

Official natural food store bread tip number one: Don't look for a bread rack. Because most of the breads here don't contain preservatives, they're kept on ice in the freezer. An exception: Space-age packaging and a half-dollar-size "oxygen absorber" allow at least one brand of brown rice bread to reside in the store refrigerator.

But locating these whole-grain feasts isn't nearly as much fun as sampling them. Most natural food stores stock a flavorful selection of whole-grain, rye, sourdough and sprouted breads that are so heavy and dense you'll need a steak knife to carve off a slab. And nobody has to feel left out: most stores stock wheat- and yeast-free loaves for those with allergies.

Whole-grain breads also retain more vitamins and fiber than those using refined ingredients—a healthful plus of which cancer experts approve. Some breads combine as many as 12 grains; others, like macrobiotic brown rice bread, are made from organically grown grain.

Sprouted breads are made from grains like rye or wheat that have been sprouted just before baking. "You know the grains are wholesome if they're able to sprout a plant," says Whittekin.

Most breads available in natural food stores contain baking powder free of aluminum for those concerned about a possible link between high amounts of that metal and Alzheimer's disease. And sourdough preparations allow many people with yeast allergies to enjoy bread worry-free, Whittekin says.

Flat, round, whole-wheat chapatis—often sold by the dozen—look like tortillas, but they're actually unleavened breads; they do not contain any yeast.

And if you can't find a bread you like, why not bake your own? A wide variety of flour is generally available, including organic barley, buckwheat, millet, oat, rice, rye and teff.

Used to make injera, an Ethiopian flat bread, teff is the smallest grain in the world. Yet it has more bran ounce per ounce than any other grain.

Multigrain flour combines the goodness of wheat, barley, pinto beans, green lentils, millet, rye and other ingredients.

And what about bake mixes that make oat bran, blue corn and seven-grain pancakes? There's even high-lysine corn flour that has a nutty flavor, crunchy texture and a naturally sweet taste along with its enhanced protein content.

CEREALS: SOMETHING NEW FOR YOUR BOWL

They may come in boxes similar to those on supermarket shelves, but these cereals usually contain fewer additives, not to mention less sugar and salt. "Some cereals on the market today have more salt than a bag of potato chips," says Whittekin.

Varieties range from oatmeal and millet to crispy brown rice and muesli. You'll find corn, wheat and other flakes, too. The sweeteners of choice: fruit juice concentrate and honey.

Once the darling of the natural foods industry, granola has also enjoyed mainstream success in supermarkets. To fight back, health food stores are now stocking fat-free granolas that claim to be the best you can buy.

Amaranth cereal, often with whole wheat and barley added as well, is a tasty, high-protein breakfast alternative made from this newly rediscovered grain.

First introduced in Europe, muesli is the cereal with a strong following in natural food stores. It's easy to see why: Muesli is a rich, tasty collection of unsweetened, whole grains like oats, wheat, millet and barley, combined with nuts and dried fruit.

Organic brown rice cereal brings the benefits of minimally processed rice to breakfast. Because the thick outer bran layer has not been removed, brown rice cereal offers more fiber per spoonful than traditional rice cereals.

And for those with a taste for all, there are multigrain cereals that combine amaranth, barley, buckwheat, corn, millet, oats and rye. Some are even sprouted.

REDISCOVERING THE GREAT GRAINS

Some grains increasingly popular in natural food stores have been used for centuries by other cultures, says Burton Kallman, Ph.D., director of science and technology for the National Nutritional Foods Association.

Amaranth. Very high in protein, this ancient grain is now appearing in everything from cereals and cookies to cake mixes. The Spaniards eradicated amaranth farming after conquering Mexico because the Aztecs thought the grain had mystical powers.

Barley. An excellent source of complex carbohydrates, barley has been shown to have some effective cholesterol-lowering properties, Dr. Kallman says.

Millet. Used extensively in China, millet is a hardy grain that is high in fiber, Dr. Kallman says. Millet is now found in cereal mixes and can also be ground for use in baking.

Quinoa. Another increasingly popular South American grain, quinoa (pronounced *KEEN-wa*) is unusually high in protein. Often sold as a hot cereal or as a substitute for rice, it can also be blended in flour for baking.

MILK SUBSTITUTES: BETTER THAN BETSY?

Cow's milk offers unsurpassed portions of protein and calcium in a no-muss, no-fuss liquid. But what if you're like two-thirds of the world's population—that is, unable to digest milk—or simply don't like milk's taste?

How about a glass of soy or rice milk, two popular dairy substitutes. Soy milk is made from—you guessed it—the tiny, but dependable soybean, plus water. But soy milk tastes remarkably like skim milk—without the cholesterol.

Eight ounces of a popular soy milk, made with filtered

water, organic soybeans, barley malt and pearl barley, has 110 calories and contains seven grams of protein, ten grams of carbohydrates and just five grams of fat. It supplies just 6 percent of the Recommended Dietary Allowance (RDA) of calcium. A popular rice milk, made from filtered water and brown rice, is 99 percent fat-free and contains no cholesterol. A serving provides just 2 percent of the RDA for calcium and protein.

Processing techniques have inflated prices of these products, making them an expensive dairy alternative. If the price is too high, you might consider making your own.

Both soy and rice milk are available in a variety of flavors.

ENERGY BARS: SNACK OF CHAMPIONS?

Weekend warriors searching for the competitive edge have caused a "bar war" of sorts in natural food stores. Over a dozen brands of energy bars grace store shelves, nearly all purporting to supply the energy you need to fuel your workout or replace a missed meal. And while some are on target when it comes to delivering the requisite amount of complex carbohydrates and protein in a low-sugar, low-fat package, others are less healthy.

Your best bet: Grab a bar that's packed with complex carbohydrates like maltodextrin, glucose polymers, oats, wheat flour or rice—with over 60 percent of calories from carbs and less than 30 percent from fat, according to *Runner's World* magazine sports nutrition columnist Liz Applegate, Ph.D. Because many bars are also fortified with vitamins and minerals, they may contain as many nutrients as a bowl of fortified breakfast cereal, says Dr. Applegate, who is author of *Power Foods*.

But they don't always taste as good. One bar contains 50 grams of carbohydrate, 15 grams of protein and just 3 grams of fat but has the consistency of frozen salt water taffy—not exactly the best snack for someone in a hurry.

MAKE YOUR OWN SOY MILK

If you find commercial soy milk too expensive for everyday use, you can prepare your own at home for a fraction of the cost. It's a little time-consuming because the beans need soaking, but it's not really difficult. You may use the milk as is for cooking and baking. But for drinking, you'll probably want to flavor the batch with about ⅓ cup honey.

Start with 1 cup dry soybeans. Rinse well and place them in a large bowl. Cover with cold water and allow to soak for 4 to 16 hours (refrigerate the beans if you soak them for more than 6 hours). Drain. You'll have about 2¼ cups beans.

Place half the beans in a blender and add 1½ cups cold water. Process on high speed for at least two minutes, or until the beans are well pureed. Transfer the mixture to a four-quart saucepan. Repeat the process with the remaining beans and another 1½ cups water.

Add an additional 4½ cups water to the pan. Bring to a slow rolling boil, stirring frequently to minimize sticking. After the mixture reaches the boiling point (the foam on top will rise up suddenly, threatening to overflow), reduce the heat so the mixture simmers. Cook for 10 to 15 minutes.

Line a colander with several layers of cheesecloth and place it over a large bowl. Ladle the bean mixture into the colander. Strain out as much of the soy milk as possible, pressing with a spoon to extract the liquid. When the mixture has cooled sufficiently, you can also squeeze the cheesecloth with your hands. You'll end up with about 1½ quarts of soy milk.

Bars that get most of their energy from simple sugars like corn syrup will almost certainly leave you with an energy crisis after the sugar rush wears off. Also be wary of those that claim a boost from such ingredients as bee pollen: It's never been proved to enhance performance, says Dr. Applegate.

SPORTS NUTRITION'S PUMPED-UP EXPECTATIONS

Soaring interest in fitness has sent sales of sports nutrition supplements surging. As a result, most health food stores stock everything from weight-gain shakes to electrolyte-replacement drinks.

Some bodybuilding supplements are more sophisticated than ever, with ingredient blends supposedly based on advanced research in muscle fatigue and recovery. Others simply tout their protein content.

But be wary of products like bee pollen that claim to instantly boost energy or performance. None of these supplements have been proven to enhance sports performance, according to Ann C. Grandjean, Ed.D., chief nutrition consultant for the U.S. Olympic committee.

In fact, bee pollen can cause severe allergic reactions in some people, Dr. Grandjean says. Brewer's yeast, pangamic acid and bioflavanoids, also widely touted, have no value as performance aids. And no studies have demonstrated that individual amino acids boost performance, she says.

Many carbohydrate-rich sports drinks however, have been shown to benefit performance.

HERBS: A SPRIG A DAY KEEPS DISEASE AWAY?

Of all the unusual products stocked in health food stores, few carry the aura of herbs. Rows of jars stocked with the leaves, roots and bark of obscure plants conjure images of ancient healers working their magic arts. And yet, few realize that, today, herbs are still the primary medicines of much of the world's population. And over 25 percent of modern prescription drugs are actually made with synthesized versions of the active ingredients in herbs, says Mark Blumenthal, executive director of the American Botanical Council.

Most stores carry a broad range of herbal products for medicinal purposes—from alfalfa to witch hazel. But be advised: Many herbal healing claims have yet to be verified by scientific research. And because herbal products can vary widely in potency and sometimes cause undesirable side effects, they probably shouldn't be used without first consulting a doctor.

Here are some of the herbs most commonly found in natural food stores.

Chamomile. One of the nation's best-selling herbs, chamomile in tea is often recommended by herbalists as a digestive aid and tranquilizer.

Echinacea. Traditionally used to fight infections and stimulate the immune system, modern research suggests that echinacea may also combat arthritis.

Ephedra. This herb contains an amphetamine-like compound called ephedrine, which works as a nasal decongestant and a bronchial dilator. Ephedra has also been used by people attempting to lose weight.

Garlic. One of the world's oldest medicines, garlic is undergoing a revival that has supporters advocating its use for preventing colds and flu, enhancing immune function and helping lower blood pressure and cholesterol. Garlic is also one of several foods under investigation by the National Cancer Institute for its cancer-fighting properties. If you do decide to try it, don't worry about scaring friends and loved ones away with the smell—garlic supplements in capsule form are often deodorized.

Ginger. A digestive aid, ginger, studies suggest, allays nausea and mild motion sickness.

Ginkgo. The biggest-selling over-the-counter remedy in Europe in 1989, ginkgo is thought to improve short-term memory and boost circulation.

Goldenseal. Considered one of the most useful herbs by contemporary herbalists, goldenseal is thought to be helpful as an antibiotic, an immune stimulant and a digestive aid.

Juniper. Herbalists claim that this herb helps combat high blood pressure, congestive heart failure and arthritis.

Valerian. This herb is frequently used as a sleep aid.

MEAT SUBSTITUTES: FAKE FLESH

For years, those following a vegetarian diet for ethical or religious reasons were the primary buyers of meat substitutes. But today, an even broader audience is waking up to these products' health advantage: far less saturated fat and cholesterol than the real thing. A variety of soy-based, grain and vegetable meat substitutes are now available. Among the most popular: tofu pups. These aptly named creations mimic the All-American hot dog, but with less fat and no chemical additives.

Meatless cold cuts, often made from wheat and tofu, come close to copying corned beef, ham, pastrami, turkey and roast beef. Soy is also used to replicate sausage, burgers and even chicken.

Tempeh, a pressed, fermented soybean cake popular in Indonesia, is also gaining increasing acceptance here as a beef or chicken substitute. And with good reason: Tempeh has almost as much protein as beef and chicken, without the saturated fat or cholesterol. Produced by exposing soybeans to harmless bacteria, tempeh can be used in recipes that call for everything from baking to frying.

JUNK FOOD AS HEALTH FOOD

Our tour is nearly complete. But before you haul all your goodies to the cash register, here's some closing advice: You may want to check the ingredient labels one last time, suggests Dr. Bland. "In the present state of regulation, consumers do need to be informed label readers in natural food stores just as they would be in traditional stores," he says.

In fact, "natural" may be the most abused word in the English language. "It's become a nonsense term in the absence of a standard identity. It can be used and misused in any way possible," Dr. Bland says.

Some of the worst offenders: sports and weight-loss beverages, breakfast foods, snack foods, dairy substitutes and confections. Just because these and other items are being sold in a natural foods market, you should not assume they are all healthier, says Dr. Bland.

Some items, he contends, may not even belong in natural food stores. Candy is candy, for example. And some chips, crackers and cookies sold in health food stores have as much or more fat and salt as supermarket snacks.

Over the years other products of dubious value have appeared on natural food shelves. One product billed as a natural herbal energizer, for example, became a hit with customers and retailers—until it was discovered that it was loaded with caffeine, says Danny Wells, a natural food store consultant in Pleasant Hill, California.

In an attempt to head off such problems, some natural food markets like Mrs. Gooch's simply refuse to stock items containing questionable ingredients.

A "standards and criteria" worksheet sent to all Mrs. Gooch's suppliers says: "We only stock items meeting these criteria: no artificial flavorings, no artificial colorings, no artificial sweeteners, no refined sweeteners, such as sucrose, fructose, corn syrup, glucose, maltose, brown, raw or

---

SOMETHING TO MUNCH ON

The snacks found in natural food stores may appear to be more healthy than those found elsewhere. But read labels carefully because some are still loaded with fat and salt: "Junk food disguised as health food," says clinical nutritionist Jeffrey Bland, Ph.D. A one-ounce serving of a popular carrot chip, for example, has nine grams of fat.

But you'll also discover a number of items that make snacking virtually guilt-free. A one-ounce serving of a light, crunchy (and addicting, according to taste testers) corn snack actually had *no* fat and 21 grams of carbohydrate.

And when was the last time you had a supermarket-bought raspberry muffin so flavorful that the exceptional nutritional value—five grams of fiber and less than one gram of fat—was an afterthought?

---

turbinado sugars, no MSG, no caffeine, no chocolate, no hydrogenated oils, no alcoholic beverages, no white flour (including unbleached), no irradiated foods, no harmful preservative agents, no harmful chemical additives."

"In the natural foods industry we're finding greater and greater numbers of foods that adhere to our standards," says Gooch. "My advice is: If it's so chemically preserved that it can't spoil, then don't buy it."

Gooch's quest for good health began in a hospital bed. She says she nearly died from a seizure indirectly caused by the food additive, bromated vegetable oil, hidden in a diet soda. So the former teacher and housewife stopped buying processed food and started looking for fresh, natural products free from artificial anything. As she discovered after opening her hugely successful stores: A lot of other people are looking for the same thing.

CHAPTER 31

Supplements

A Smart Buyer's Guide

If there's anything nutrition experts agree on, it's that the preferred source of vitamins and minerals is food, not tablets or capsules. And no, they're not just trying to make things hard for you. "There are good reasons nutritional supplements should not be used as a substitute for a balanced diet," says Jacqueline Charnley, R.D., of the U.S. Department of Agriculture's (USDA) Human Nutrition Research Center on Aging at Tufts University in Boston.

"We don't know everything there is to know about nutrition, so no vitamin pill is perfect," Charnley says. "There may be unknown components of food, necessary for good health, that just aren't found in a multivitamin. There may be interactions or balances between particular nutrients that depend on food sources. And certainly you need to eat foods to get protein, carbohydrates, fiber, essential fatty acids and some trace minerals that aren't usually found in vitamin pills."

One more good reason to focus on diet first: If you're not eating well, you're probably eating pretty poorly, and vitamins can only go so far to make up for a lifetime of dietary indiscretions.

But many experts *also* agree there is a place for nutritional supplements.

"Dietary surveys consistently show that a certain percentage of people come up short when it comes to meeting the RDA for all nutrients," Charnley says. "Even when they know what they need to do to improve their eating habits, some people may choose not to do it."

Dieticians admit it's hard to get people to eat better. It takes time, effort and desire. You need to know how to shop for and prepare good food and how to choose wisely when you eat out. The old notion among dietitians was that supplement use should be discouraged, supposedly because it encourages people to eat poorly. But an increasing number of experts say it doesn't have to be an either/or situation. "You can improve your diet, *and* you can take supplements, if and when it's appropriate," Charnley says. In fact, some studies show that people who take vitamin supplements tend to eat better than those who don't take supplements.

In real life, experts say, many people seem to go through a natural evolution of "nutrition consciousness raising" that involves supplement use and improved eating habits—often in conjunction with health or weight problems, pregnancy or just plain getting older.

"People often work on a number of things at once—they may take supplements, improve their diets and begin to exercise," Charnley says. "And even as their diets improve, they may continue to take supplements."

SUPPLEMENT QUESTIONS ANSWERED

WHO TAKES SUPPLEMENTS?

About half the people in the United States take nutritional supplements regularly or occasionally, according to a large survey by the USDA. That includes men and women, children and adults, young and old, dog owners and cat owners and people with and without VCRs and CD players.

From surveys, experts have developed a profile of the person most likely to take vitamins. *She* lives in a western state, is well educated (high school or beyond) with a higher-than-average income and a better-than-average diet.

WHY DO PEOPLE TAKE NUTRITIONAL SUPPLEMENTS?

According to a review of studies by the National Research Council Food and Nutrition Board, people are most likely to say they take supplements because they're uncertain about the nutritional adequacy of their diets, because they desire better health than they perceive to be obtainable from medical consultation or because they've decided to treat themselves for an illness.

In one study, the most frequently given reasons for taking supplements were "to prevent colds and other illnesses," "to give me energy" and "to make up for what is not in food." (At least two studies show that vitamin users tend to have a low opinion of today's food quality.)

DO PEOPLE WHO TAKE VITAMINS FIND THEM HELPFUL?

For some reason, most studies haven't posed this question. In one that did ask, 59 percent reported that supplements were of "some benefit" to their health; another 34 percent found them to be of "great benefit."

WHAT VITAMINS ARE PEOPLE TAKING?

A survey by the Council for Responsible Nutrition (a vitamin manufacturers' trade group) shows that multiple vitamin and mineral supplements make up nearly 42 percent of all vitamin sales, followed by vitamin C (with 12 percent), B-complex (9 percent), vitamin E (9 percent), calcium (7.5 percent) and iron (7 percent). Sales of nutritional supplements have increased steadily and dramatically over the years—from $500 million in 1972 to $3.3 billion in 1990.

ARE NATURAL VITAMINS BETTER THAN SYNTHETIC VITAMINS?

For those who pefer cotton to polyester and carrot juice to cola, the word "natural" may have special meaning. It sym-

HOW TO READ A VITAMIN LABEL

It may look like a secret code, but with a little practice, you can decipher all the information on a supplemental label.

A typical label first lists the brand name of the supplement—such as Centrum, Theragran or Os-Cal. Under that is the name of the supplement—multivitamins with iron, for example, or calcium carbonate.

Behind the name of the supplement may be the letters "U.S.P." This means the supplement meets manufacturing standards set by the U.S. Pharmacopeia, an independent, nonprofit organization that sets the official standards of strength, quality, purity, packaging and labeling for medical products used in the United States. To a vitamin consumer, the U.S.P. mark guarantees a quality product that dissolves properly in the stomach and delivers the goods.

Next comes the list of active ingredients (the nutrients) and their potencies or amounts, in micrograms (mcg.), milligrams (mg.) or International Units (I.U.).

Next to that is each active ingredient's percentage of the U.S. RDA. If an active ingredient has no RDA, the label may say "RDA not established."

Beneath that comes a complete list of ingredients. This includes the chemical names of the active ingredients. Vitamin C may be listed as ascorbic acid; vitamin E as vitamin E acetate; vitamin D as ergocalciferol. If the product is marked U.S.P., this list will also include ingredients such as fillers and coatings.

bolizes purity: Mother Nature with nothing missing and no added extras. When it comes to vitamins, though, experts at the Food and Drug Administration (FDA) say that natural and synthetic vitamins are virtually identical. Any slight differences are insignificant.

Always check the expiration date. As long as the product is properly stored, it's guaranteed to meet the potency listed on the label up to the expiration date. After that time, the product begins to degrade, and its potency slowly drops. An expiration date may be two to four years from the date of manufacture, depending on the nutrient. Experts say it's best not to buy or to use "expired" vitamins.

Look for information that tells you how many tablets you need to take daily to achieve the recommended dosage. Having to take three or four tablets a day to reach the RDA levels listed on the label may make the product seem like less of a bargain.

By the time you read this, vitamin manufacturers are expected to be operating under a new Nutrition and Education Labeling Act. This act requires calories, fat and sodium to be listed on a supplement label where appropriate. For instance, a product like sodium ascorbate, a form of vitamin C, will have to list milligrams of sodium per dose, and oil-containing tablets will have to list their calories and fat content.

"This new act does allow health benefits to be mentioned on the label, provided the Food and Drug Administration [FDA] had determined there is enough scientific evidence to make that claim," says Edward Scarborough, Ph.D., director of the FDA's Office of Nutrition and Food Sciences. So far, the only health claim the FDA has permitted that pertains to supplements is that calcium may reduce the risk of osteoporosis.

Some supplements are made from natural materials. Most minerals, for instance, are derived from natural mined substances. Calcium may be derived from limestone, oyster shells or naturally occurring beds of calcium carbonate.

Most manufactured vitamins are "built" from organic molecules found in an array of substances. Why? Because vitamins are found in such small quantities in foods (even foods rich in a particular nutrient) that the cost of isolating any vitamin from food in bulk quantities is prohibitive. "Take beta-carotene, for example," says Frank Girardi, pharmaceutical business unit director for Hoffmann-La Roche in Nutley, New Jersey, one of the world's largest bulk vitamin manufacturers. "You can get it from carrots or algae, but supplement makers would need tons of carrots to come up with enough beta-carotene for their products, and a lot would go to waste because this particular micronutrient isn't very stable. Besides, the natural form could be two to ten times more expensive."

So what's most beta-carotene made from? Ultrapure byproducts of petroleum and mined calcium carbide. If that seems strange to you, consider that most of our lifesaving drugs, even aspirin, are concocted from this same soup of organic molecules. These complex molecules are isolated, purified and then precisely rearranged into many different substances. Chemically, the beta-carotene made from petroleum derivatives is exactly the same as that derived from a carrot. And experts insist it works the same way in your body. These synthetic vitamins are also the same material used in the very complex, long-term clinical trials to show the health benefits of vitamins and minerals in our diet.

Vitamin C is made from dextrose, a sugar found in corn. After it's purified, the dextrose is put through the same sort of chemical process that occurs in those animals that are capable of synthesizing vitamin C in their bodies. Chemically, the final product is exactly the same as the vitamin C derived from an orange. How does the manufacturer know that? "Years of testing, on both animals and humans, have established that the natural and synthetic versions of most nutrients are exactly the same—chemically and biologically," says David Roll, Ph.D., professor of medicinal chemistry in the College of Pharmacy at the University of Utah in Salt Lake City.

GOING DOWN EASY

Having a hard time swallowing that vitamin tablet or capsule? Relax. Take a few deep breaths. Then, try these suggestions from Bronwyn Jones, M.D., director of Johns Hopkins Medical Center Swallowing Center in Baltimore, which treats people with swallowing problems from around the world.

Keep your head level. You might also tuck your chin in just a bit. "Many people who take pills toss their heads back as they swallow, and that, in fact, is the worst thing they can do," Dr. Jones says. "It puts tension on the neck and makes it harder for the muscles of the esophagus to push the pill down to the stomach. It also makes it easier for pills or fluids to move toward the lungs as the extended position makes it harder for muscles to elevate the larynx and protect the airway."

Sit up—or stand up. It makes sense, and a study shows that tablets move more quickly through the esophagus when this mouth-to-stomach passageway is vertical, not horizontal. "If you take pills before bed, take them sitting up, with at least half a cup of water, and continue to sit up for a few minutes longer," Dr. Jones advises. Pills that stay in your throat all night long can cause irritation.

If you must take pills lying down, crush them or chew them, or ask your doctor for a liquid form. Just make sure it's okay to crush the pill. Timed-release tablets should not be crushed. It also helps to take them with plenty of water.

Try cold, carbonated water. For some people, carbonated, bottled water works better than regular water to speed pills down to the stomach. Researchers speculate that carbonation provides an air cushion around tablets, easing their passage.

Some, like vitamin E, have synthetic versions that are different from the natural versions. Natural vitamin E (d-alpha-tocopherol) is isolated from soybean oil. Synthetic vitamin E (*dl*-alpha-tocopherol) is made from petroleum derivatives. The natural version has slightly more of what's called "biological activity" than the synthetic version.

What does that mean? "In essence, all it means is that you have to take slightly more of the synthetic version of vitamin E to match the effects of the natural version," says Dr. Roll.

ARE PEOPLE TAKING VITAMINS SAFELY?

One Food and Drug Administration study showed that many supplement users took most nutrients in amounts that seldom exceeded one to two times the Recommended Dietary Allowance (RDA), an amount most experts consider safe. But 50 percent of respondents took more than double the RDA of vitamin C, thiamine, riboflavin or pantothenate. And some people took up to several hundred times the RDA of vitamins E, C, B_6, B_{12}, thiamine, riboflavin and pantothenate. Those amounts should be used only with medical guidance, experts say.

Some studies show vitamin users as independent thinkers when it comes to medical care. One revealed that "heavy" users (those taking 440 percent of the RDA) and "very heavy" users (those taking 777 percent of the RDA) tend not to involve their doctor in their decisions about supplements. That's an unwise move, experts say.

But one study suggests doctors exert the most influence on the public (in this case, their patients) in making decisions to take supplements. Most likely to consider dietary supplementation important are obstetricians, gynecologists, female doctors and doctors interested in continuing their medical education courses in nutrition.

DO HEALTH PROFESSIONALS TAKE SUPPLEMENTS THEMSELVES?

Several studies show supplements are popular among health professionals, including dietitians. In one study, 60 percent of dietitians who responded to a mail survey admitted they regularly took supplements—usually multivitamins/minerals, vitamin C and iron—for personal health. And several studies demonstrate that supplement use among doctors and medical students is not infrequent.

CHOOSING A MULTIVITAMIN

With so much interest in supplements, it's important that people know what to look for—and what to avoid—when buying these products. Multiple vitamins and minerals are by far the most often purchased nutritional supplements, so let's look at them first.

A multiple combines many nutrients into one tablet or capsule. It's for people who want to take vitamins or minerals or both, but don't want to take five or six, or more, different pills each day.

A good multivitamin/mineral can act as a sort of "dietary insurance policy." It can fix some of the common failings in a typical diet, Charnley says.

What should you look for in a multivitamin/mineral supplement?

Find a multi that supplies about 100 percent of the RDA for most, but not necessarily all, nutrients. "Most Americans get more than they need of phosphorus and iodine, so there's no reason to put these nutrients in a supplement," says Walter Mertz, M.D., director of the USDA Human Nutrition Research Center in Beltsville, Maryland. And vitamin K deficiency is so rare, this nutrient is not necessary in a multi, most experts say.

Look for a multi that also supplies the nutrients with an "estimated safe and adequate" daily dietary intake. Those include biotin, pantothenate acid, copper, manganese, fluoride, chromium and molybdenum.

Look for a multi that supplies some vitamin A as beta-carotene. In the body, beta-carotene can convert to vitamin A without the danger of an overdose.

SPECIAL FORMULATIONS—
TOO NARROW A FOCUS?

Some nutritional supplements are designed to treat a particular ailment or are geared toward a specific group of people. They may contain vitamins, minerals, herbs, essential fatty acids, amino acids and just about anything else a manufacturer thinks might be helpful.

Since Food and Drug Administration regulations restrict manufacturers' claims about potential health benefits, most of these products' names merely hint at their purpose. They include stress formulas and formulas aimed at older people, dieters, athletes, men and women. Some are formulated to address eye problems or prostate problems. Others are meant to improve immune function or prevent osteoporosis.

If you are considering buying one of these products, what do you need to know?

First, special formulas tend to offer fewer nutrients than a multiple, perhaps only three or four. "And they tend to be less balanced than a multiple, which means they have more potential to cause imbalances in your body," says David Roll, Ph.D., of the University of Utah. A premenstrual formula, for instance, may offer many times the Recommended Dietary Allowance of vitamin B_6, but contain very little of other B vitamins. A men's formula may contain large amounts of zinc. Geriatric formulas may be top-heavy in antioxidants—vitamins C and E, beta-carotene and selenium. An osteoporosis formula may contain calcium but not much of other nutrients important for bones.

Just like single-nutrient supplements, special formulas are best used with medical supervision. Dr. Roll says "a better choice might be a good multivitamin/mineral."

Don't fall for a long list of ingredients. More is not necessarily better, says Dr. Roll. "All sorts of fringe substances find their way into nutritional supplements," he says. "For instance, choline, PABA, inositol, lecithin, glutamic acid—these substances are not proven to be necessary in the diet of humans. Our bodies make these substances internally. All they add to a supplement is cost."

Note where a multi falls short. Some contain only vitamins, not minerals. That's easy enough to detect by scanning the label. Even those that do supply minerals tend to be low in calcium and magnesium, two bulky minerals that add substantially to the size of a pill. A multi seldom contains potassium. Because potassium is considered "ubiquitous" in the diet—it's found in many foods—potassium deficiency is considered rare.

Many multis lack essential trace minerals like selenium, copper, manganese and chromium. Some contain iron, some don't.

If a multi falls short here or there, and you can't make up for it in your diet, it's easy enough to supplement with additional individual nutrients.

CHOOSING SINGLE-NUTRIENT SUPPLEMENTS

Individual vitamin or mineral supplements can correct specific nutrient shortfalls, address special needs and provide protection above and beyond the RDAs, Charnley says.

If, for example, you're concerned about developing osteoporosis but dislike milk, calcium supplements can supply extra amounts of this bone strengthener. Or if you've decided you want to take more than the RDA of nutrients that appear to help protect against cancer—vitamins C and E, beta-carotene, perhaps selenium—you might consider single-nutrient supplements.

Single-nutrient supplements do carry some risk, though. While reputable manufacturers offer supplements that stay

VITAMIN AND MINERAL SUPPLEMENT GUIDELINES

In this table, you'll find two sets of numbers—one for the Recommended Dietary Allowance (RDA) and the other for the "preventive amount." The numbers in the RDA column simply tell you how much supplement you'd need to reach the high range of the Recommanded Dietary Allowance. In the "preventive amount" column is a ballpark number that early research findings suggest should put you in the right range for preventive purposes. If you stay at this level or below, you can supplement nutrients that may be lacking in your diet without taking excessively high (and perhaps dangerous) amounts of those nutrients.

Nutrient	RDA*	Preventive Amount
Vitamins		
Vitamin A	5,000 I.U.	5,000 I.U.
Beta-carotene	6 mg.‡	15-30 mg.
Thiamine (vitamin B$_1$)	1.5 mg.	1.5 mg.
Riboflavin (vitamin B$_2$)	1.8 mg.	1.8 mg.
Niacin	20 mg.	20 mg.
Vitamin B$_6$	2 mg.	2-1 mg.
Vitamin B$_{12}$	2 mcg.	2-1 mcg.
Folate	200 mcg.	400-800 mcg.
Vitamin C	60 mg.	100-500 mg.
Vitamin D	10 mcg. (400 I.U.)	10 mcg. (400 I.U.)

within a safe range, FDA officials say, for most nutrients there is no set ceiling.

Don't go overboard. Because supplements may provide many times the RDA of a nutrient in one dose, it's easy to get large amounts, especially if you take several tablets.

Nutrient	RDA*	Preventive Amount
Vitamins		
Vitamin E	15 I.U. (10 mg. αTE)	100-400 I.U. (67-268 mg. αTE)
Minerals		
Calcium	1,200 mg.	1,200-1,500 mg.
Chromium	50-200 mcg.§	100-200 mcg.
Iron‖	15 mg.	15 mg.
Magnesium	400 mg.	400 mg.
Selenium	70 mcg.	70-200 mcg.
Zinc	15 mg.	15 mg.

NOTE: Don't take more than the upper limit of the preventive amount unless prescribed by a licensed health professional. Supplements are best taken with meals, particularly calcium, which needs the stomach acid produced by eating to enhance digestion.

*Represents the highest Recommended Dietary Allowances for all ages and sex groups except pregnant and lactating women.

†Vitamin A is best taken in the form of beta-carotene.

‡6 milligrams of beta-carotene provides 100 percent of the RDA for vitamin A.

§Range for chromium is an Estimated Safe and Adequate Daily Dietary Intake.

‖Men should not take supplemental iron without checking first with their doctors.

"Some nutrients, such as vitamins C and E, appear to be quite safe, at least for healthy people, even in large amounts," says John N. Hathcock, Ph.D., of the FDA's office of Experimental Nutrition. Others, including most trace minerals and vitamins A and D, have a narrower range of safety. "If you are taking amounts that are several times more than the RDA or estimated safe range of any nutrient, you are essentially using it as a drug, and you should have the guidance of a health-care professional," Dr. Roll says.

Stay in balance. Too much of one nutrient can interfere with your body's ability to use other nutrients, Dr. Mertz says. "Too much zinc interferes with your body's ability to absorb copper, and too much calcium affects the absorption of many trace minerals," he says. "And too much B_6 or folate will increase the body's requirement for riboflavin," says John Pinto, Ph.D., director of the Nutrition Research Laboratory at Memorial Sloan-Kettering Cancer Center in New York City.

THE PROBLEM OF ABSORPTION

Nobody absorbs 100 percent of all the vitamins and minerals they take, nutritionists say, but most people do pretty well, as long as a supplement is manufactured properly. (Exception: Low stomach acid, a problem that's not uncommon in older people, can cause absorption problems.) To improve absorption:

Buy supplements with "U.S.P." on the label. U.S.P. after a supplement name means the product has been manufactured according to U.S. Pharmacopeia standards in a way that makes it disintegrate and dissolve properly and assures that it contains the amount of nutrients stated on the label.

Take your vitamins with or right after a meal. "The very sight of food begins to stimulate the appetite, triggering the release of various enzymes that aid digestion and increase intestinal blood flow," Dr. Pinto says. And taking supplements with meals makes them unlikely to upset your stomach, Dr. Roll adds.

If you are taking iron, choose a ferrous, not ferric, compound. Ferrous iron is easier to absorb and causes less stomach irritation, experts agree.

Take iron with orange juice. The vitamin C in the orange juice makes absorption of the supplemental iron easier.

If you're taking large amounts of a vitamin, divide it into smaller doses, taken at each meal. Your body can absorb only a certain amount of a nutrient at any one time. By dividing the dose throughout the day, you increase the amount absorbed.

PROTECTING YOUR STASH

"Store in a cool, dry place." That's what it often says on the supplement label. But what's considered a cool, dry place?

Well, it's definitely not your bathroom, experts say. And it's not the cupboard above your stove. Other than those two spots, a cool, dry place might be found almost anywhere in your house.

"A kitchen pantry, away from direct sunlight, humidity or heat, is probably the best area to store vitamins," says V. Srinivasan, Ph.D., a scientist with the U.S. Pharmacopeia.

Do you buy large amounts of vitamins on sale, then store them? You can keep them in the refrigerator or freezer until you start using them, Dr. Srinivasan says, but let the container warm up to room temperature before you open it. Otherside, moisture may condense inside.

Some additional tips: Don't leave vitamins in a hot car. Always keep the cap on tight, and keep supplements out of the reach of children. Discard any product that begins to look or smell strange.

PART 5

HEALING DIETS

CHAPTER 32

Weight Loss

What Really Works

Are you a prisoner of war in the battle of the bulge? Held hostage by bad eating habits? So was Kathy Biggerstaff of Evansville, Indiana—until some no-nonsense nutritional concepts helped her lose nearly 100 pounds.

Kathy's quest to escape from her dietary torture is a tale repeated from San Francisco to St. Petersburg. "Because I never ate breakfast, I'd start eating potato chips or other junk by about 10:00 A.M.," she says. "Then I'd have a big lunch, more junk at 3:00 P.M., and, of course, red meat and fried potatoes for dinner."

When it came time to shed the weight, something that an estimated 35 percent of Americans try to do each month, Kathy chose the parallel American obsession: miracle weight-loss programs, Her favorite: diet shakes.

"I always looked at it like 'Now I have to go on a diet—I can't eat what I want anymore,'" she says.

The weight came off, but like a criminal who returns to the scene of the crime, it always came back. By age 30, Kathy was lugging 200 pounds on her tiny 5'5" frame.

Depressed about her condition, Kathy finally abandoned diets and instead developed a low-fat eating plan based on nutritional information she got from her doctor and Weight Watchers—tips like trading away burgers for broiled chicken, eating more vegetables (*without* coating them with butter) and packing her own low-fat salad dressing. She also started walking regularly.

From the results, you'd think she had a body transplant. In two years, Kathy dwindled from a size 20 to a size 3 and reached her dream weight of 107 pounds. Now she even teaches exercise classes.

But she's also the first to admit that if she can do it, anyone can: "You just have to recognize the fact that eating right and exercise are the only solutions," she says. "You can't diet your way around it."

Kathy's discovery confirms the conclusion reached by weight-loss experts: Whether you're trying to lose 10 or 100 pounds, restrictive diets that dramatically cut calories don't work in the long run. Healthy, low-fat eating, combined with moderate exercise, is the only way to lose weight and keep it off.

"Only long-term lifestyle changes make weight loss permanent," says C. Wayne Callaway, M.D., associate clinical professor of medicine at the George Washington University Medical Center in Washington, D.C., and author of *The Callaway Diet*. "Starvation, formulas and gimmicks just don't work."

Forget Fad Diets

Each year literally hundreds of new diets appear on bookstore shelves, magazine stands and grocery check-out racks, each claiming to melt pounds quickly and permanently.

Unfortunately, most weight-loss gimmicks on the market will only make your wallet lighter, according to Judy Goffi, R.D., a staff nutritionist who's counseled hundreds of overweight women at the Francis Stern Nutrition Center at the New England Medical Center Hospital in Boston. "It's sad because the people who try these diets are the ones who are the most desperate," she says.

Among the worst methods, according to Goffi: single-food diets that insist items like grapefruit have some newly discovered power to burn fat. Aside from the absurdity of those claims, single-food diets are nearly impossible to sustain beyond a few weeks, she says.

And some diets aren't just laughable—they can be downright dangerous. At least 60 people died while on the aptly named Last Chance Diet, an 880-calorie liquid protein fast sold during the early 1980s, says Goffi.

Ignoring your body's normal hunger signals while on a diet ordinarily won't kill you—most people give in before they starve. But severely restricting your eating can damage your natural ability to control eating, according to Peter Herman, Ph.D., a psychology professor at the University of Toronto in Ontario. "You can tolerate more hunger, but when you start eating, you can't stop—you lose your brakes as well as your accelerator," says Dr. Herman.

At the heart of his theory on the hazards of severe calorie cutting: the milk shake study. Under the guise of an ice cream taste test, dieters and nondieters were fed a milk shake before being allowed to sample ice cream. To his amazement, Dr. Herman found that once they got started, the self-described dieters actually ate 30 percent to 40 percent more ice cream than the nondieters. Apparently, once the dieters allowed themselves to down that milk shake, they felt they might as well go on and indulge to their heart's content—a familiar theme among those trying to starve themselves thin.

"Dieters have a strange way of keeping score," says Dr. Herman. "They think if they're good then they're good, but if they're bad, it doesn't matter how bad. It does matter. Overeating today will count against you tomorrow," he says.

MANAGE YOUR METABOLISM

Whether you overeat because you're addicted to ice cream or because you're unhappy, gaining weight is simply a matter of eating more calories than you burn for energy.

Think of your body as a roaring fire. Every bite of food above your body's energy needs stacks fat cells on different parts of your body just out of reach of the hungry flames. And you don't need marathon sessions at an all-you-can-eat buffet to get the fat collection started. An extra 50 to 100 calories a day—roughly a handful of potato chips—could add 5 to 10 pounds a year! That's because 3,500 calories are equal to a pound of fat.

To get rid of that lumpy surplus, you have to do at least two things: Stop the accumulation of new fat and start throwing some of what's already there on the fire. The best way to do that: Keep your body's built-in fat burner, your metabolism, burning intensely.

"This will effectively improve your body's ability to use body fat as fuel, regardless of your genetic endowment," according to Herman M. Frankel, M.D., an obesity expert and director of the Portland Health Institute in Oregon.

Although experts still have a lot to learn about metabolism, they know it's generally efficient when left alone, ravenously consuming calories to help fuel circulation, digestion, body temperature, muscle repair and all your other bodily functions. The problem begins when you interfere with your body's natural metabolic setting by dieting.

Drastic calorie cutting *will* make the pounds drop off. But unfortunately, your body doesn't just harmlessly burn fat and water to quickly shed those pounds. It also burns muscle. The problem with that is that muscle tissue—even when not in use—is a very efficient calorie burner. So when you lose muscle because of drastic dieting, you're damping the flames of your metabolism.

But starvation dieting creates another, even more severe, problem: Your body hoards calories as if it were trying to endure an Ethiopian famine. The result: Your once-fiery metabolism merely flickers.

A sluggish metabolism isn't bad—if you intend to eat like a bird for the rest of your life. But once you begin putting food on your plate again, all those extra calories will begin piling up as fat even faster than before, says Dr. Frankel.

"The body clings tenaciously to any fat and tries to build up more, anticipating the next famine situation," says Dr. Frankel. "And that makes it even harder to lose weight the next time."

A landmark University of Pennsylvania study of laboratory animals dramatically illustrates the dilemma. Obese rats on a starvation diet needed only 21 days to lose the excess weight. It was a different story during the second phase of the experiment. After the animals regained the weight, it took more than twice as long for them to lose the same amount of weight while on the same starvation diet.

The effects on chronic human dieters can be even more severe. "I've seen people gain 5, 10 or even 15 pounds within 24 to 48 hours after going off a very low calorie diet," says Dr. Callaway.

Little wonder that starvation dieting has been linked to binge eating as well as anxiety and other stress-realted psychological problems.

"Sometimes I feel like the body's rebellion against dieting is just the natural consequence of trying to fight the forces of nature. The dieter tries desperately to keep the lid on, but the pressure to eat builds and then, when the lid blows off, and you gorge, you end up weighing more than you did in the first place," says Dr. Herman.

EATING THROUGH THE AGES

It's probably just another of life's little surprises. But by the time you're ready to retire, move to Orlando and finally take advantage of some of those early-bird dinner specials, something has happened to your body: It actually needs less food.

Chalk it up to age—and inactivity. As you exercise less, your muscle mass shrinks, causing your metabolism to slow. Doctors believe that after age 30, metabolism slows at a rate of 5 percent every ten years, cutting your need for calories still further.

"If your muscle mass has decreased over the years, you're just going to need less food," says Susan Kayman, R.D., of the Kaiser Permanente Medical Group in Oakland, California.

In fact, while the average adult male needs 2,700 calories a day and the average adult female needs 2,000 calories a day, a man over the age of 50 needs just 2,400 calories a day. And a woman over the age of 50 needs just 1,800.

PLAN PERMANENT CHANGES

By now you should be getting the message: When it comes to weight loss, never, ever, say diet. "Weight management is not a one-shot attempt to lose weight. It is a lifelong adoption of healthy eating and physical activity habits," says John P. Foreyt, Ph.D., director of the Nutrition Research Clinic in the Department of Medicine at the Baylor College of Medicine in Houston.

Both factors are important—in fact, moderate exercise will give your weight-loss efforts a significant boost. But we're going to focus here on nutritionally sound eating recommendations and food-related behavioral tips that doctors say can help you lose at the safest and most sustainable rate—at least

But here's the problem: While you need *fewer calories* than you did when you were younger, you still need all the essential nutrients—protein, vitamins and minerals.

So to avoid gaining weight yet make sure you're getting all of the nutrients you need, you actually have to make smarter food selections, says Kim Galeaz-Gioe, R.D., a spokesperson for the American Dietetic Association.

"There's just no room for junk food in your diet," says Galeaz-Gioe. "If you choose junk food, you're getting the calories you need—and more—but none of the nutrients."

One of the best ways to fulfill your vitamin and mineral quota is by eating more fruits and vegetables. "They're loaded with vitamins and minerals but are low in calories," she says.

You can also beat nature's clock by muscling up your metabolism with moderate exercise. Not only does exercise burn calories, some forms—like weight training—build muscle mass, a key calorie consumer.

½ to 1 pound a week. An eating plan that's 55 to 60 percent complex carbohydrates, 25 percent fat and 15 percent protein is generally recommended for weight loss.

But before we show you how to arrange your dinner plate down to the last lima bean, consider the encouraging results of a University of California study of 30 women who were able to lose weight and keep it off for at least two years without starvation diets or gimmicks.

A few of the women credited their success to learning a package of strategies through a special program. But most simply said they made a decision to lose weight and then devised their own realistic weight-loss plans—based on sound nutritional principles—to fit their lives, according to Susan

MIND OVER MUNCHING

Engage your brain before you put your mouth in gear. This grade school maxim was usually directed toward kids who answered without thinking. But it's also good advice for people who are trying to lose weight. The right mental preparation and behavior can play a key role in your weight-loss efforts long before you put a fork to your mouth, say doctors.

"In many ways, awareness and control over your eating behavior can increase your options, improve how you deal with food situations and keep you from being a victim of old behaviors," says F. Matthew Kramer, Ph.D., research psychologist with the U.S. Army's Research, Development and Engineering Center in Natick, Massachusetts.

What follows are some behavioral techniques developed by Dr. Kramer and Kelly D. Brownell, Ph.D., professor of psychology at Yale University.

Get ready. Before you start your weight-loss program, you should feel ready to do it and aware of why you want to do it, Dr. Brownell says.

Kayman, R.D., coauthor of the study and senior consultant for Kaiser Permanente Medical Group in Oakland, California.

Needless to say, the plans they implemented didn't include grapefruit-topped pizza—or any other wacky weight-loss scheme. In fact, they all used several practical techniques found in this chapter, including getting regular exercise, cutting fat and eating more fruits and vegetables. The successfully trim also reported being patient, setting small goals they could meet and sticking to their personally devised weight-loss plans.

"If you're eating turkey breast instead of salami, using less

Never say never. Don't swear off pizza or other tempting favorites for good. "It's important not to set absolutes—it's not very realistic," says Dr. Brownell.

Tuck away treats. You can reduce temptation by storing food out of sight. Reducing food handling and preparation can keep you from excess sampling.

Dine only where (and when) designated. Eating should be limited to specific times and places each day. Not reading or watching television while eating may also help you eat less.

Give yourself a hand. Treat yourself to a movie or a new outfit as a reward for sticking to your program.

Enlist an ally. Several studies have shown that active support by your spouse can help you stay on your new low-fat eating plan.

Ditch your self-doubt. Having a bad eating day—downing a bag of potato chips at lunch, for example—doesn't doom your program to failure. Simply resolve to lay off the fat for the duration and do better tomorrow. "It's important to keep slips in perspective," says Dr. Brownell."One slip doesn't ruin the whole program."

oil when you cook, using low-fat dairy products, we're not talking about dieting any more. We're talking about a sensible, easy way of eating that's going to pay off in weight loss," says Kayman.

WRITE YOUR WEIGHT DOWN

Before you can start eating smart, you have to figure out where you're going wrong. The best way, doctors say: Keeping a detailed food dairy.

A daily log that records what, when and where you eat as

well as the circumstances is probably the best approach, says Barbara Scott, assistant professor of the Nutrition Education and Research Program at the University of Nevada School of Medicine.

After a week of faithfully recording everything you eat, take a good look at the results. See lots of chocolate bars, cookies, croissants and other high-fat goodies—accompanied by weight gain? Target the junk for dietary termination—or at least start looking for low-fat alternatives, says Scott.

GO ON A FAT ATTACK

Lots of food favorites over the past half-century have been falsely branded as weight-gain villains—bread, potatoes and pasta—to name a few. But doctors now agree at least one truly guilty party belongs on your most unwanted eating list: fat.

And even the slickest team of Washington lawyers couldn't beat this case: Several studies conducted by the nation's top dietary sleuths show eating less fat can drop pounds effortlessly—without eating less food!

"If you're eating a high-fat diet and you cut the amount of fat you're eating, you'll lose weight. It's as simple as that," says Alan Kristal, Dr. Ph., a researcher at the Fred Hutchinson Cancer Research Center in Seattle.

For proof, consider the results of Dr. Kristal's groundbreaking study on the *unintended* effects of a low-fat diet. Half the 300 women in the study maintained their regular diets, which averaged 39 percent of calories from fat. The rest were shown how to slash their dietary fat to 21 percent of calories by creating low- and nonfat versions of high-fat favorites, using less fat for cooking and eating more fish, chicken, fruits and vegetables.

Even though the study was designed simply to determine whether eating a diet so low in fat was realistic, something remarkable happened. The lean food eaters quickly began losing weight—even though they were filling their fat void by actually eating more complex carbohydrates and protein! In fact, for every percentage point of fat the women cut from their diet, $\frac{1}{4}$ to $\frac{1}{2}$ pound of flab dropped off their bodies during the six-month study. And an impressive number of the women kept the weight off: Two years later, 50 percent of the participants were still lean.

The reason that cutting fat works for weight loss: A single gram of fat is equal to nine calories, while a gram of protein or complex carbohydrates is equal to just four calories. In short, eating less fat means eating fewer calories. What's more, dietary fat is quickly stored in the body as fat, while carbohydrates are more readily burned as fuel, says Dr. Kristal. Call it the one-two punch for taking off pounds: "You have two things going for you—not only do you take in fewer calories, but the calories that are going in are more readily used by the body," he says.

So how much fat should you drop from your plate? The average American gets about 37 percent of calories from fat. But folks who still eat bacon and eggs for breakfast and meat for lunch and dinner are getting closer to 40 to 45 percent of calories from fat, according to David Levitsky, Ph.D., professor of nutrition and psychology at Cornell University in Ithaca, New York.

As a result, one of the most successful weight-loss methods is simply eating no more than 25 percent of calories from fat. Based on a daily calorie intake of 2,700, that means most men need no more than 75 grams of fat a day. For every 200 calories above or below 2,700, add or subtract 5 to 6 grams of fat.

If you're a woman eating an average of 2,000 calories a day, that's a goal of just 56 grams of fat for the entire day. Bad news for fast-food fans: You'd blow the day's fat budget with a burger and fries.

The good news, says Dr. Levitsky: "Learn where the fat is, make low-fat selections instead, and you're going to lose weight automatically."

THE BATTLE OF THE BULGE:
MEN VERSUS WOMEN

He occasionally has a beer with his burger and still manages to drop his paunch. She counts every calorie—but the bathroom scale refuses to budge. Don't give him a gold star or hold her accountable—weight loss often occurs at a different rate for men and women.

Although doctors aren't exactly sure what causes this documented discrepancy, several solid theories have emerged. Perhaps the best is that women just naturally store more fat than men, a phenomenon linked to the woman's unique role as child bearer, according to Rose Frisch, Ph.D., associate professor of population sciences at the Harvard University School of Public Health in Boston.

The average man's body is 12 percent fat, while the average woman's is 26 percent fat, she says. Where does the extra fat come from? During adolescence, young women generally experience a whopping 120 percent gain in body fat, while boys' gains are nearly all muscle—a significant calorie burner.

"There's a metabolic cost to reproduction," says Dr. Frisch. "A woman's body apparently tries to build up and keep fat at a certain level to cover the cost of a potential pregnancy." It's easy to see why this fat savings plan is so ambitious: During pregnancy, a woman generally needs 50,000 calories above her own body's needs to keep the baby inside her healthy.

In fact, the need for fat is so great that a woman's reproductive system will actually shut down if she drops below 15 percent of her natural body weight, Dr. Frisch says.

Still, women can safely *and* successfully lose weight if they eat a low-fat diet, says Dr. Frisch. "That seems to be the best approach," she says.

To help make those low-fat choices, try these tips, suggested by obesity experts.

Become a fat detective. No entrée should contain more than 10 grams of fat, no snack or side dish more than 5 grams per serving. Using this approach, a plate of spaghetti with cheese (9 grams) gets a thumbs-up, while half a batter-dipped chicken breast with skin (18 grams) gets a thumbs-down. For a lean snack, choose a cup of low-fat fruit yogurt (2 grams) over a small slice of apple pie (18 grams).

Live and learn. Buy a new low-fat cookbook and learn ten alternative low-fat recipes that you'll enjoy cooking and eating.

Banish boring bites. Low-fat food doesn't have to be flavorless. Spice up good-for-you fare with herbs like basil, oregano, thyme and marjoram. Swirl chili peppers, dill or coriander into cottage cheese or sprinkle nutmeg or cinnamon on fruit plates.

Say adios to oil. Fat-free broth, fruit or vegetable juice also works fine for cooking meats or sautéing vegetables.

Make lemons your aide. Substitute lemon juice for butter or margarine on vegetables.

Say "yo" to yogurt. Drop fattening sour cream and top potatoes and vegetables with nonfat yogurt.

Make a deal. Trade in high-fat dairy, like 2 percent milk, for an alternative—like skim.

CALL IN THE CAVALRY: COMPLEX CARBOHYDRATES

Now that fat has been relegated to a low profile in your dietary picture, you'll need a replacement. But don't settle for expensive pre-made shakes or diet bars. Call in the cavalry: complex carbohydrates.

Found in such foods as pasta, potatoes and bread, complex carbohydrates can play a significant role in your weight-loss plan by rescuing your faltering willpower.

PLANNING YOUR SNACK ATTACKS

If you're a nibbler at heart, keeping your hand out of the cookie jar may be setting you up for a Cookie Monster-size snack attack . . . unless you satisfy yourself with healthy alternatives.

Rather than fighting cravings with refusenik diets, Herman M. Frankel, M.D., of the Portland Health Institute in Oregon says he encourages his patients to eat as many as six small meals throughout the day. The caveat: All meals must be low in fat.

"A lot of our patients find they get hungry if they go more than four hours without food," he says. "We say 'Go ahead and eat as much as you want just as long as the items are low in fat.' "

Dr. Frankel says his recommendation is based on studies that show people who cut out the fat—yet eat far more complex carbohydrates than ever—can still lose weight.

If you like the sound of Dr. Frankel's approach, but you don't trust yourself with unlimited calories, here's a sample menu for a 1,500-calorie, low-fat, six-meals-a-day eating

Once digested, complex carbohydrates are turned into a substance called glycogen that is used by the muscles, brain, liver and kidneys for fuel.

Let those glycogen reserves run low by not eating enough carbohydrates, and the results are predictable: You'll feel grumpy, headachy, restless and perhaps worst of all, downright ravenous. And that can have devastating consequences on your weight-loss efforts, says Dr. Frankel.

"You won't push the cheese and the eggs out of the way in the refrigerator on your way to the cold rice or cold macaroni," says Dr. Frankel. "You'll *eat* the cheese and the eggs."

plan. You can also create new combinations by trying any of the many fat-free foods now available in supermarkets.

Breakfast: Bran-type cereal, 1 serving with skim milk (150 calories, 1 gram fat); half a grapefruit (40 calories, 0 grams fat); 8 ounces tomato juice (40 calories, 0 grams fat); white or whole-wheat toast with 1 teaspoon all-fruit spread (80 calories, 1 gram fat)

Mid-morning snack: Banana (105 calories, 0 grams fat); 7 vanilla wafers (130 calories, 4 grams fat)

Lunch: Tuna pita pocket sandwich with lettuce and tomato slices (215 to 230 calories, 1 gram fat); two gingersnaps (60 calories, 1 gram fat)

Mid-afternoon snack: 2 fig bars (110 calories, 2 grams fat)

Dinner: Half a chicken breast, baked or broiled (140 calories, 3 grams fat); plain baked potato (145 calories, 0 grams fat); 1 cup red cabbage with apple slices (60 calories, 0 grams fat); medium salad with 2 tablespoons oil-free dressing (37 calories, 0.5 gram fat)

Evening snack: 3 cups air-popped popcorn (90 calories, 0 grams fat)

To beat the low-carb, gotta-eat blues:

Take six. Eating six daily servings of complex carbohydrates like beans, cooked whole grains, breads and pasta will keep your glycogen levels—and dietary resolve—high.

Sneak a high-carb snack. Dr. Frankel says his patients are able to lose more weight when they snack on complex carbohydrates like a bagel or banana between meals, rather than starving until lunch or dinner—and then overeating.

Play nutritional scientist. The best way to determine whether you'll benefit from eating complex carbohydrates between meals is by experimenting, Dr. Frankel says. "You might discover that you're not starving just an hour after dinner anymore," he says.

FILL UP WITH FIBER

Boosting your complex carbohydrate consumption adds another benefit to your weight-loss routine: higher fiber.

Your mouth gets satisfaction from high-fiber foods because of the chomping needed to break them down, says George L. Blackburn, M.D., Ph.D., associate professor of surgery at Harvard Medical School and chief of the Nutrition/Metabolism Laboratory at the Cancer Research Institute of New England Deaconess Hospital in Boston. Another bonus is that your stomach takes longer and needs more gastric juices to break down fiber, giving your tummy a full feeling, says Dr. Frankel.

What's the best way to fiber up?

Get your daily dose. Don't bother measuring fiber by the gram or sprinkling it on your lunch with a teaspoon. By eating the recommended six servings of whole grains, three to five servings of vegetables and two to four servings of fruit, you'll be ahead of the game, says Dr. Frankel.

And after eating all that fiber, you simply won't be as hungry for fattening foods, says Dr. Frankel.

Backing up that theory is a study from the Veterans Administration Medical Center in Minneapolis that suggests eating high-fiber foods in the morning may help you reduce how much food you eat the rest of the day.

Fourteen volunteers were given their choice of cereals for breakfast—from high to low fiber. About 3½ hours later, the volunteers were invited to a high-fat buffet with burgers, peanut butter, corn chips and other foods.

The result: Those who ate the highest-fiber cereal put the smallest dent in the delectables, devouring about 45 fewer calories, say researchers.

Fine-tune your fiber feast. Once you're getting enough servings of fiber, increase portion size and focus on the highest-fiber foods, especially legumes (beans and peas) and other fiber-rich fruits like apples, prunes, raspberries and pears.

TIME YOUR MEALS

When you eat can also have some bearing on the size of your bottom line. Breakfast skippers take heed; you may be reducing your metabolic rate 25 percent by not eating a morning meal, says Dr. Callaway.

Again, think of your body's metabolism as a fire, but one that dies down while you sleep. Waking up, moving around and eating breakfast stokes the fire, enhancing your body's calorie consumption.

Dr. Blackburn agrees: "Breakfast serves as a metabolic kicker. The body needs fluids and a range of nutrients in the morning to get started. And breakfast will ward off the afternoon munchies."

To keep your metabolism ticking like a Rolex:

Eat a good breakfast. In addition to mangling your metabolism, skipping breakfast may actually sabotage your eating plan for the rest of the day. Without breakfast, you're more likely to succumb to a midmorning sugar fix—like a doughnut or a candy bar, doctors say. And the sugar can make you hungrier at lunch, weakening your willpower and increasing the chances you'll order a high-fat meal.

Never dine after nine. Eating a big meal after 9:00 P.M. can also set you up for dietary disaster: Not only will your body more readily store the calories as fat, but you'll be too full to eat breakfast, resuming the fattening cycle.

In fact, some doctors suggest making breakfast the largest meal of the day and tapering the amount of food you eat as the day goes on.

WEIGHING YOUR OPTIONS:
THREE WEIGHT-LOSS PROGRAMS

Lots of people pick a weight-loss plan as if they're buying a lottery ticket: They make their selection and hope for the best.

But you don't have to gamble with your health. It is really just a matter of finding the right plan to meet your needs, doctors say.

"Our feeling is that no single diet plan works for everyone. The trend is toward specific things for different people," says John P. Foreyt, Ph.D., of Baylor College of Medicine in Houston. Among the factors to consider, says Dr. Foreyt, are how much weight you need to lose, dieting history, genetics and metabolic rate.

To help make your decision easier, *Prevention* magazine's staff investigated several of the country's top weight-loss programs and summarized them below. As always, before beginning any weight-loss regimen, consult your doctor.

Nutri/System
    Program: A prepackaged foods diet accompanied by weight-maintenance training.
    Prerequisites: None.
    Details: No counting calories, weighing portions or worrying about fat—all meals are high carbohydrate, low fat and low sodium. In most cases, just microwave and serve or add water. Three Nurti/System meals plus three snacks tally about 1,100 calories. The program is divided into two phases: weight loss and weight maintenance. Participants eat Nutri/System foods—supplemented with fresh fruits and vegetables—seven days a week. After achieving your goal weight, you go back to regular food five days and Nurti/System meals for two.

Rate of reduction: 1½ to 2 pounds a week.

Potential problems: Some participants don't like the taste of the meals.

What a participant said: (Stewart Werley, 40 pounds lost) "I felt hungry during the first week, but that was all. We had fun playing around with the meals, doctoring them up here and there."

Cost: Moderate to high priced—based on how much you lose. Nutri/System will refund half the program cost if you successfully complete the year-long maintenance program.

Location: Available nationwide at free-standing centers. Check the white pages of the telephone directory.

Overeaters Anonymous (OA)

Program: Group fellowship of men and women dedicated to recovering from compulsive overeating. No diet or food plans offered.

Prerequisites: Participants must want to stop eating compulsively; an OA survey showed that the majority of members were 50 to 100 pounds overweight when they started.

Details: This 12-step program is modeled after Alcoholics Anonymous. A recurring theme in OA literature: Compulsive overeaters are driven by forces they don't understand to eat more than they need, and they eat in ways that aren't rational. Steps include admitting you're powerless over food, turning your life over to a "higher power" to get better, making amends with people you've harmed through compulsive eating and helping other compulsive overeaters. Anonymity is retained by use of first names only.

Rate of reduction: Varies.

Potential problems: No instruction on correct nutritional choices.

What a participant said: (Earl, 300 pounds lost) "The meetings have taught me to live life on its own terms and not to take things so personally."

Cost: No fee or dues.

Location: Check the white pages in the telephone directory under "Overeaters Anonymous."

Weight Watchers

Program: Low-calorie food plan with wide range of choices. Stresses lifestyle change.

Prerequisites: For men, woman and children (ten years or older) who are five or more pounds overweight.

Details: In the full-choice plan, you get a 1,075- to 1,465-calorie-a-day food plan consisting of most common foods. During week three, new foods are added. Portion control is the key. Slogan: "Moderation, not deprivation." Daily servings are chosen from a food list with seven categories: fruits, vegetables, fats, protein, breads, milk products and diet products. You're allowed to substitute a specific amount of any item for an equivalent amount of any other food in the same group.

Rate of reduction: Generally three to five pounds the first week; one to two pounds thereafter.

Potential problems: Leaders are experts in the Weight Watchers system, not nutritionists.

What a participant said: (Kevin Connolly, 63 pounds lost) "The food plan was very simple, and I never felt hungry on it. I lost 63 pounds in 14 weeks."

Cost: Inexpensive.

Location: Nationwide and 23 foreign countries. 19,000 weekly meetings in United States. For the nearest location, check the white pages of the telephone directory.

KEEP AN EYE ON CALORIES

You've reduced your fat, added complex carbohydrates and fiber, and done it all before 9:00 P.M. But that *still* doesn't mean that you can give yourself carte blanche with calories.

Even twins burn calories at a different rate. So, short of a doctor's visit, it's nearly impossible to determine just how many calories you need to eat each day. There are, however, two methods you can use at home to give you a general idea, according to Kris Etherton, a researcher with the Nutrition Department at the University of Pennsylvania in Philadelphia and coauthor of several weight-loss studies.

Do your math. First, take your weight and multiply it by 10. If, for example, you weigh 120, that's 1,200 calories. But you're not done yet—you need to figure in your activity level. If you're sedentary, you're considered a 3; if you're moderately active, you're a 5; if you're very active, you rate a 7. Take this number, multiply it by 100, and then add it to your first calorie level. According to this formula, a sedentary 120-pounder needs to eat about 1,500 calories a day. To get a more accurate number, consult your doctor or a dietitian, says Etherton.

Step on a scale. Another way to determine whether you're eating too many calories is to weigh yourself, Ehterton says. "If you're gaining weight, then you're eating too many calories."

But whenever you are ready to lose weight permanently, take a tip from Kathy Biggerstaff: Drop the diets and stick to a sensible, low-fat, high-carbohydrate eating plan. You'll like the results.

"I don't even feel like the same person anymore," she says. "That overweight woman who hated herself is long gone."

High-Nutrition Recipes

BREAST OF CHICKEN ITALIAN

Chicken breast is a longtime favorite among weight watchers. With the skin removed, it is very low in fat. Surprisingly, pasta is also a good choice for dieters. It's virtually fat free and has lots of hunger-appeasing complex carbohydrates. This recipe was created by Houston chef Raymond Potter for the American Cancer Society.

4 boneless, skinless chicken breast halves	2 teaspoons grated Parmesan cheese
½ cup fat-free Italian dressing	8 ounces angel hair pasta
4 thick (½") tomato slices	1 cup frozen peas
¼ cup seasoned dry bread crumbs	

Combine the chicken and dressing in a 9" × 9" shallow baking dish; turn to coat the chicken on all sides. Cover and marinate at room temperature for 1 hour. (If marinating longer, refrigerate the pan.)

Bake at 400° for 10 minutes. Top each breast with a tomato slice. Sprinkle with the bread crumbs and Parmesan. Bake for 10 minutes, or until the crumbs are brown and the chicken is cooked through.

Just before serving, cook the pasta in a large pot of boiling water for 3 minutes. Add the peas and cook for another 2 minutes, or until the pasta is just tender. Drain. Serve topped with the chicken.

Serves 4
Per serving: *406 calories, 3.2 g. fat (7% of calories), 3.4 g. dietary fiber, 67 mg. cholesterol, 217 mg. sodium*

HUEVOS RANCHEROS

A good breakfast is essential for a successful weight-loss program. This Mexican casserole is a favorite breakfast of guests at the Heartland Spa in Gilman, Illinois. It would also make a delicious lunch or light dinner. Serve it with chunky salsa and nonfat sour cream or yogurt.

2	eggs or ½ cup fat-free egg substitute	⅛	teaspoon ground black pepper
8	egg whites	5	large corn tortillas
¼	cup nonfat cottage cheese	1½	ounces reduced-fat Monterey Jack cheese, shredded
¼	cup skim milk		
¼	teaspoon ground cumin	6	thin tomato slices
¼	cup snipped chives		
1	tablespoon chopped fresh coriander		

Place the egg, egg whites, cottage cheese, milk and cumin in a blender. Process for about 5 seconds to mix well. Add the chives, coriander and pepper. Blend for 5 seconds.

Wrap the tortillas in a damp paper towel and microwave on high for 25 seconds to soften.

Coat a 9" pie plate with no-stick spray. Line the pan with the tortillas, overlapping them to completely cover the bottom (allow the edges to stick up a little over the top of the pan). Sprinkle with the Monterey Jack. Gently pour in the egg mixture.

Bake at 350° for 40 minutes, or until puffed and golden brown. Remove from the oven, top with the tomato slices and let stand for 5 minutes. Slice into wedges.

Serves 4
Per serving: *211 calories, 6 g. fat (25% of caloriese), 2.5 g. dietary fiber, 113 mg. cholesterol, 295 mg. sodium*

BLACK-EYED PEA SALAD

Foods that are high in fiber and low in fat—like black-eyed peas and other legumes—are a boon to dieters. This easy salad makes a satisfying low-cal lunch.

4	cups cooked black-eyed peas	1	tablespoon minced fresh sage
2	cups finely shredded spinach or kale	3	tablespoons lemon juice
2	carrots, finely diced	4	teaspoons olive oil
½	cup minced scallions	2	teaspoons red-wine vinegar
1	tablespoon minced fresh basil	¼	teaspoon dry mustard

In a large bowl, toss together the peas, spinach or kale, carrots, scallions, basil and sage.

In a small bowl, whisk together the lemon juice, oil, vinegar and mustard. Pour over the salad. Toss to combine.

Serves 4
Per serving: *277 calories, 5.8 g. fat (18% of calories), 7 g. dietary fiber, 0 mg. cholesterol, 61 mg. sodium*

WARM FRUIT SOUFFLÉS

You don't have to forgo all desserts when watching your weight. These soufflés will satisfy a sweet tooth without adding a lot of fat or calories to your diet. Other equally delicious soufflés can be made with dried apricots, cherries or peaches.

1¼ cups water
4   ounces pitted prunes
1   teaspoon vanilla
3½ tablespoons brown
     sugar

3   egg whites, at room
     temperature

In a 2-quart saucepan, combine the water and prunes. Bring to a boil, then reduce the heat to medium-low, cover the pan and simmer for about 25 minutes, or until most of the liquid has been absorbed.

Transfer to a food processor. Add the vanilla and 2 tablespoons of the sugar. Process until pureed. Place in a large bowl and let cool to room temperature.

Place the egg whites in a medium bowl. Using an electric mixer, beat until soft peaks form. Sprinkle in 1 tablespoon of the remaining sugar and continue beating until stiff glossy peaks form.

Stir about ⅓ of the whites into the prune puree to lighten it. Then fold in the remaining whites.

Coat four 8-ounce soufflé dishes or custard cups with no-stick spray. Take the remaining ½ tablespoon of the sugar and sprinkle it in the dishes to lightly coat them.

Spoon the prune mixture into the cups and smooth the tops with a rubber spatula. Place the cups in a baking dish and add enough hot water to come about halfway up the sides of the soufflé dishes. Bake at 375° for 20 to 25 minutes, or until the soufflés are puffed and browned. Serve warm.

Serves 4
Tip: *You may make the prune puree ahead and refrigerate or freeze it until needed. Bring it to room temperature before proceeding with the recipe.*

Per serving: *129 calories, 0.1 g. fat (1% of calories), 1.9 g. dietary fiber, 0 mg. cholesterol, 48 mg. sodium*

CHAPTER 33

Vegetarianism

A Healthy Life Without Meat

At the age of 43, Pennsylvania artist Wayne Michaud became a vegetarian.

"It was the health thing, mostly," explains Michaud, whose father, grandfather and great-grandfather were all—either as restaurateurs or meat brokers—in the business of selling meat. "And it was actually unintentional.

"I'd pick up the paper, read an article about diet and heart disease, then stop eating eggs and hot dogs and start eating more chicken and fish." Then a couple of months later I'd pick up the paper, read an article about diet and cancer and I'd cut back on chicken and fish so that I could eat more whole grains and vegetables.

"Then, next thing you know, I'd hear a news report about diet and high blood pressure and I'd start to eat more fruit.

"Pretty soon," he adds with a chuckle, "I was a vegetarian almost by default. I hardly even noticed the change."

A KILL-IT-AND-COOK-IT PAST

Michaud is not alone in his evolution toward a vegetarian lifestyle. Food industry reports indicate that consumption of meat is down and consumption of fruits and vegetables is up all across the country. Sales of broccoli alone have soared 800 percent over the past two decades, reports the United Fresh Fruit and Vegetable Association. And the United States Department of Agriculture reports that meat consumption has dropped 10 percent in the last decade.

Although only 3 or 4 percent of us have actually taken a pledge of allegiance to the vegetarian flag, enough folks like living under its protection that, according to one survey, roughly 20 percent of us routinely search for vegetarian meals whenever we go out to eat. We may not define ourselves as vegetarians, but we're no longer major meatheads either. You might even say that we're in transition from our kill-it-and-cook-it past to a more thoughtful mode of eating in our future.

Igniting the movement are studies indicating that, compared with meat eaters, vegetarians are more likely to live longer and avoid such debilitating conditions as heart disease, stroke, cancer, high blood pressure, osteoporosis, gallstones, kidney stones, diverticular disease, constipation, overweight, rheumatoid arthritis, gallstones and the life-threatening complications of diabetes.

In a landmark study of more than 25,000 Seventh-Day Adventists between the ages of 30 and 84, for example, researchers at Loma Linda University in California discovered that eating meat even once a day *tripled* the risk of fatal heart disease in men between the ages of 45 and 64. Or to put it another way, vegetarians had one-third the risk of dying from heart disease of their meat-eating counterparts.

Then, in an 11-year study of 1,904 vegetarians conducted by the German Cancer Research Center in Heidelberg, scientists confirmed the cardiovascular protective effects of a vegetarian diet when their research revealed that deaths due to heart attacks or strokes were *50 percent* lower in vegetarians than in a comparable group of so-called normal eaters.

To top it all off, a subsequent study of 44 Dutch vegetarians between the ages of 65 and 97 revealed that the vegetarians had healthier hearts than meat eaters who were *ten years younger.*

WHAT KIND OF VEGETARIAN ARE YOU?

Although the basic vegetarian diet consists of fruits, vegetables, whole grains and legumes, some vegetarians include eggs or dairy products in their diets and some do not, says Suzanne Havala, R.D., of The Vegetarian Resource Group in Baltimore.

An *ovolactovegetarian,* for example, excludes meat, poultry and fish, but includes both eggs and dairy products in his diet. A *lactovegetarian* follows exactly the same diet, but won't eat eggs. And a *vegan* excludes meat, poultry, fish, eggs, milk, cheese and other dairy products.

"Only a small percentage of the vegetarians in the United States are vegans," says Havala. Most vegetarians are ovolactovegetarians.

HEALTHY DIET OR HEALTHY LIFESTYLE?

Most of those who participated in the American, German and Dutch studies had been vegetarians over a long period of time. And since vegetarians are generally considered to have a healthier lifestyle than the general population—they tend to smoke less, drink less and exercise more—the scientists really weren't sure how much of the astonishing health benefits they were seeing was due to a meatless diet and how much was due simply to the fact that vegetarians are pretty healthy people to begin with.

So to see whether or not a sudden switch to a vegetarian diet would produce the same kind of beneficial effects on people who were not only meat eaters, but meat eaters who were in pretty bad shape, a group of World Health Organization (WHO) researchers collaborated with doctors at the Medical Hospital and Research Centre in Moradabad, India. They divided a group of 406 men who had suffered heart attacks within the past 48 hours into two groups. One group received a normal hospital diet of meat, eggs, vegetables, fruits and grains for six weeks. The other received a similar diet, but with the meat and eggs replaced by fish, nuts and a vegetarian meat substitute.

The result? Even though all their other hospital care remained the same, the meat eaters subsequently had 66 percent more heart attacks and nearly 48 percent more complications than the vegetarian group over the next six weeks. There were also 43 percent more deaths among the meat eaters.

Scientists are still trying to figure out *why* a vegetarian diet appears to have such a healthy effect on the heart. Researchers involved with the WHO study in India thought that their spectacular results might have been due to the fact that the diet helped them lose weight—a 7½-pound average weight loss. They also speculated that it could be the result of a drop in their cholesterol, which averaged 20 points in the vegetarian group. (Cholesterol is only found in animal foods.) Those who continued eating meat only experienced about a 3-pound drop in weight, the researchers noted, with a 10-point drop in cholesterol.

Taking a closer look at the cholesterol levels in a group of 31 strict vegetarians in New Jersey, researchers from the American Health Foundation in New York found total cholesterol levels averaged 23 percent lower than those of so-called normal eaters. Moreover, the vegetarians' LDL (low-density lipoprotein) cholesterol—usually referred to as the bad kind of cholesterol—was 30 percent lower than that of the meat eaters, while their HDL (high-density lipoprotein) cholesterol—the "good" kind—was 8 percent higher. Triglyceride levels—an indicator of how much fat is being stored in the body and frequently also a predictor of heart disease—were 27 percent lower in the vegetarian group.

GETTING THE DROP ON FAT

When Fat and Skinny had a race around the dinner plate, as the childhood ditty goes, this is what they might have seen after a week's worth of plate-racing. It compares the totals for fat, calories, carbohydrates and fiber that two different dinners—one vegetarian, one with meat—would provide if eaten for seven consecutive nights.

Meal	Fat (g.)	Calories	Carbohydrate (g.)	Fiber (g.)
Beans, rice and broccoli	3.5	1,790	365	40
Beef, rice and broccoli	51.1	2,480	208	15

NOTE: Serving amounts per dinner equal 4 ounces black beans or lean, top round beef roast, ½ cup white rice and ½ cup broccoli.

WIDER ARTERIES IN WEEKS

Markedly lower cholesterol levels among vegetarians are pretty good evidence that something healthy is going on inside their bodies. But what exactly *is* it?

To answer that question, a group of scientists from the University of Texas Medical School at Houston, the University of California at San Francisco and the University of California at Berkeley got together to figure out a way that they could peek inside people's coronary arteries and then quantify the changes that occurred after adopting a vegetarian lifestyle.

They took 40 men and women between the ages of 35 and 70 with a combined total of 192 disease-narrowed sections in their coronary arteries, hooked them up to special x-ray machines and computers, ran thin wires through their arteries, and—like a bunch of ancient cartographers—mapped the topography of their arteries. How big were the arteries? How small were the narrowed sections? How much blood could get through to transport its precious oxygen cargo throughout the body? How big a blood clot would it take to block one of those narrowed sections and cause a heart attack?

Once they had their measurements, the scientists put about half the group on a vegetarian diet—with instructions to stop smoking, start exercising and reduce stress as well—and half remained on their usual diet.

One to 1½ years later, the team of scientists remeasured everybody's arteries. The result? The worse a person's arteries had been before adopting a vegetarian lifestyle, the more improved they were afterward. But coronary arteries in those on their usual diets continued to narrow at a rapid rate. Forty percent of the vegetarian group had literally *remolded* their coronary arteries to create better blood flow throughout the heart. Those who had adhered fairly well to their vegetarian pledge stopped arterial disease cold. Those who had adhered perfectly to the program actually widened their arteries—and narrowed their chances of having a heart attack.

VEGETABLES UP, PRESSURE DOWN

The powerful effect a vegetarian diet has on arteries may also explain why vegetarians tend to have lower blood pressures than the general population. After all, the top (systolic) number on the readout from your doctor's blood pressure gauge actually reflects the amount of force your heart has to use to pump and circulate blood. And it's only common sense that the heart will have to exert far less pressure if your arteries are open and flexible from a healthy lifestyle rather than narrowed and stiff from disease.

But how effective is a vegetarian diet in actually lowering blood pressure? A six-week study of 26 Australian men between the ages of 28 and 64 found that the top number on their blood pressure readings dropped an average of six points when they consumed a vegetarian diet. The bottom (diastolic) number—which essentially measures the amount of pressure in your blood vessels when your heart is at rest—decreased by four points.

Since a similar group of lean-meat-eating Australians had pretty much the same results, researchers are beginning to wonder if at least some of the healthy effects of a vegetarian diet owe more to the abundant presence of fruits and vegetables, rather than simply to the absence of meat.

LOWER CANCER RISK

Besides documenting the cardiovascular effects of a vegetarian diet, research supporting other health benefits continues to accumulate at a rapid pace. The German Cancer Research Center, for example, found that the incidence of cancer among vegetarian men was *half* that of meat eaters, and the incidence of cancer among women vegetarians was roughly 25 percent lower.

Further studies of Seventh-Day Adventists demonstrate that the risk of fatal lung cancer among these nonsmoking vegetarians is about *half* that of a nonsmoking but meat-eating group. And still other studies indicate that colorectal cancer is also significantly less likely to occur among vegetarians, possibly because of the way a vegetarian diet alters bile acids and digestive enzymes.

Prostate cancer and pancreatic cancer may also be less

likely to occur in vegetarians, says Paul Mills, Ph.D., an associate professor of public health and preventive medicine who studies Seventh-Day Adventists at Loma Linda University. In fact, his studies reveal that "the people with the most copious consumption of fruits and vegetables encounter the lowest risk of cancers at many sites in the body."

As far as cancer is concerned, it's apparently not just the absence of meat that makes a vegetarian diet so healthful, concludes Dr. Mills. The presence of so many fruits and vegetables seems to have a protective effect in and of itself.

In any case, scientists are beginning to get an inkling of how a vegetarian diet goes about building cancer defenses. German researchers, for example, found that the immune system's white blood cells in vegetarians are *twice* as deadly to tumor cells as those of meat eaters.

PROTECTION FOR DIABETICS?

Although most of us tend to take our kidneys for granted, the fact is that we can't live without them. They're responsible for filtering metabolic leftovers out of the bloodstream and sending them to the bladder for disposal. Allowed to hang around, these leftovers would otherwise turn our bodies into toxic waste dumps.

Unfortunately, serious kidney damage is a common, life-threatening complication of Type I, or insulin-dependent, diabetes. Doctors frequently try to at least slow onset of kidney damage by recommending a low-protein diet. But although a low-protein diet does slow other types of kidney disease, it has not been helpful when kidney damage is caused by diabetes.

Those on a vegetarian diet might fare better, however. Scientists have discovered that the kidney reacts differently to vegetable protein than it does to meat protein—so much so that a preliminary study at the Ysbyty Gwynedd Renal Unit in

THE ROAD TO VEGETARIANISM:
A DOCTOR'S JOURNEY

Thirty-nine-year-old Washington, D.C., psychiatrist and health activist Neal Barnard, M.D., was raised on pork chops and roast beef in Fargo, North Dakota, in a family that included several cattle ranchers.

He hunted ducks and geese, and even worked one summer in a fast-food restaurant serving burgers. Yet despite his hoof-heavy background, Dr. Barnard always leaned more toward vegetarian cuisine.

"From an aesthetic standpoint, my favorite food was always Mexican food," he says. "We had the world's best Mexican restaurant in Fargo. They made beans mixed with jalapeños, wrapped in tortillas and served with a wonderful sauce."

Yet despite his preferences, Dr. Barnard didn't actually become a full-time vegetarian until a part-time job gave him an insider's view of what heavy meat consumption can do to the body.

"I worked in a hospital where, as an autopsy assistant, I

Wales indicates that a vegetarian diet (which includes milk and eggs) might help to prevent kidney disease in people with diabetes.

The researchers first measured kidney function in seven men and women with diabetes who ate a conventional diet over an eight-week period. Then they switched the group to a vegetarian diet for the next eight weeks, and back to a conventional diet for a third eight-week period.

Kidney function tests conducted over the entire 24-week study revealed that the vegetarian diet apparently cut the kidney's workloads in half—thus protecting them from the in-

saw what killed people," he says. "And what I saw was lots of colon cancers, strokes and heart disease.

"Then, when I started medical school, I became more sensitive to the pain and suffering that animals experience. All these things added up," says the psychiatrist, "and I began to eat less and less meat until, finally, I didn't eat any at all. Seven or eight years later, I stopped eating dairy products and eggs, too."

How did he feel as he made the transition? "The one thing I really noticed was that my endurance was better and I didn't feel sleepy after meals. Before that, I would have lunch and later feel like nodding off. I now know the reason for that: After fatty meals, the viscosity of blood is increased and the blood doesn't circulate as well. The theory is that the brain doesn't get as much oxygen from the thicker blood," he explains.

As for his future prospects, says Dr. Barnard: "I hope to spread the message about the surprising power of vegetarian foods to as many people as possible. With the current epidemics of heart disease and cancer, we can't keep it a secret."

creased work caused by diabetes. Although further research is necessary to substantiate this effect, it may well be that a vegetarian diet will help those with renal disease caused by diabetes to live longer.

Fewer Arthritis Symptoms

Doctors have known for years that fasting seems to relieve the pain and swelling of rheumatoid arthritis, but they also have known that the minute someone with arthritis resumes a normal diet, their joints begin to ache and swell once again.

To see if they could help people with arthritis maintain the therapeutic effect of a fast, researchers from the University of Oslo and the Norwegian National Hospital in Oslo set up an experiment involving 53 people with arthritis. After documenting arthritic symptoms—pain, swelling, morning stiffness, grip strength, number of tender joints—with lab tests and physical exams, they divided participants into two groups. One group was sent for a month-long stay at a health farm, while the other was sent to a nursing home. The health farm group was told to fast, while the nursing home group was told to eat their usual diet.

The health farm group's fast—which lasted from seven to ten days—included herbal teas, garlic, vegetable broth, water in which potatoes and parsley had been cooked, various vegetable juices from carrots, beets and celery.

Once the fast was complete, the group added a new food to their diet every other day. If they developed any increase in pain, stiffness or joint swelling within 48 hours, the food was then omitted from their diet. If they had no reaction, it was added back on a permanent basis. The group was asked not to include any foods that contained meat, fish, eggs, dairy products, gluten, refined sugar, salt, strong spices, preservatives and citrus fruits.

The fast and restricted diet produced a dramatic reduction in symptoms within the first month: the number of tender joints dropped by a third, morning stiffness duration was reduced from about three hours to a little more than an hour. Grip strength was considerably increased, and pain was considerably decreased.

After keeping to this kind of an eating regime for three to five months, the health farm group was then allowed to gradually reintroduce milk, other dairy products and gluten-containing foods until their menu evolved into a well-balanced vegetarian diet. They maintained this diet until the study's conclusion, 13 months after it had started.

While the health farm group was fasting and then moving toward a vegetarian diet, the nursing home group was still eating what researchers felt was an ordinary diet. So, at the study's conclusion, the researchers were able to measure the pain, swelling, grip strength and number of joints affected in both groups and compare those numbers with the measurements taken at the beginning of their study.

The result was astounding. The arthritic symptoms of the ordinary group either stayed the same or got worse. But the arthritic symptoms of the vegetarian group, which had been dramatically reduced within the first month, stayed nearly as low as long as they were still on the vegetarian diet. And lab tests confirmed the researchers' observations.

WHY PEOPLE VEG OUT

Although health is clearly the major reason why people become vegetarians, there are a few others. "Many people feel it is against their ethical beliefs to kill an animal for food when there are other alternatives," points out Baltimore nutritionist Reed Mangels, R.D., Ph.D. Plato, Horace, Virgil, Pythagoras and—more recently—Albert Schweitzer, Albert Einstein, Leo Tolstoy and Mahatma Gandhi are a few of the people who became vegetarians because they didn't believe in killing animals.

Other vegetarians cite the huge amounts of land needed to produce meat. "An acre of grain yields five times as much protein as an acre devoted to livestock," says Rudolph Ballentine, M.D., director of the Himalayan Institute in Honesdale, Pennsylvania. An acre of beans produces ten times more. And as feeding the world becomes increasing more difficult, people are asking whether it's better to cultivate ten acres to feed perhaps 1,000 people, or to cultivate ten acres to feed a single steer—especially when the steer will only feed a half-dozen people.

Money is another reason why people choose a vegetarian diet, adds Dr. Mangels. "I had friends who wanted to take a trip out West, for example, but they didn't have enough

---

WHAT'S FOR DINNER?

Making the switch from an omnivorous to a vegetarian lifestyle can give your meal-planning imagination a good daily workout. But if racking your brain to healthfully answer the question, "What's for dinner?" sounds torturous, you may need the kind of help that's found in a basic vegetarian food guide.

The table below, which tells you how much of each food type you should eat, was adapted from a complete, practical guide developed by Ella Haddad, R.D., D.H.Sc., assistant professor in the School of Public Health at Loma Linda Univeristy in California. All servings are per day, unless otherwise noted.

Food Group	Servings
Breads, grains, cereals	6-11 (4 or more should be whole grain)
Legumes (dry beans and peas)	1-2
Nuts and seeds	102
Vegetables and fruits	5-9
Milk products	203
Eggs	2-3 *per week*
Fats or oils	3-6 (small amounts)
Sweets	Eat in moderation

NOTE: Adolescents and very active adults may require the larger number of servings from each group per day.

money. So for a year they ate a vegetarian diet and banked the difference between that and what they usually spent on groceries. By the time they were ready to travel, they had enough to take a trip to the Tetons for two weeks."

Religion is also a motivating factor for some people, says Dr. Mangels. Seventh-Day Adventists are encouraged to become vegetarians. Hindus and Buddhists are commonly vegetarians, and observant Jews will sometimes turn to vegetarianism if a kosher butcher is not available.

THE GRADUAL VEGETARIAN

Whatever motivates you to make the switch, there are a few helpful strategies that experts say can make the transition from meat eater to vegetarian an easy experience.

Take your time. Although some people feel the need to go cold turkey, most people who successfully part with meat make the transition gradually over the course of a year or so, says Dr. Ballentine.

Start with red meat. Most budding vegetarians seem to make the transition in three moves, says Dr. Ballentine, who has adapted this natural tendency into a more structured three-phase program at the Himalayan Institute. Phase one calls for gradually eliminating red meats while adding grains and legumes to your diet. Phase two calls for slowly eliminating poultry and increasing the number of cooked green vegetables that appear on your plate. And phase three means increasing fruits as you cut back on fish, eggs and dairy products—or eliminate them altogether.

Make a day of it. Some nutritionists suggest you kick the first phase into gear by scheduling a "Meatless Thursday" or "Meatless Friday." Not only is it an easy way to effortlessly slip into a new way of eating, but it also gives your digestive system a preview of what's about to come down the pipe on a regular basis.

THE MEAT OF IT ALL

Here are three ways to get the flavor and texture of meat in your diet.

Discover soy. "I'm using more and more foods that come from soy, like textured soy protein," says Nancy Rutherford, chef and owner of the vegetarian Bluegrass Spa and Resort in Stamping Ground, Kentucky. "When I use it in chili, it can look and seem so much like meat that I've had people send it back, thinking meat was mistakenly added."

Potentiate taste with tofu. "I'm also crazy about tofu because it's a high-protein food that takes on the flavor of whatever it's cooked with," Rutherford says. A plateful of spaghetti with tofu really projects the exquisite taste of the sauce.

Serve seitan. A wheat product that can be formed into loaves like meat loaf, seitan is a tried-and-true people pleaser that Rutherford uses at her spa. It gives people in transition the sensation of eating meat, and its flavor blends easily with all kinds of sauces and vegetables. It also slices well for sandwiches. Seitan is available at health food stores.

IT'S EASY IF YOU FOLLOW THE RULES

"A vegetarian diet is very easy to plan," says Suzanne Havala, R.D., a nutrition consultant and adviser for the Vegetarian Resource Group in Baltimore. "It doesn't take meticulous planning that researchers thought it once took to meet your nutritional needs. In fact, it's easier to meet the Dietary Guidelines for Americans on a vegetarian diet than it is on a typical Western diet."

There are just a few simple rules to good, nutritious vegetarian eating: Eat a variety of foods, including fruits, vegetables, whole grains and legumes. Be sure that you get an adequate number of calories per day to meet your energy needs—the average woman, for example, needs about 2,000 calories per day to maintain her weight. And keep calorie-dense, nutrient-poor foods such as sweets and snack foods to a minimum.

It was once believed that strict vegetarians could not get enough protein. "Today we know this isn't true," says Havala. "In fact, most vegetarians meet or exceed recommended protein intake levels."

Proteins from meat, fish, poultry and milk are considered complete proteins—they have all of the essential amino acids in balanced proportions. Vegetable sources of protein do not. To ensure that you get all of the amino acids, you need to eat foods that will compensate for each other's shortcomings. Sound complicated? It's not. Basically, all you need to remember is that the proteins in whole grains, vegetables and legumes complement each other. You're sure to come up short if all you eat is pasta, pasta and more pasta. But, if during the course of a day or two you eat a variety of foods and enough calories to meet your energy needs, it's almost impossible to not get enough protein, Havala says.

AVOID THE FAT TRAP

Most vegetarian diets are high in fiber and low in fat. But when the novice vegetarian begins to replace meat with other foods, he may have a tendency to substitute cheese, eggs and other high-fat foods, says Havala. Here's how to stay on a healthy course.

De-fat your casseroles. Almost any meatless casserole is easily modified into a healthier low-fat dish, says Havala. Two egg whites, or the recommended portion of a commercial egg substitute, can be used in place of one whole egg. You not only eliminate fat but cholesterol, too.

Choose your cheeses wisely. Hard cheeses like sharp Cheddar and Parmesan are generally lower in fat than soft cheeses. They're still pretty high though, so, whenever possible, use the new reduced-fat versions of some of your favorite cheeses such as Swiss and Cheddar. Nonfat yogurt can be a great alternative to cream cheese. Simply place the yogurt in a sieve lined with cheesecloth or a paper coffee filter, refrigerate and allow to drain overnight. The next day, you'll have a healthier version of cream cheese ready for spreading.

Use full-bodied seasoning. Cookbook author Mollie Katzen of Berkeley, California, used to rely on rich ingredients like sour cream to give her vegetarian cooking so much excitement. Now she leaves the sour cream in the refrigerator and reaches instead for her spice shelf. "My current favorite ingredient is garlic," Katzen says. "I'm learning to use it so that it's a really full-bodied seasoning, but not overpowering. I'm also using other herbs and seasonings very intensely."

BOOST YOUR IRON INTAKE

Since iron from vegetable sources is absorbed less efficiently than iron from meats, vegetarians—especially vegetarian women—should be sure to include enough high-iron foods like whole or enriched grains, legumes, dried fruits and vegetables such as broccoli, turnip greens, kale and collards.

Add some vitamin C. To increase the ability of your body to absorb and use iron, nutritionists say you should eat foods rich in vitamin C—citrus fruits, green peppers or onions, for example—when you consume iron-rich foods. And, skip the tea or coffee—it seems to interfere with iron absorption.

COVER YOUR VITAMIN NEEDS

Since there are no plant sources of vitamin D or vitamin B_{12}, vegetarians—particularly those who do not eat eggs or dairy products—must make a little extra effort to make sure that they get enough.

In an Israeli study, for example, researchers found that vegetarians who did not eat any animal products had half the amount of vitamin B_{12} in their bodies as their meat-eating counterparts. The vegetarians were not actually deficient in the vitamin, researchers reported, but they certainly didn't have enough in reserve in case it was needed.

Get a blood test. An inadequate amount of vitamin B_{12} circulating through your body can result in serious neurological, cerebral or psychitraic problems, doctors say. And the damage is irreversible. That's why the Israeli researchers recommend that all strict vegetarians, those who eat no animal products, periodically have a blood test to check the amount of B_{12} available to their bodies.

Take advantage of fortified foods. If you eat no fish, eggs or dairy products at all, nutritionists say that fortified foods such as fortified cereals can provide a solid source of vitamin B_{12}, as can vitamin supplements. Be sure to check the labels.

Walk in the sunshine. Exposure to sunshine can also give you a dose of vitamin D, since this nutrient is actually made right on the surface of your skin. But whether or not the dosage is adequate may depend on how far north you live and the amount of sunshine available. In a study at the University of Kuopio in Finland, for example, blood levels of vitamin D among vegetarians were adequate in the late spring and summer. In the long Finnish winter, however, they dropped below the levels needed to maintain strong bones and teeth.

Some nutritionists feel that it's difficult for vegetarians to get enough calcium if they decide not to eat cheese or drink milk. Studies have shown, however, that vegetarians absorb and retain more calcium and have a lower rate of osteoporosis than nonvegetarians, says Havala.

Add extra calcium. Fortunately, calcium is plentiful in many plant sources, so adding just a few extra servings of calcium-rich foods on a daily basis—two cups of beet greens, a cup of broccoli and three pieces of cornbread, for example—will go a long way toward keeping your bones healthy.

Zero in on zinc. Zinc levels can be marginal in a vegetarian diet since meat, poultry and seafood are the richest sources of this mineral. The problem can be complicated by the fact that fiber normally present in vegetables will grab hold of some of the zinc and prevent it from being absorbed by your body. This could be a double whammy in those who don't eat enough good sources of zinc. To counteract the effect of this, nutritionists suggest you boost your zinc intake by adding regular servings of wheat germs, whole grains and dried yeast to your diet.

High-Nutrition Recipes

SPINACH PIE

Brown rice, egg substitute and low-fat dairy products all contribute protein to this easy entrée.

1½ cups skim milk	2 cups cooked brown rice
1 cup nonfat cottage cheese	½ cup shredded reduced-fat Cheddar cheese
¾ cup fat-free egg substitute	½ cup minced sweet red peppers
2 teaspoons Dijon mustard	1 teaspoon dried dill
¼ teaspoon hot-pepper sauce	1 tablespoon grated Parmesan cheese
1 box (10 ounces) frozen chopped spinach, thawed and squeezed dry	

In a blender, process the milk, cottage cheese, egg, mustard and hot-pepper sauce until smooth. Pour into a large bowl.

Stir in the spinach, rice, Cheddar, peppers and dill.

Coat a 10" pie plate with no-stick spray. Add the rice mixture. Sprinkle with the Parmesan.

Bake at 350° for 45 to 50 minutes, or until set and golden on top. Cool for 10 minutes before serving.

Serves 4
Per serving: *258 calories, 4.4 g. fat (15% of calories), 3.6 g. dietary fiber, 12 mg. cholesterol, 406 mg. sodium*

THREE-BEAN SALAD

Adding dried beans, such as chick-peas and kidney beans, and low-fat cheese to your vegetarian salads gives them an extra dash of protein.

1   can (19 ounces) chick-peas, rinsed and drained

1   can (19 ounces) kidney beans, rinsed and drained

12   ounces wax beans, cut into 1" pieces and steamed

⅔   cup diced cucumbers

½   cup thinly sliced scallions

¼   cup minced fresh parsley

4   ounces nonfat mozzarella cheese, cubed

⅓   cup basil vinegar or white-wine vinegar

3   tablespoons olive oil

1   clove garlic, minced

1   tablespoon minced fresh basil

½   teaspoon ground black pepper

    Endive or watercress

In a large bowl, mix the chick-peas, kidney beans, wax beans, cucumbers, scallions, parsley and mozzarella.

In a small bowl, whisk together the vinegar, oil, garlic, basil and pepper. Pour over the salad and toss. Serve on a bed of endive or watercress.

Serves 4
Per serving: *249 calories, 8.8 g. fat (26% of calories), 10 g. dietary fiber, 5 mg. cholesterol, 817 mg. sodium*

BARLEY SOUP

This hearty soup will satisfy your hunger and help keep you warm on cold days. Serve it with crusty whole-grain bread.

1	large onion, diced	1	teaspoon
1	sweet red pepper, diced		Worchestershire sauce
1	clove garlic, minced	½	teaspoon dried thyme
1	teaspoon olive oil	½	teaspoon ground black
4	cups vegetable stock		pepper
1	cup quick-cooking barley		Pinch of celery seeds
1	cup thinly sliced		Pinch of ground red
	mushrooms		pepper

In a 3-quart saucepan over medium heat, sauté the onions, diced peppers and garlic in the oil for 5 minutes. Add the stock, barley, mushrooms, Worcestershire sauce, thyme, black pepepr, celery seeds and ground red pepper. Bring to a boil.

Cover and simmer for 20 minutes.

Serves 4
Per serving: *212 calories, 3.3 g. fat (13% of calories), 5 g. dietary fiber, <1 mg. cholesterol, 33 mg. sodium*

SPAGHETTI WITH TOFU SAUCE

Tofu acquires a meaty texture if you freeze it before using it in a recipe. When crumbled into a spaghetti sauce, such as this, it looks just like ground beef.

8	ounces firm tofu	1	cup tomato sauce
1	cup finely chopped	½	teaspoon dried basil
	mushrooms	½	teaspoon dried oregano
1	cup finely chopped onions	½	teaspoon dried thyme
1	clove garlic	½	teaspoon ground black
1	teaspoon olive oil		pepper
2	cups canned plum	8	ounces spaghetti
	tomatoes, drained		
	and chopped		

Rinse the tofu and place it in a freezer bag. Freeze until solid, about 4 hours, then thaw. Using several layers of paper towels, press out excess moisture. Crumble the tofu into a bowl and set aside.

In a large no-stick frying pan over medium heat, sauté the mushrooms, onions and garlic in the oil for 5 minutes. Add the tofu and sauté for 5 minutes. Stir in the tomatoes, tomato sauce, basil, oregano, thyme and pepper. Cover and simmer for 20 minutes. Remove the lid and cook for a few minutes until slightly thickened.

Meanwhile, cook the spaghetti in a large pot of boiling water for 10 minutes, or until just tender. Drain. Serve topped with the sauce.

Serves 4
Per serving: *416 calories, 10.4 g. fat (22% of calories), 3.3 g. dietary fiber, 0 mg. cholesterol, 339 mg. sodium*

CHAPTER 34

Dietary Controversies

Going to Extremes

Dietary debate probably first started when one daring caveman chased down a different type of game and brought it home. He and his family happily cooked it and ate it, although most of the other cavepeople thought he was crazy and refused to try it.

Food controversies have raged ever since.

For every new discovery or concept, there are doctors or dietitians who refuse to consider it. And for every well-founded, well-researched new program, there are haphazard, unfounded, even dangerous ones.

"Many people who promote extreme fad diets or associated programs are quacks," says Maurice E. Shils, M.D., adjunct professor in the Department of Public Health Sciences at the Bowman Gray School of Medicine of Wake Forest University in Winston-Salem, North Carolina. Unfortunately, many people—expecially those confronted with a serious disease such as cancer—are all too quick to embrace such programs.

One problem, according to Jack Zeev Yetiv, M.D., Ph.D., is

that most doctors aren't well trained in nutrition. Many physicians too quickly dismiss *any* different idea as a fad, says Dr. Yetiv, author of *Popular Nutritional Practices: A Scientific Appraisal.* It's not surprising that many patients turn to supermarket tabloids for their nutritional information.

How can you tell if a concept is a flaky, possibly dangerous fad or an innovative, effective program?

Separating fact from fantasy in the nutrition field can be tricky. "Be wary of programs that advise completely rejecting standard health and nutrition principles or programs that promise a quick, painless solution to a major health problem," says Bettye J. Nowlin, R.D., Los Angeles dietitian and a spokesperson for the American Dietetic Association.

And before you try a new program, consult your doctor— a doctor you're comfortable with and whose opinion you trust. "There has to be a relation with your physician based on mutual respect and understanding," says Dr. Shils.

Some dietary controversies burn themselves out and others smolder on, while some concepts eventually become acceptable to the medical community. Here are a variety of controversial topics and how professionals view them today.

DOUBTS ABOUT YOUR MORNING JOLT

You can't believe it's time to get up. You're groggy and wobbly and your eyelids feel glued shut. And then you smell it, wafting invitingly from the kitchen.

Coffee.

Minutes later, with half your first cup downed, you begin to feel invigorated, alert and alive, and you start to think that maybe life isn't so bad after all.

But as you're flipping through your morning paper you see a headline, "The Hazards of Coffee." What? Coffee linked to heart disease? Cancer? High cholesterol? High blood pressure? Could the stuff that makes you feel so good be this bad for you?

Maybe, say some doctors. Not a chance, say others.

What we *do* know is that the caffeine in coffee packs a potent punch, giving us energy by releasing adrenaline into the bloodstream and raising blood sugar levels. The caffeine we get from one to two cups of coffee increases alertness, reduces fatigue and speeds reaction time.

Caffeine also tends to be addictive, and cutting out your regular dose can lead to withdrawal symptoms such as headache, drowsiness, lethargy, irritability and nausea. One study at Johns Hopkins Hospital in Baltimore found that people who drink the equivalent of just one cup of coffee (or two to three cans of caffeine-containing soda) a day are addicted. All seven people in the study suffered withdrawal symptoms ranging from fatigue to severe headaches and vomiting when taken off caffeine for even *one day*.

And it's also possible that the lift you get from caffeine is "borrowing" energy rather than creating it, according to Dean Ornish, M.D., director of the Preventive Medicine Research Institute in Sausalito, California. "The increased energy level that you feel after you drink coffee will eventually fall even lower than it was when you started," says Dr. Ornish.

But what about serious diseases?

"There's never been any evidence linking moderate coffee drinking with any form of cancer or heart disease," says coffee expert Manfred Kroger, Ph.D., a food science professor at Pennsylvania State University in University Park. He considers "moderate" to be two to three cups of coffee a day. That's about 200 to 250 milligrams of caffeine. But different people can react differently. Two cups of coffee for a person who drinks coffee regularly may have no effect on cholesterol, blood sugar, metabolic rate, respiration, blood pressure and heart rate—but that same dose can raise all these things in a person who doesn't regularly drink coffee.

Although some studies have suggested links between caffeine consumption and pancreatic cancer, heart disease and fibrocystic breast disease, other studies have not substantiated those findings. The American Cancer Society considers that there has been no definite connection established with cancer.

Caffeine's link to certain diseases can be muddied by the fact that people who drink lots of coffee also tend to have *other* habits that can also affect their health, say experts. One study found that coffee drinkers tended to drink more alcohol, smoke more, exercise less and eat more saturated fat and cholesterol than people who don't drink coffee. And the people who drank the most coffee had the worst smoking and exercise habits.

Research has found that caffeine fed to rats caused birth defects and slowed fetal bone development when amounts equal

HOW MUCH CAFFEINE ARE YOU GETTING

Before you belt down that cup of steaming beverage or can of cola, check out just how much caffeine you're getting. It may be more—or less—than you think.

All coffees are not created equal: A cup of drip coffee has around 110 to 150 milligrams of caffeine, a cup of percolated coffee, 60 to 125 and a cup of instant java, 40 to 105. If your beverage of choice is tea, the amount of caffeine depends on how long you let it steep: Three minutes yields only 20 to 50 milligrams, while five minutes ups the ante to 40 to 100. A cup of cocoa weighs in at a meager 2 to 10 milligrams, while a 12-ounce can of cola has about 45. Don't assume that your orange- or citrus-flavored pop doesn't have caffeine, however: Some varieties do, so check the label.

You can also get caffeine from chocolate: about 20 to 30 milligrams in a slice of cake and 1 tp 15 milligrams in an ounce of milk chocolate. Other unexpected sources of caffeine include some headache remedies, diuretic and weight-control pills. Always read labels carefully.

to 18 cups or more of coffee a day were consumed. A study at the National Institutes of Health showed that women consuming more than 100 milligrams of caffeine (about one cup of coffee) a day were only half as likely to become pregnant in a given month as those consuming less caffeine. While caffeine's role in infertility, miscarriages and birth defects is still being debated, the Food and Drug Administration (FDA) recommends that pregnant women avoid caffeine or limit the amount they drink.

THE RAW FOODS MYSTIQUE

You probably never thought of a raw apple or carrot as *alive,* but some people believe that raw foods have living enzymes crucial to good health.

Enzymes are used in digesting food, and according to this theory, the enzymes in raw foods are superior to those produced by your body. By eating raw fruits, vegetables, nuts, grains and legumes, say the authors of *The Raw Foods Diet*— who advocate eating 60 to 75 percent of your foods raw—you supply enzymes that allow each food to digest itself. Cooked foods, on the other hand, with their "dead" enzymes, strain your body and result in breakdown. Or so the theory goes.

Nutritionists, in general, don't support the vital enzyme theory. It's true that raw foods have more *nutrients* than cooked ones, but that doesn't mean that cooked foods are somehow second-rate. And you can minimize the damage. Vegetables that are steamed, baked or stir-fried retain most of their nutrients. When foods are cooked at high temperatures, more nutrients are lost. The best strategy is to cook food as briefly as possible, keep temperatures low and use as little cooking water as possible (reusing it later in soups or gravies).

Even though raw foods may not have any magical enzymes, some studies have indicated that certain raw vegetables may help prevent health problems as diverse as cancer and cavities.

Eating lots of cruciferous vegetables such as cabbage and broccoli has been linked to lower rates of cancer of the digestive system. The protection may come from certain chemical compounds in these vegetables, but researchers at the University of Manitoba in Winnipeg think that cooking may break down these chemicals into other forms that aren't as beneficial.

And what about cavities? Raw vegetables require lots of chewing, which increases the flow of saliva in your mouth. This helps rinse away food particles. And most vegetables leave your teeth cleaner than other foods. "Raw celery and carrots give your body nutrients without leaving debris in your mouth after they're chewed," says Warren Lesmeister, D.D.S., past president of the Academy of General Dentistry.

Eating *everything* raw isn't a good idea, however. Eggs, for instance, should be thoroughly cooked to avoid the possibility of food poisoning from salmonella. This means no runny eggs or Caesar salad dressing—and even soft-boiled eggs and French toast are questionable. And don't keep batter that contains raw eggs in your refrigerator more than a week.

Have a penchant for steak tartare and sushi? "I wouldn't eat them," says Barbara Harland, R.D., Ph.D., associate professor of nutrition in the Department of Nutritional Sciences at Howard University in Washington, D.C. "I think it's too risky." Raw meat can harbor potentially harmful bacteria and parasites, and eating raw fish has caused parasite infections in some cases.

Finally, raw (unpasteurized) milk can be a source of harmful bacteria that can cause serious illness. Health professionals agree there is also no evidence that raw milk is any healthier than other kinds of milk.

Food Combining: To Mix or Match?

If you take a glance at the basic rules of food combining, you may think this system should more accurately be called "food separating." The basic idea here is that certain foods interfere with the digestion of other foods and therefore must not be eaten at the same time.

According to this theory, you shouldn't eat starches, protein, fats, sugars and acids at the same time, or drink beverages with your meals. Yes, this sort of puts the kibosh on dining out with friends and having Thanksgiving dinner with Cousin Charlie.

The reasoning is that if you eat, say, meat (protein) and potatoes (starch) together, the digestion of the meat will halt the digestion of the potato, according to Jeffrey Mannix, author of *Food Combining*. The potato will putrefy in your stomach before it passes into your intestines, according to this theory, and here's where the problem arises. "Food that putrefies in the digestive tract gives off toxins [poisons] . . . that contaminate everything in their environment while they paralyze the intestines, preventing them from eliminating waste," Mannix writes.

It's tough to find medical support for this theory. One doctor points out that food putrefying in the stomach would pretty quickly be regurgitated. And nutritionists just don't buy the theory, either.

"The body actually digests foods very efficiently, regardless of what order they're consumed in," says Nowlin. "Most health professionals look on food combining as a myth with no validity."

What *is* true, Nowlin points out, is that some vitamins in foods can change the rate of absorption of other vitamins or minerals—although this doesn't interfere with the digestion process. Foods high in vitamin C increase absorption of iron, for example, and vitamin D can increase absorption of calcium. A huge amount of fiber in the diet can interfere with absorption of some trace minerals.

For the most part, however, this all balances out. "Your best bet is a balanced, varied diet," says Nowlin.

The Pros and Cons of Irradiated Foods

Listen to a proponent of irradiated foods, and you'll think this is the greatest discovery since the wheel. An opponent, however, may convince you that this process is an accident waiting to happen.

If you use dried spices, you may already be using irradiated products. The FDA has also approved the irradiation of grain, flour, fresh fruits, vegetables, pork and poultry.

What exactly is food irradiation? It's the bombardment of food by x-rays and gamma rays, which can kill mold, bacteria and insects, inhibit germination or sprouting and extend the shelf life of fruits and vegetables. It could also reduce the need for chemical insecticides and preservatives and might reduce risks of salmonella contamination in poultry.

So what's the truth about this process? Irradiation under strictly controlled conditions does not, as many people fear, make food radioactive or leave a radioactive residue. The consensus from a 1980 meeting of the Food and Agriculture Organization, International Atomic Energy Agency and World Health Organization was that no toxicologic studies showed adverse effects of irradiation and that irradiated foods did not harm lab animals, cattle or people.

The disadvantages of irradiation? "Irradiation reduces levels of certain vitamins in certain foods," says Michael Jacobson, Ph.D., executive director of the Center for Science in the Public Interest. That's not a problem with the small amount of food now irradiated, he says, but if, as predicted, 40 percent of the food supply is eventually irradiated, it could *become* a problem.

Dr. Jacobson believes that pro- and anti-irradiation forces exaggerate both the potential benefits and problems from irradiation. "The consumer is getting caught in the cross-fire between the two camps," he says. His opinion? "We shouldn't have to build multimillion-dollar facilities with radioactive cobalt at their cores to kill bacteria or flies," he says.

THE CASE OF THE NAUGHTY NIGHTSHADES

What are nightshades? They're plants that belong to the Solanaceae family, and according to Norman F. Childers, Ph.D., they are the primary culprit in many cases of arthritis.

Nightshades include tomatoes, potatoes, eggplant, all peppers except black pepper, and tobacco. Toxins in these, according to Dr. Childers, a retired professor of horticulture, cause aching joints. By eliminating nightshades, he says, chances are better than seven out of ten that you'll improve.

The 1986 edition of Dr. Childer's book *The Nightshades and Health,* which was first published in 1977, cites page after page of case histories of people who reported significant reductions in arthritis pain from eliminating nightshades.

Subsequent studies have shown that certain foods *can* affect arthritis. A study at Albany Medical College in New York found that doses of fish oil helped arthritis sufferers, and other research suggests that some arthritis flare-ups are triggered by allergic reactions to certain foods. A study in Norway suggested that food allergy or intolerance could be at the root of rheumatoid arthritis.

Is there any connection between *nightshades* and arthritis? "There's no concrete substantiation," says Barbara Harland, R.D., Ph.D., of Howard University in Washington, D.C., although at least one physician points out that there's certainly no harm in *trying* a no-nightshade diet.

Many professionals agree that not enough research has been done to declare irradiated foods and the irradiation process perfectly safe. "If the FDA says an irradiated food is safe, I would eat it. The foods that have been tested so far are okay," says Dr. Shils. "But I'm impressed with the arguments that we just don't know enough about irradiated foods yet. We don't have sufficient information on each individual food."

You can make your own decision about purchasing irradiated foods—in most cases they will be marked with a special symbol that resembles a plant within a circle.

THE MACROBIOTIC LIFESTYLE

When you think of macrobiotics, you may think of a diet based on Asian philosophy and consisting of brown rice and tea—but it's more complicated than that.

Macrobiotics has been promoted as a cure-all for just about every disease. According to Michio Kushi, author of many books on the topic, a macrobiotic diet can treat infertility, diabetes, allergies, stress, arthritis and obesity. Macrobiotic advocate George S. Ohsawa stated in his book *Zen Macrobiotics:* "I have seen thousands of incurable diseases such as asthma, diabetes, epilepsy, leprosy and paralysis of all kinds cured by . . . macrobiotics in ten days or a few weeks." Anthony Sattilaro, M.D., asserted in his 1978 book *Recalled to Life* that a macrobiotic diet helped cure him of advanced prostate cancer.

What exactly is a macrobiotic diet? The Kushi Institute in Becket, Massachusetts, recommends eating 50 to 60 percent whole-grain cereals, 25 to 30 percent organically grown vegetables, 5 to 10 percent soup made from vegetables, seaweed, grains or beans and 5 to 10 percent cooked beans and sea vegetables. Fish, fruit, nuts and seeds are allowed occasionally, but meat, eggs, dairy products, chocolate, coffee and some other foods are not allowed. The diet varies according to age, sex, activity, special requirements or conditions, cultural background and the season.

But macrobiotics is more than what you eat. The aim, according to proponents, is to achieve balance between two basic forces of the universe, yin (expansion) and yang (contraction) as well as a balance among five basic elements: water, earth, wood, fire and metal.

Most nutritionists take a decidedly dim view of macrobiotic diets—particularly when promoted as a cure for a disease such as cancer. "No diet or combination of foods has the ability to cure cancer," says Nowlin. "What can be harmful to people is when they decide to substitute a macrobiotic diet for effective treatment." She adds that a macrobiotic diet can also cause malnutrition or weight loss, which can interfere with treatment or weaken a patient. Another problem is that macrobiotic diets tend to be high in sodium.

It can also be difficult to obtain adequate nutrients on a macrobiotic diet, which is stricter than most vegetarian diets. One study concluded that some children following a macrobiotic diet were deficient in some nutrients and experienced slowed growth. Other work turned up severe malnourishment in macrobiotic children.

Dr. Shils advises caution if you decide to try a macrobiotic diet: "Definitely consult with a doctor or nutritionist to review your diet."

How Much Aluminum Is Okay?

No one debates that aluminum buildups are found in the brains of Alzheimer's patients—what is argued is whether the aluminum is a *cause* or an *effect* of the disease. Many researchers, however, now believe there is enough evidence to point to aluminum as a significant factor in the development of Alzheimer's.

Studies in areas with high levels of aluminum in the water supply, for instance, have shown high levels of Alzheimer's or diseases similar to Alzheimer's. Theodore Kruck, Ph.D., member of a leading team of aluminum-investigating scientists at the University of Toronto in Ontario, says nine drinking water surveys in various countries have shown higher rates of Alzheimer's in people who drank water with high aluminum levels.

Where else do you get aluminum? From foods that naturally take up aluminum from the soil, from acidic foods cooked in aluminum cookware and from many products such as cosmetics, antiperspirants, antacids, certain pickles and commercially baked foods like doughnuts, muffins, cookies and pound cakes. In healthy people, most of the aluminum is excreted: Most of us consume 10 to 15 milligrams a day but have only 30 to 45 milligrams in our bodies.

Although there is no evidence proving definitely that the aluminum we ingest causes Alzheimer's—and some doctors scoff at the very idea—most agree it doesn't hurt to play it safe. Dr. Kruck and other researchers at the University of Toronto believe people should try to limit their intake of aluminum to less than 10 milligrams a day, as a first step, while the final goal should be 3 milligrams or less.

How do you cut your intake? Several participants in a Royal Society of Medicine discussion panel held in London said they avoid using aluminum cookware, drink bottled water and avoid aluminum-containing aerosols.

You can reduce the amount of aluminum in your diet by never cooking acidic foods such as tomatoes, cabbage, sauerkraut, cranberry sauce, applesauce or rhubarb in aluminum pots and pans. Dr. Kruck also suggests avoiding using aluminum foil under meats when grilling.

Other products with aluminum include some baking powders (check the label), soft drinks (if made from water with high aluminum levels), certain beauty and grooming products and antiperspirants. You can select nonaluminum forms of most of these products, however.

THE YEAST BEAST

It's a common little microorganism, *Candida albicans,* that quite commonly resides happily in our bodies along with bac-

DOES MILK PRODUCE MUCUS?

"Don't drink that milk—it'll make your nose more stopped-up," a father tells his child, clogged up with a bad cold.

Well, Father knows best. Or does he?

The milk-produces-mucus theory has been around for a long time, and some people swear by it. Most experts, however, discount it completely.

"It's a myth," says Bettye J. Nowlin, R.D., of the American Dietetic Association. "There's no connection."

In one study exploring this fabled cause and effect, 60 volunteers—who drank amounts ranging from none to 11 glasses of milk a day—were infected with a cold virus and records kept of their nasal secretions. Those who *believed* that milk produced mucus reported that they coughed and were more congested when they drank milk, but they actually produced no more mucus than others. In fact, no association between milk and mucus production was found.

Another study, however, suggests that fat in milk *can* interfere with airflow, at least in people with asthma. Airflow in healthy people wasn't affected by either whole milk or skim milk. In the asthmatic group, however, airflow decreased after drinking whole milk but *not* after water or skim milk.

The conclusion? If you aren't asthmatic, milk should present no problem. Because the fat in whole milk may make your mouth feel gummy when you have a cold, however (and also because low-fat milk is wiser from a nutritional standpoint), give the whole milk a miss. Dietitians recommend not cutting out milk but switching to low-fat or skim milk, Nowlin says.

teria and other microorganisms. But when things get out of whack, many of the other "bugs" can get killed off and allow the yeast population to explode.

The out-of-control yeast population, according to one theory, releases toxins that circulate in your body and weaken your immune system—and that can make you vulnerable to a variety of health problems, including fatigue, depression, joint pain, digestive problems, hypoglycemia and hyperactivity.

That's the theory that William G. Crook, M.D., has promoted in his many books, including *The Yeast Connection* and *Solving the Puzzle of Your Hard-to-Raise Child.*

If a physical exam shows no other cause for your symptoms, your problems may be yeast-caused, suggests Dr. Crook. To keep the monster at bay, he prescribes a sugar-free, yeast-free diet that excludes foods that contain yeast or molds, including cheeses, fermented liquors, coffee, tea, melons and many condiments and sauces.

Many health professionals will tell you, however, that most of us seldom have to worry about yeast. Yeast infections are liable to occur only when your immune system is weakened or when you've been taking antibiotics that "knock out" the good germs holding *Candida albicans* in check.

Is the yeast connection overblown? Most doctors say yes, a few doctors say no. Dr. Shils is one of many physicians who don't buy the yeast theory. "I've talked to my colleagues about this," he says. "I don't know of anyone who takes it seriously. The evidence is against this being a hazard for the average, relatively healthy person. Yeast infections can be serious, though, for those people whose immune system is seriously compromised."

Many dietitians tend to think the problem is less prevalent than the popularity of Dr. Crook's books would imply. "The physicians or books that advise you to stay away from all yeasts are doing you a disservice," says Dr. Harland. "Yeasts are a valuable part of our food supply."

CALMING HYPERATIVE KIDS

The late Ben Feingold, M.D., a California allergist and pediatrician, probably didn't realize what a storm he was provoking in his 1974 book *Why Your Child Is Hyperactive* when he promoted a diet free of artificial colors and flavorings to help calm overly wound-up kids.

Some doctors and researchers say the diet is completely unsubstantiated, others support it, and some prescribe it for their patients. Thousands of parents swear by it.

Who's right?

Much of the support for the Feingold diet has come from doctors who have seen children in their practice respond favorably. But early studies didn't meet strict scientific standards—because of the nature of the diet, it's difficult to carry out a study in which children and parents don't know what foods they're getting. And most double-blind, placebo-controlled studies (where no one knows which type of food they're getting) did not show significant results from the diet. But even in most of the double-blind studies, 10 to 15 percent of the hyperactive children studied *did* benefit from the diet, notes Dr. Yetiv.

And some studies have shown significant results from the diet. One ten-week study in Calgary, Alberta, found that more than half of 24 hyperactive preschool boys showed improvement on a diet free of artificial colors as well as chocolate, preservatives and caffeine.

Jane Hersey, executive director of the Feingold Association in Alexandria, Virginia, and doctors who support the program believe it's a mistake to focus exclusively on studies, which may have little in common with the practical application of Feingold's program. Hersey says she doesn't see why the diet spawns such controversy.

"Certain chemicals in food appear to have the capacity to cause certain reactions in some people," she says. "And what can it hurt to try the diet?"

The Feingold diet is basically an elimination diet: You avoid foods with synthetic dyes and flavorings and certain antioxidants used as preservatives. When you first start the program, you also remove foods naturally high in salicylate, an aspirin-like substance that is found in many fruits, coffee, tea and a few vegetables. Later, the salicylate-containing foods are reintroduced one at a time.

Hersey admits she wasn't eager at first to try the diet on her five-year-old daughter. "I was a convenience-food freak," she says. "It seemed like too much trouble." After a few days on the diet, however, her daughter's behavior improved drastically and her husband's migraine headaches disappeared.

Now she doesn't think of it as much trouble. "When you re-

CAN SUGAR TURN LITTLE ANGELS INTO LITTLE MONSTERS?

"Johnny goes crazy after he's had sugar," the hapless mom says, watching her six-year-old career around the room.

Despite such observations, many researchers view claims that link sugar intake and behavior problems as having no basis in fact, and a 1987 Food and Drug Administration task force concluded that sugar was not addictive and couldn't be linked to criminal behavior (what a relief for Johnny's mom!)

In a study at Yale University School of Medicine, however, the adrenaline levels of 14 children and 9 adults were monitored after they were fed sugar. The pediatricians directing the study found that the adrenaline levels of the children increased dramatically, while those of the adults did not move. All but one of the children also complained they felt "shaky and weak" after ingesting the sugar.

This suggests, says one of the researchers, that children are more sensitive to sugar than adults, and that the adrenaline surge from sugar *could* affect behavior in some children.

alize that a package of commercial gelatin dessert has synthesized dyes made from petroleum, several kinds of acid, no juice
and 82 percent sugar, it's not a question of, 'Gee, why do I have
to give this up?' but 'Why would I *want* to eat it?' " she says.

Dr. Yetiv concludes that hyperactivity may have many
causes, and some hyperactive children do seem to be sensitive
to the substances eliminated by the Feingold diet.

DO WE NEED TO EAT AT ALL?

For most of us, the idea of fasting doesn't have much appeal: We get grumpy, headachy and listless after one skipped
breakfast or worked-through lunch.

Many people, however, devoutly believe that going without food for an extended period can cleanse your system,
clear your mind and even cure some diseases. Morton Walker,
D.P.M., author of *The Healing Powers of Elderberry Internal
Cleansing,* advocates a seven-day "detoxification" program
that involves drinking only a concentrate of elderberry and
honey. Dr. Walker claims that this fast cleans mucus from
your system, helps you stay younger, cures constipation,
forces wastes out of your body, removes unnecessary fat and
helps you lose weight.

Allan Cott, M.D., author of *Fasting: The Ultimate Diet,*
promotes fasting to lose weight, feel better, look younger,
lower blood pressure and cholesterol and relieve tension. He
recommends an occasional fast of a day or two but claims that
fasts of up to a month will benefit specific health problems.

Most medical experts, however, doubt that, with the exception of weight loss, fasting can accomplish what its advocates say. But it could have harmful effects. Long-term
interruption of needed nutrients is one obvious problem, but
it's possible that even a relatively short fast could have negative effects. A study by the National Institutes of Health reported increased risks of gallstone disease among women
who fasted longer than 14 hours between the last meal at night
and the first one the following day.

One condition that fasting *does* seem to benefit is arthritis, although the effect is only short term. A study of 27 patients in Norway found fasting, followed by a vegetarian diet, to be an effective treatment for rheumatoid arthritis. A Swedish study also involving a seven- to ten-day fast found that improvement occurred by the fourth or fifth day of fasting. The effect ended as soon as the fast was over, however, and according to Lars Skoldstam, M.D., author of the study, there is no reason for doctors to recommend fasting to persons with rheumatoid arthritis.

The bottom line? If you just need a change of pace or have no appetite for some reason, a "modified fast"—cutting your food intake in half—is okay for three to five days, according to George L. Blackburn, M.D., Ph.D., associate professor of surgery at Harvard Medical School and chief of the Nutrition/Metabolism Laboratory with the Cancer Research Institute at New England Deaconess Hospital in Boston. Be sure, however, to drink plenty of fluids.

FOOD ALLERGY: AN OVERRATED PROBLEM?

Food allergies *exist*—what's controversial about them is how many people actually do have allergies and how effective some testing systems are.

The Asthma and Allergy Foundation estimates that less than 1 percent of the population is allergic to food, while the U.S. Department of Agriculture says 10 to 15 percent—but you can find figures in the media as high as 60 percent.

What's going on here?

The concept that food allergies can cause certain problems such as fatigue and depression was seized on by the media, according to Dr. Yetiv, despite little scientific documentation. Only a small percentage of suspected food allergies can actually be confirmed, he says.

A number of studies have shown that some people only *think* they're allergic. In one study of 23 patients, persons whose allergies could not be scientifically documented reported symptoms from "nonallergic" foods as often as they did from the foods they were supposedly allergic to. In another case, a woman who thought she was allergic to milk was fed milk and a nonmilk substance via a tube to her stomach. When she was told she was receiving milk (although she wasn't), she experienced abdominal contractions, a rapid heart rate and a drop in blood pressure. When she was told she was receiving the nonmilk placebo (actually milk), she showed no symptoms.

A problem that impedes accurate diagnosis of allergies is possibly faulty diagnostic techniques. Cytotoxic testing, in which white blood cells that have been incubated with the suspected allergen are studied for signs of disintegration, is considered useless by the FDA and many professionals. Even when the suspected allergen is introduced in a water solution through a skin puncture, only a *negative* test (showing no reaction) is considered reliable, according to Raymond Slavin, M.D., of St. Louis University School of Medicine. A positive test—showing redness and swelling—doesn't always prove that you're allergic.

Food allergy is also not the same as food *intolerance,* such as when a person cannot digest milk. A true food allergy results from a reaction within your immune system, just as ragweed or cat dander triggers reactions in persons allergic to them.

In people who *are* allergic to food, symptoms range from annoying to life threatening. What are people most commonly allergic to? Eggs, wheat, peanuts, fish, milk and soybeans account for more than 90 percent of food allergies in children. Common problem foods for adults are shellfish, fish, peanuts and other nuts, and eggs. Chocolate and strawberries, contrary to popular belief, are not common allergens. If you suspect an allergy, check with your physician, or try eliminating the suspect food on your own.

PART 6

IMPROVING YOUR EATING STYLE

CHAPTER 35

Quiz Time

Does Your Diet Measure Up?

You can't put together a healthy nutrition plan without taking a close look at your diet and the foods you actually put into your mouth every day. Just how much fiber are you really getting? Have you trimmed the fat from your diet as much as you think you have? Is your sodium intake under control?

The self-tests in this chapter put your diet under the microscope and examine every detail so you can identify your nutritional strengths as well as the weak spots that need improvement.

"Dietary self-tests can be entertaining but at the same time incredibly revealing," says Rebecca S. Reeves, R.D., chief dietitian with the Nutrition Research Clinic at Baylor College of Medicine in Houston. "These tests are like a mirror. They help reflect back to you that you are what you eat—in terms of your health, at least. If a quiz reveals that you're eating lots of salty, fatty food, for example, chances are your waistline and blood pressure are going to reflect this."

Self-tests, of course, can't track your diet nearly as precisely as a professionally supervised analysis. And they don't take the place of blood tests, physical exams and a de-

'

tailed health and genetic history. So don't hesitate to consult your doctor or a professional dietitian/nutritionist, especially if you have a health problem, are on a restricted diet or uncover some dietary trouble spots when you take these tests.

So now, if you're ready to fine-tune your diet, grab a notebook, sharpen your pencil and go to it. Your answers could yield important clues that will point you to the right nutritional track for a healthier life.

DIAGNOSE YOUR DIET

The following 32 questions adapted from a test developed by nutritionists at the Center for Science in the Public Interest in Washington, D.C., will give you an overall idea of how well you're eating. The (+) or (–) numbers after each set of answers instantly pat you on the back for good habits or alert you to problems you may not realize you have.

The scoring section at the end rates your diet on a scale from super to critical and suggests changes to bring your diet up to an optimum level.

Instructions. After each answer is a number for you to circle. That is your score for the question.

In most cases, you'll circle only one number for each question. If the instructions tell you to "average scores, if necessary," add the two scores and then divide by 2. (If the average gives you a fraction, round it off to the nearest whole number.)

Pay attention to serving sizes. For example, a serving of vegetables is ½ cup. If you usually eat 1 cup of vegetables at a time, count it as two servings.

1. How many times per week do you eat unprocessed red meat (steak, roast beef, lamb or pork chops, burgers, etc.)?

    a. 1 or less   +3

    b. 2–3   +2

    c. 4–5   −1

    d. 6 or more   −3

2. Do you trim the visible fat from red meat?

    a. yes   +3

    b. no   −3

    c. don't eat red meat   +3

3. What kind of ground meat do you usually eat?

    a. regular ground beef   −3

    b. lean ground beef   −2

    c. extra-lean ground beef   −1

    d. ground round   0

    e. ground turkey   +1

    f. don't eat ground meat   +3

4. How many times per week do you eat deep-fried foods (fish, chicken, vegetables, etc.)?

    a. none   +3

    b. 1–2   0

    c. 3–4   −1

    d. 5 or more   −3

5. How many servings (½ cup) of vegetables and non-fried potatoes do you eat per day?

    a. none   −3

    b. 1   0

    c. 2   +1

    d. 3   +2

    e. 4 or more   +3

6. How many servings of cruciferous vegetables (kale, broccoli, cauliflower, cabbage, brussels sprouts, greens, bok choy, kohlrabi, turnips and rutabagas) do you usually eat per week?

    a. none   −3

    b. 1–3   +1

    c. 4–6   +2

    d. 7 or more   +3

7. How many servings of vitamin A–rich fruits or vegetables (such as sweet potatoes, cantaloupe, spinach, winter squash, greens, apricots, and broccoli) do you usually eat per week?

    a. none   −3
    b. 1–3   +1
    c. 4–6   +2
    d. 7 or more   +3

8. How many times per week do you eat at a fast-food restaurant? (Don't include meals of only baked potato, broiled chicken or salad.)

    a. never   +3
    b. less than 1   +1
    c. 1   0
    d. 2   −1
    e. 3   −2
    f. 4 or more   −4

9. How many servings of grains rich in complex carbohydrates do you eat per day? (1 serving = 1 slice of bread, 1 large pancake or ½ cup cooked cereal, rice, pasta, etc. Heavily sweetened cold cereals don't count!)

    a. none   −3
    b. 1–2   0
    c. 3–4   +1
    d. 5–6   +2
    e. 7 or more   +3

10. How many times per week do you eat seafood? (Do not include deep-fried items, tuna packed in oil, shrimp, squid, or tuna salad with mayo.)

    a. never   −2
    b. 1–2   +1
    c. 3–4   +2
    d. 5 or more   +3

11. How many servings of fresh fruit do you consume per day?

    a. none   −3
    b. 1   0
    c. 2   +1
    d. 3   +2
    e. 4 or more   +3

12. Do you remove the skin before eating poultry?

    a. yes   +3
    b. no   −3
    c. don't eat poultry   +3

13. What do you usually put on your bread or toast? (Average scores, if necessary.)

    a. butter or cream cheese   −3
    b. margarine   −2
    c. diet margarine   −1
    d. jam   0
    e. fruit butter   +3
    f. nothing   +3

14. Which of these beverages do you drink on a typical day? (Average scores, if necessary.)

    a. water or club soda   +3
    b. fruit juice   +1
    c. diet soda or coffee or tea   −1
    d. soda or fruit drink or ade   −3

15. Which flavorings do you most frequently add to your foods? (Average scores, if necessary.)

    a. garlic or lemon juice   +3
    b. herbs or spices   +3
    c. soy sauce   −2
    d. margarine   −2
    e. salt   −3
    f. butter   −3
    g. nothing   +3

16. What do you eat most frequently as a snack? (Average scores, if necessary.)

    a. fruits or vegetables   +3
    b. sweetened yogurt   +2
    c. nuts   −1
    d. chips   −2
    e. cookies   −2
    f. granola bar   −2
    g. candy bar   −3
    h. pastry   −3
    i. nothing   0

17. What is your typical breakfast? (Subtract an extra 3 points if you also eat bacon or sausage.)

    a. croissant, Danish or
        doughnut   −3
    b. eggs   −3
    c. pancakes or waffles   −2
    d. nothing   0
    e. cereal or bread   +3
    f. yogurt or cottage cheese   +3

18. What do you usually eat for dessert?

    a. pie, pastry or cake   −3
    b. ice cream   −3
    c. yogurt, ice milk or sorbet   +1
    d. fruit   +3
    e. nothing   +3

19. What dressings or toppings do you usually add to your salads? (Add scores together if you use more than one.)

    a. nothing, lemon or vinegar   +3
    b. reduced-calorie dressing   +1
    c. regular dressing   −1
    d. croutons or bacon bits   −1
    e. coleslaw, pasta salad or
        potato salad   −1

20. What sandwich fillings do you eat most frequently? (Average scores, if necessary.)

    a. luncheon meat   −3

    b. cheese or roast beef   −1

    c. peanut butter   0

    d. tuna, salmon, chicken or

        turkey   +3

21. What do you usually spread on your sandwiches? (Average scores, if necessary.)

    a. mayonnaise   −2

    b. light mayonnaise   −1

    c. mustard   0

    d. catsup   0

    e. nothing   +3

22. How many times per week do you eat canned or dried soups? (Don't count low sodium, low fat.)

    a. none   +3

    b. 1–2   0

    c. 3–4   −2

    d. 5 or more   −3

23. How many servings of a rich calcium source (⅔ cup milk or yogurt, 1 ounce cheese, 1½ ounces sardines, 3½ ounces salmon, 5 ounces tofu, 1 cup greens or broccoli or 200 milligrams of calcium supplement) do you eat per day?

    a. none   −3

    b. 1   +1

    c. 2   +2

    d. 3 or more   +3

24. What kind of pizza do your order? (Subtract 1 extra point if you order extra cheese.)

    a. no cheese w/nonmeat

        toppings   +3

    b. cheese w/nonmeat toppings +1

    c. cheese   0

    d. cheese w/meat toppings   −3
    e. don't eat pizza   +2

25. What kind of cookies do you usually eat?
    a. graham crackers   +1
    b. gingersnaps   +1
    c. oatmeal   −1
    d. chocolate coated, chocolate
        chip or peanut butter   −3
    e. sandwich cookies (like Oreos)−3
    f. don't eat cookies   +3

26. What kind of frozen dessert do you usually eat? (Subtract 1 extra point for each topping—whipped cream, hot fudge, nuts, etc.)
    a. gourmet ice cream   −3
    b. regular ice cream   −1
    c. sorbet, sherbet or ices   +1
    d. frozen yogurt or ice milk   +1
    e. don't eat frozen desserts   +3

27. What kind of cake or pastry do you usually eat?
    a. cheesecake, pie or any
        microwave cake   −3
    b. cake with frosting or filling   −2
    c. cake without frosting   −1
    d. angel food cake   +1
    e. unfrosted muffin, banana
        bread or carrot cake   0
    f. don't eat cakes or pastries   +3

28. How many times per week does your dinner contain grains, vegetables or beans and little or no animal protein (meat, poultry, fish, eggs, milk or cheese)?
    a. none   −1
    b. 1   +1
    c. 2   +2
    d. 3   +3

29. Which snacks do you typically eat?
   a. potato chips or packaged
      popcorn   −3
   b. tortilla chips   −1
   c. light potato chips   −2
   d. salted pretzels   −1
   e. unsalted pretzels   +1
   f. homemade air-popped
      popcorn   +3
   g. don't eat snacks   +3

30. What kind of cereal do you usually eat?
   a. hot, whole-grain (like
      oatmeal or Wheatena)   +3
   b. cold, whole-grain (like
      Shredded Wheat)   +3
   c. cold, low-fiber (like corn
      flakes)   0
   d. sugary, cold, low-fiber
      (like Frosted Flakes)   −1
   e. granola   −2

31. With what do you make tuna salad, pasta salad, chicken salad, etc.?
   a. mayonnaise   −2
   b. light mayonnaise   0
   c. low-fat yogurt   +2
   d. nonfat yogurt   +3

32. What do you typically put on your pasta? (Add 1 point if you also add sautéed vegetables. Average scores, if necessary.)
   a. tomato-based sauce   +3
   b. tomato sauce with a little
      Parmesan   +3
   c. white clam sauce   +1
   d. meat sauce   −1
   e. tomato sauce w/meatballs   −2
   f. Alfredo or other creamy
      sauce   −3

Scoring: Total (+): _____

Total (–): _____

GRAND TOTAL: _____

+59 to +98 = Super. You're a nutrition superstar. Give yourself a big (nonbutter) pat on the back.

+24 to +58 = Good. It wouldn't take much to put you in the superstar category and boost your health even more.

–10 to +23 = Fair. There are more than a few places where you need to trim the fat from your diet.

–11 and below = Critical. Your diet needs major surgery and a transfusion of healthy nutrition tips. Clean out the refrigerator and pantry and start over based on the information in this book.

Copyright © 1992, Center for Science in the Public Interest

FOCUS ON FAT

Knowing the importance of a low-fat diet is one thing. Eating a low-fat diet is quite another.

Does your own diet meet the current recommendations for limiting fat to a third of your calories? To help you get the straight skinny on your diet, take this quiz developed at the Northwest Lipid Research Clinic at the University of Washington in Seattle.

Check the answer that best describes how you have been eating recently.

1. How many ounces of meat, fish or poultry do you usually eat?*

____**1.** I do not eat meat, fish or poultry.

____**2.** I eat 3 ounces or less per day.

____**3.** I eat 4–6 ounces per day.

____**4.** I eat 7 or more ounces per day.

*3 ounces of meat, fish or chicken is any *one* of the following: 1 regular hamburger, 1 chicken breast, 1 chicken leg (thigh and drumstick), 1 pork chop or 3 slices of pre-sliced lunch meat.

2. How much cheese do you eat per week?
   ___**1.** I avoid cheese altogether.
   ___**2.** I use only low-fat cheese (ricotta, low-fat cottage cheese).
   ___**3.** I eat whole-milk cheese (such as Cheddar, Swiss, Monterey Jack) once or twice per week.
   ___**4.** I eat 3 or more servings of whole-milk cheese per week.
3. What type of milk do you use?
   ___**1.** I use only skim or 1 percent milk or don't use milk.
   ___**2.** I usually use skim milk or 1 percent milk, but use others occasionally.
   ___**3.** I usually use 2 percent or whole milk.
4. How many egg yolks do you use per week?
   ___**1.** I avoid all egg yolk and/or use only the egg substitutes.
   ___**2.** I eat 1–2 eggs per week.
   ___**3.** I eat 3 or more eggs per week.
5. How often do you usually eat lunch meat, hot dogs, corned beef, spareribs, sausage, bacon, braunschweiger or liver?
   ___**1.** I do not eat any of these meats.
   ___**2.** I eat them about once per week.
   ___**3.** I eat about 2–4 servings per week.
   ___**4.** I eat more than 4 servings per week.
6. How many commercial baked goods and how much ice cream do you usually eat? Examples: cake, cookies, sweet rolls, doughnuts, etc.
   ___**1.** I avoid baked goods and ice cream.
   ___**2.** I eat baked goods or ice cream once a week.
   ___**3.** I eat 2–4 servings of baked goods or ice cream per week.

____**4.** I eat more than 4 servings of baked goods or ice cream per week.

7. What is the main type of fat you cook with?

____**1.** I don't use fat in cooking.

____**2.** I use safflower oil, sunflower oil, corn oil or soybean oil.

____**3.** I use olive oil, peanut butter or margarine.

____**4.** I use shortening, butter or bacon drippings.

8. How often do you eat snack foods such as chips, fries or party crackers (Triscuits, Wheat Thins, Ritz, etc.)?

____**1.** I avoid these snack foods.

____**2.** I eat 1 serving of these snacks per week

____**3.** I eat 2–4 servings of these snacks per week.

____**4.** I eat more than 4 servings of these snack foods per week.

9. What type of butter/margarine do you usually use on bread, vegetables, etc.?

____**1.** I don't use butter or margarine.

____**2.** I use soft (tub) or diet margarine.

____**3.** I use stick margarine.

____**4.** I use butter.

Scoring: Add up the numbers from each of your answers. If you score 15 or less, congratulate yourself. You're eating a low-fat diet. A score of 16 to 18 qualifies as a moderate-fat diet, roughly equivalent to the Step One diet the American Heart Association recommends. Anything higher than 18 can be considered high fat.

If your number's too high, start incorporating the 1 and 2 answers into your diet as much as you can. Note that you can still get away with one or two 4s, but only if you balance them out with enough 1s.

Are You Meeting Your Fiber Quota?

Next to low fat, fiber is one of the most talked about features of a healthy diet. Despite the fact that fiber is relatively

1ance from nutrition lecturer Liz Applegate,
Ph.D., and nutrition professor Judith Stern, Sc.D., R.D., both
at the University of California, Davis.

1. What type of bread (including rolls and muffins) did
you usually eat?
   - **a.** whole-wheat or whole-grain +4
   - **b.** white or partial whole-wheat +2

2. How many servings of oat products did you average
daily? (1 serving = 1 cup cooked oatmeal or oat bran.)
   - **a.** 2 or more   +4
   - **b.** 1   +3
   - **c.** ½   +2
   - **d.** none   0

3. How many times during the last three days did you eat
beans (legumes), such as kidney beans, pintos, garbanzos, soybeans, lentils, and split peas?
   - **a.** 3 or more   +4
   - **b.** 2   +3
   - **c.** 1   +2
   - **d.** none   0

4. How many times during the three-day period did you
eat high-fiber breakfast cereals?
   - **a.** 3 or more   +4
   - **b.** 2   +3
   - **c.** 1   +2
   - **d.** none   0

5. How many times during the three-day period did you eat cooked whole-grain side dishes, such as brown rice or barley?

    a. 3 or more   +4
    b. 2   +3
    c. 1   +2
    d. none   0

6. Approximately how many servings of canned or fresh fruits and vegetables did you eat daily? (Use an average from the previous three days. 1 serving = ½ cup cooked or 1 cup or 1 piece raw.)

    a. 7 or more   +5
    b. 5–6   +4
    c. 3–4   +2
    d. 1–2   +1
    e. none   –2

Scoring: If your overall score is over 20, your fiber intake is probably adequate. If you scored lower, see chapter 7 for help.

CHECK YOUR CALCIUM INTAKE

If you are not a fan of dairy products, you may be coming up far short of your calcium needs. But even if you are a milk lover, how much calcium your body actually absorbs depends upon your genetic makeup. And how much you retain depends upon your intake of salt and protein. This duo increases the elimination of calcium, causing your body to steal calcium it needs from your bones.

The following quiz was developed with the assistance of Robert P. Heaney, M.D., professor of medicine at Creighton University School of Medicine in Omaha, Nebraska. It can tell you how close your diet comes to providing the appropriate amount of bone food. Just check the answer that applies to you.

1. I eat a serving of yogurt (8 ounces), milk (1 cup) or cheese (1 ounce) at least once a day.

    ___True   +3
    ___False   −1

2. Dairy products give me gas and bloating, so I avoid them.

    ___True   −1
    ___False   +1

3. I make sure I eat one or more of the following nondairy sources of calcium at least three times a week: leafy green vegetables (kale, bok choy or broccoli), shellfish (oysters or clams) or canned fish with bones (salmon or sardines).

    ___True   +1
    ___False   0

4. I make an effort to slip dairy foods into my diet whenever I can (grating cheese over salads, for example).

    ___True   +1
    ___False   0

5. I eat calcium-enriched forms of products (such as breakfast cereal or fruit juice) whenever possible.

    ___True   +1
    ___False   −1

6. When given a choice, I drink carbonated soft drinks over low-fat dairy drinks or water.

    ___True   −1
    ___False   0

7. I tend to get my protein from meats.

    ___True   −1
    ___False   +1

8. I usually salt foods automatically without tasting them.

    ___True   −1
    ___False   +1

Scoring: If you scored between 7 and 9, you are laying the dietary foundation for a rock-solid skeleton. (Remember, though, that even if you scored a perfect 9, you may still have a bone deficit if you are inactive, underweight or postmenopausal, have a family history of osteoporosis or take aluminim-based antacids or other calcium-robbing drugs.)

If you scored between 4 and 6, try to include more low-fat dairy products and go easy on the calcium bandits.

If you scored below 4, your skeleton may be becoming perilously porous. Learn to love low-fat yogurt and make friends with skim milk. Ask your doctor about taking a calcium supplement.

THE EASIEST WAY TO TEST YOUR WATER LEVEL

You may be getting enough vitamins, minerals and fiber, but still be starving your body of one important nutrient: water.

Unfortunately, you can't always rely on thirst to indicate a water deficit, especially as you get older, according to studies conducted by Barbara Rolls, Ph.D., of Johns Hopkins University School of Medicine in Baltimore.

A rough indicator to determine your water level? Check the color of your urine, says Dr. Rolls. If it's dark amber or has a strong odor, it means the kidneys have concentrated wastes in urine and you're not drinking enough water. Passing a full bladder of colorless or pale yellow urine at least four times daily means you're getting enough water. "You should always be looking for change in volume, color and odor," Dr. Rolls says. "If these changes persist, see a doctor."

CAN YOU FIND THE HIDDEN SALT?

If you've already banned the saltshaker from the table and sworn off salty snacks—good for you! But to keep your intake at the recommended one-teaspoon-a-day limit takes a bit more vigilance. Three-fourths of your dietary sodium is hidden in already-prepared foods, experts say. And many salt-laced foods like cereal, diet soda and instant pudding don't taste a bit salty.

Just how good are you at avoiding this hidden salt? If you're eating more potassium-rich fresh fruits and vegetables than packaged convenience foods, for example, you're probably doing great. (Potassium helps rid your body of excess sodium.)

Take this quiz to find out where you stand on the hidden salt scale.

1. When barbecuing meat or fish, I'm more likely to brush on herbs or homemade marinara sauce than commercial catsup, barbecue sauce or soy sauce.

   ___True   +1
   ___False   –1

2. The fresh fruits and vegetables and lean meats in my grocery cart usually crowd out the canned, frozen and processed food.

   ___True   +1
   ___False   –1

3. I buy only the low-salt type of margarine

   ___True   +1
   ___False   –1

4. I usually have dehydrated, instant versions of soups, sauces, salad dressings, oatmeal or other foods on hand.

   ___True   –1
   ___False   +1

5. I steam, microwave, broil or stir-fry vegetables rather than boil them.

___True   +1

___False   −1

6. Processed cheese never passes my lips.

___True   +1

___False   −1

7. I rinse canned foods such as tuna, ham and beans before preparing them.

___True   +1

___False   −1

8. I'm a sucker for deli food—cold cuts, prepared salads, pastrami, ham, smoked fish and so on.

___True   −1

___False   +1

9. I usually order my hamburger with the works—cheese, pickles, catsup, mustard and special sauce.

___True   −1

___False   +1

10. When dining out, I usually order oil and vinegar dressing for my salad, and ask for gravies and sauces on the side.

___True   +1

___False   −1

Scoring: 8–10: You're a top-notch salt sleuth.

5–7: There's room for improvement. Scan food labels closely for the key phrases "sodium-free" or "very low sodium."

Below 5: You're probably relying on too many prepared condiments and packaged convenience foods. See chapter 10 for help.

WHAT'S YOUR OVEREATING STYLE?

At one time or another, we've probably all used food as first-aid for wounded emotions. Jelly doughnuts become a security blanket for a bruised ego; cherry-vanilla ice cream becomes a sedative when you're stressed out; nachos become Saturday night entertainment when you're bored or lonely.

But if you *frequently* use a bag of chips or other food as an emotional bandage, it's likely that you also carry around more than a few unwanted pounds. According to studies conducted by Maria Simonson, Ph.D., and staff at the Health, Weight and Stress Clinic at Johns Hopkins Medical Institutions in Baltimore, 85 percent of overweight people turn to food when something is eating them. Psychological overeaters, they say, fall into several distinct categories like the ones listed here.

Finding yourself in one of these categories is no cause for panic. Becoming aware of when, why and where you overeat can help you avoid the triggers that lead to nonstop nibbling.

To find out where you fit in, answer the questions below as follows:

0 = never
1 = once in a while
2 = fairly often
3 = regularly

The category with the highest score gives you your basic overeating style.

Nervous Night Eater
—I often skimp on meals until nightfall, then I stuff my
   face non-stop.
—I crave sweet, salty or high-fat snacks.
—I often munch in front of the boob tube, starting with the
   evening news on through the late show.
—I often conduct midnight raids on the refrigerator.
—I have trouble getting to sleep or staying asleep.
—I drink more than 3 cups of coffee a day.
—On a scale of 1 to 10, I'd say my stress level rates a 9 or
   10.
—I've been called a worrywart.

HAIR ANALYSIS TESTS: A HELP OR A HOAX?

Could elevated levels of lead or depressed levels of zinc in your hair be warning flags of internal trouble?

Some alternative health practitioners think so. That's why these practitioners routinely run hair analysis tests on their patients. Supposedly, a lock of hair unlocks nutritional secrets other tests fail to find.

Several laboratories now offer mail-order hair analysis tests to anyone who sends in a snip of hair and about twenty bucks. In return, you get a computer printout summarizing the levels of metals and minerals detected in your hair. Typically, you'll also get a detailed interpretation of the findings along with specific dietary recommendations to detoxify your body or correct a deficiency.

Is hair analysis worth the money? "Probably not," says Leslie M. Klevay, M.D., research leader of the Clinical Nutrition Laboratory with the U.S. Department of Agriculture's Human Nutrition Research Center at the University of North Dakota in Grand Forks.

Hair follicles contain a trace of the same minerals and metals that are in your bloodstream. As hair grows, it also incorporates elements from the environment such as lead, mercury and aluminim.

Compulsive Eater
—I often skip sit-down meals and usually eat on the run.
—I'm rarely without some type of food in my mouth.
—I'd rather eat food—even when I'm not hungry—than waste it.
—I crave foods that are sweet, starchy and soft (but I'll eat anything).

Analyzing your hair content might tell you if toxic exposure to these minerals has taken place and reveal cumulative exposure over a period of time—but that's probably the extent of it.

"If you suspect lead or mercury poisoning or want to monitor environmental pollutants, a hair analysis test might be worthwhile for these specific situations," says Dr. Klevay. But, he adds "I would never rely solely on hair analysis as a diagnostic tool for, say, lead poisoning. Hair analysis tests should be viewed as a complement to standard blood, urine and physical tests."

As far as using hair analysis for detecting mineral deficiencies and diagnosing early metabolic diseases, there isn't a strand of evidence that it works for this purpose.

Hair analysis is fraught with other problems. Results can be tainted from hair dyes, shampoo, tap-water impurities—all factors that can alter the mineral composition of hair.

Furthermore, since there are no standardized procedures for analyzing hair, results are unreliable. One expert sent three hair samples from the same person to three different labs. He got back three different results—"that were not even close."

—I usually sneak food when no one is around to see me eat it.
—My favorite beverage is diet soda—lots of it.
—I'm cheery on the outside, but inside, I feel lonely and blue.
—My love life is either stressful or nonexistent.

Closet Binge Eater

—About three times a month, I suddenly pig out uncontrollably.
—When I binge, I gobble food fast and steadily, easily polish off an entire bag of cookies.
—I binge in private and usually at night.
—My binges are usually triggered when I'm upset or stressed out.
—Immediately after bingeing I feel calm, but later ashamed and furious at myself.
—After a binge, I often fast or crash diet.
—Often after bingeing, my stomach aches or I have trouble sleeping.
—I often feel angry and depressed but don't know why.

Hand-Me-Down Eater

—My family devours king-size portions of rich food at every meal.
—My parents and siblings are overweight.
—My family frequently snacks together in front of the TV.
—The most exercise my family gets is reaching for seconds on pie.
—Both my mother and I love to cook.
—Having a well-stocked pantry makes me feel secure and loved.
—My mother always serves an extravagant dinner with rich desserts.
—My family celebrates even minor occasions with lavish feasts.

Thin/Fat

—I was overweight as a teenager and am now deathly afraid of gaining weight.
—It's a never-ending battle to stay thin.
—I eat nothing but low-calorie meals.

—I nag my husband and children if they gain even a pound or two because I detest fat people.
—My life would be ruined if I gained weight.
—I can tell you the fat and calorie count of every food on God's green Earth.
—Fat people are weak and have no willpower.
—Bingeing is the furthest thing from my mind.

Chronic Dieter
—I've tried all the latest diets and read all the diet books, but none of them are any good.
—Within a few months of losing weight, I'm back to my former fat self.
—I often crash diet before a party or important social event.
—I know more than most people about diets, nutrition and psychological causes for weight gain.
—I can tell you exactly how and why I lost and regained every pound.
—I've memorized the calorie count for foods from A to Z.
—Don't try to recommend a weight-loss group or doctor—they've all failed me.
—I'm into quick and easy weight loss.

Environmental Eater
—I can't resist the aromas emanating from a bakery.
—Just reading about luscious dessert recipes makes me drool.
—TV food commercials send me to the refrigerator.
—Eating food goees along with the territory of my job—power lunches, social dinners, etc.
—I eat more than most people at meals.
—When dining out, I rarely pass up the pastry dessert cart.
—I've begun to develop love handles on my waist and batwings under my arms.
—I rarely turn down an extra helping or a meal, even if I'm not hungry—if it's there, I'll eat it.

Couch Potato

—I prefer curling up with a bag of chips to physical activity.

—The most exercise I get these days is lifting a fork to my mouth.

—It takes fewer and fewer calories to maintain the same weight.

—I wouldn't be caught dead in workout gear.

—It's an effort to even walk to stores at the mall.

—I'm stressed and anxious most of the time.

—I sit behind a desk all day.

—Once I could have danced all night, but since I've gained weight, I can barely shuffle to the TV.

ARE YOU COMMITTED TO FOOD SAFETY?

More than half of all food-borne illness is caused by sloppy food handling habits in preparing, cooking and storing food in home kitchens, experts say. Are you taking unnecessary risks in your own kitchen? Take this test to find out. Simply circle the appropriate answer.

1. I usually keep my refrigerator thermostat set below:
    a. 32°F
    b. 15°F
    c. 40°F
    d. 30°F

2. I would probably select the items below in the following order as I move through the grocery store.
    a. strawberries, shrimp, eggs, canned soup, paper towels
    b. eggs, shrimp, strawberries, canned soup, paper towels
    c. paper towels, canned soup, strawberries, shrimp, eggs

3. I assume food is safe to eat if it doesn't smell, taste or look spoiled, no matter when the expiration date.

    Yes/No

4. I would toss out a can of green beans because:

    a. the can was leaking

    b. the lid was bulging

    c. the can was badly dented

    d. all of the above

5. I usually thaw frozen raw meat, poultry or fish in the refrigerator on the lowest shelf.

    Yes/No

6. After Thanksgiving dinner, the longest I would allow turkey and other leftovers to remain at room temperature is:

    a. 3 hours

    b. ½ hour

    c. 2 hours

    d. 24 hours

7. The container I use to store a large quantity of leftover stew in my refrigerator is:

    a. several small, shallow containers

    b. a big, deep, airtight container

    c. the stewpot covered with a lid

8. My cutting board is made out of:

    a. hardwood

    b. acrylic

9. After cutting up raw ground meat for a taco salad and before using the same knife and cutting board to chop the tomatoes, I nromally do the following:

    a. wipe the knife and board with a paper towel

    b. wash the knife and board with hot, soapy water

    c. rinse the knife and board under hot water

    d. wash the knife, board and my hands with hot, soapy water

10. When preparing potato salad for a buffet table, I omit the mayonnaise to reduce the risk of spoiling.
Yes/No

11. When removing barbecued chicken from the grill, I normally use a different fork than the one used to place the raw poultry on the grill.
Yes/No

12. If I want to use milk on my cereal but the milk container reads "sell by May 14" and it's now May 17, I'd use the milk anyway.
Yes/No

13. When cooking meat, fish and poultry dishes in the microwave, I cover them to trap the steam and test them for doneness with a thermometer.
Yes/No

Answers: 1. c.; 2. c.; 3. No; 4. d.; 5. Yes; 6. c.; 7. a.; 8. b.; 9. b.; 10. No; 11. Yes; 12. Yes; 13. Yes.
Scoring: If your total number of correct answers is between:

10 and 13: You should be wearing a halo for your fastidious food handling.

7 and 9: Your food handling habits are generally well intentioned but you should do better to be on the safe side.

6 or below: You have habits that could endanger your family's health and invite food-borne illness. Review chapter 29 and take this test again in a few weeks.

IS YOUR GLOBAL GRAZING ON TRACK?

Sampling the world's bounty of ethnic foods can excite your tastebuds. Besides out-of-this-world taste, a second reason to "go ethnic" is that many of these ancient dishes have little fat, sugar and salt, but lots of fiber—exactly the dietary recommendations for health-conscious Americans.

To reap the benefits from ethnic foods, though, you also need to steer clear of Americanized and fancy versions that are meat-laden, deep-fried, crisped or smothered in high-calorie cheese, sour cream or coconut milk.

Are you making the most of your ethnic eating opportunities? Take the quiz below and find out.

1. My idea of a great Mexican meal is:
    a. nachos with Cheez Whiz or anything that comes in a bag emblazoned with a bell
    b. a beef enchilada made with a flour tortilla and garnished with guacamole
    c. chicken roasted in mole sauce with a side of black-bean soup or a soft-corn tortilla

2. When I think of Italian food, it means:
    a. a large pizza with the works
    b. stuffed pasta shells
    c. cannellini beans and arugula greens with a side of crusty bread

3. When I crave Chinese food, it's usually:
    a. chop suey, fried rice and an egg roll
    b. Hunan shrimp and steamed rice so spicy my eyes water and my nose runs
    c. A cousin cuisine, the more delicately flavored Thai foods such as peanut oil-and-papaya shrimp salad with cellophane noodles

4. If I want a light Middle Eastern-style lunch, I choose:
    a. lean roast beef stuffed in a pita pocket
    b. bits of meat skewered on a short stick
    c. baba ghannoush (pureed eggplant) with pita bread or tabbouleh (parsley salad and cracked wheat)

5. My experience with Indian food is:
    a. chutney relish on my frankfurter
    b. Mulligatawny soup
    c. Tandoori chicken marinated in yogurt, served with nan (flat-bread) and a side of cauliflower curry

CAN A COMPUTER BE YOUR NUTRITION GUIDE?

First it was computerized horoscopes, then computerized dating services and now computerized diet analysis.

"People want more control over their health, and they want to learn how food contributes to their well-being," says Rebecca S. Reeves, R.D., of Baylor College of Medicine in Houston. "Computerized diet analyses can offer a starting point in designing a healthy eating plan."

But before mailing in your diet survey and your check, ask what standards the computer-diet folks are basing their nutrient assessments on. A good analysis should be based on the Recommended Dietary Allowances (RDAs) set by the government.

Even a top-notch computerized diet analysis has its limits, though. For starters, a typical analysis based on a one-week dietary recall does not take into account your body's stores of nutrients. You may have eaten low-vitamin A foods during your surveyed week, for instance, yet the week before, you ate high-vitamin A foods. You could have an adequate store of vitamin A in your blood that is not reflected in your computer analysis. "This can be unnecessarily alarming," says Reeves. On the other hand, if you have a true nutrient deficiency, this can only be revealed with the appropriate blood and other biochemical tests.

6. Any Japanese meal I order would probably include:
   a. Teriyaki beef cooked tableside by chefs tossing knives and peppermills
   b. batter-dipped tempura shrimp and vegetables
   c. chicken yakatori broiled in gingerroot, sesame oil and chili pepper

Some experts believe that computer assessments place too much emphasis on vitamin deficiencies and ignore the behavioral issues that affect nutrition—whether you skip breakfast for example, or eat most meals in fast-food joints.

"Your body does not work like a computer," says Pittsburgh dietitian Pat Harper, R.D., a spokesperson for the American Dietetic Association. You need skilled detective work to uncover not just what you eat but how you eat. A personal nutritionist can fill in the gaps. "For example, I ask clients the type and amount of food they eat, what time they eat it and whether it's fried in fat, smothered in catsup, salted and so on."

A personal nutritionist or registered dietitian can also help you tailor nutritious meals. They'll give you tips on how to design a calcium-rich diet that won't raise your cholesterol levels, for instance, or show you how to dine sensibly on a hectic schedule. Some personal nutritionists will even peer into your refrigerator or take you on a tour of the supermarket, showing you exactly what margarine to buy.

In sum, the ideal nutritional assessment includes both a printout and a professional dietitian/nutritionist. To find an expert in your area, contact the American Dietetic Association at 1-800-366-1655. Or write to the National Center for Nutrition and Dietetics, 216 West Jackson Boulevard, Suite 800, Chicago, IL 60606-6995.

Scoring: Give yourself no points for each **a.** answer, 1 point for each **b.** answer and 2 points for each **c.** answer. If you scored between 0 and 5, you are missing the boat in your gastronomic adventures. See chapter 18 for advice. A score between 6 and 8 shows that you're making some good choices, but there's still plenty of room for improvement. If your score was between 9 and 12, give yourself a gold star—you're eating the healthiest international cuisine of all.

CHAPTER 36

Eating Light, Eating Right

A Six-Week Program

Now that you've read this far, you know that a diet that emphasizes fruits, vegetables and grains can help reduce your risk of cancer, heart attack, obesity and stroke. You know that a diet of burgers, blue cheese and baloney can kill. But how do you move from the "typical" high-fat, high-cholesteral, high-calorie American diet to an eating program that prevents disease, promotes longevity and energizes both mind and body?

How do you put together all the recommendations from the American Heart Association, the National Cancer Institute, the National Cholesterol Education Program, the National Research Council and your doctor?

How do you eat everything these experts say you should—4 servings of this, 2 of that and 11 of the other—without getting fat, going crazy or needing a computerized tracking system to analyze what you eat?

We asked two of the country's leading experts in diet modification to develop a nutrition-improvement program that would be effective yet easy to follow.

Lynne W. Scott is director of the Diet Modification Clinic and assistant professor of medicine at Baylor College of Medicine in Houston. Franca Alphin is nutrition director of the Duke University Diet and Fitness Center in Durham, North Carolina. Both are registered dietitians. And though they are far apart in miles, they stand shoulder-to-shoulder when it comes to how you should switch from the old-fashioned American diet in which a "salad" is the wimpy tomato and lettuce on top of your burger to the new American diet in which a "salad" is a full-bodied mix of greens and other nutrient-dense vegetables.

Both the experts say that you should begin the transition to healthy eating by launching an all-out attack against fat. By taking that first major step, you could actually begin to feel healthier and more energetic within five days.

Then follow the fat offensive by cracking down on cholesteral, fortifying with grains, sifting out salt, draining oil, clipping calories and decriminalizing desserts, and your body should feel as though it has been reborn.

A key point to remember while working your way through the six-week program, however, is that it is only the *beginning*. This program is designed to jump start your motivational engines and propel you toward a healthy lifestyle. Getting there is up to you. You'll probably make a slew of mistakes—both accidentally and deliberately—and, our experts warn, it may actually take up to a full year before you can trust your hand to automatically reach for an apple instead of a cookie.

The point is that you should accept those setbacks as a natural consequence of being human. Just ignore them. Pick up the program where you left off and move forward. Once you've worked your way through the entire six weeks, you'll have a solid nutritional foundation on which to build the rest of a very healthy, very long life.

Week 1: Attack Fat

Day 1: Launch Your Offensive

"Take a pad and pencil and, for a day or two, write down absolutely everything you eat and drink and include the amounts," says Alphin. "Don't change anything—just write it down."

Then go out and buy a book with a comprehensive fat-content-of-foods table, suggests Scott. One that lists every conceivable food and every single gram of fat. Because once you get a handle on what you're eating, the first step you're going to take on the path to a healthier you is the one where you ditch excess dietary fat.

Both dietitians agree that your goal is to keep daily fat intake below 30 percent of the calories you're supposed to eat in any given day. And if your eyes glaze over at the thought of figuring out how much that is, you're figuring it out the hard way.

The easy way, says Scott, is to flip to the calorie table on page 726. Based on your ideal weight—what you're *supposed* to weigh, not what you weigh now—determine your optimal daily calorie level. Then check the fat table below. Right next to the total number of calories you should eat to maintain your ideal weight, you will see the maximum number of grams of fat you dare eat in a day.

Note the operative word here is *maximum*. If your height, weight and frame size dictate that you eat, say, 1,900 calories a day, then—according to the table—you should be eating no more than 63 grams of fat, and no more than 21 grams of that should be saturated fat.

Whatever your numbers, memorize them, urges Scott. Write them on your heart and in your mind. Because by the

WHERE TO DRAW THE LINE ON FAT

After you've consulted the table on page 726 to find how many calories a day you should be eating, use this table to determine the maximum amount of fat permitted daily.

Calorie Levels	Total Fat (g.)*	Saturated Fat (g.)†
1,200	40	13
1,300	43	14
1,400	47	16
1,500	50	17
1,600	53	18
1,700	57	19
1,800	60	20
1,900	63	21
2,000	67	22
2,100	70	23
2,200	73	24
2,300	77	26
2,400	80	27
2,500	83	28
2,600	87	29
2,700	90	30
2,800	93	31
2,900	97	32
3,000	100	33
3,100	103	34
3,200	107	36
3,300	110	37
3,400	113	38
3,500	117	39
3,600	120	40
3,700	123	41
3,800	127	42

*Grams of fat equal to 30 percent of calories.
†Grams of saturated fat equal to 10 percent of calories

end of your second week on this Eating Light, Eating Right Program, you're going to have to account for every gram of fat while keeping within those limits.

DAY 2: MEET THE MEATCUTTER AT YOUR MARKET

Now that you've written down everything you ate for at least a day, bought a good fat-content-of-foods table and memorized your personal fat ceilings, head for the supermarket—the meat counter, in particular.

"Meat contains the highest concentration of fat in the American diet," says Scott. "So a major strategy in the war against fat is to learn how to select the leanest cuts."

Take a look at the ground beef, for example. And don't just look at the labeling. Despite the fact that ground beef is usually somewhere around 20 percent fat by weight, it seems as though every package claims to be lean. "Lean," "Leaner" and "Superlean," right?

There is, however, a secret code that meatcutters use to reveal the fat content of some cuts of beef (but not ground meat): Its key words are "Prime," "Choice" and "Select." Prime has the most fat. Choice is leaner, and Select is the very leanest.

"Once you've deciphered this code," says Scott, "a key strategy that will allow you to limit the amount of fat you get from ground beef, is to buy select cuts of beef and ask your meatcutter to grind them." Make sure you also choose the lean cuts of meat—top round steak, for example—and ask your meatcutter to trim all visible fat before he grinds.

If it's inconvenient to wait for your custom grind, you can buy ground turkey instead. It's lower in fat than beef and easily substituted for ground beef in cooking.

If the turkey is freshly ground, however, make sure to ask your meatcutter whether it's pure meat or meat mixed with skin and fat. "Pure meat will be lower in fat," says Scott, "so that's what you want to buy." If you buy frozen ground turkey, she adds, read the labels carefully and pick the product with the fewest grams of fat per serving. It will be least likely to contain skin and extra fat.

Fortunately, choosing pork and poultry is a little bit easier than choosing beef. Just reach for the pork tenderloin—the leanest cut—and the light-meat cuts of chicken and turkey. White meat is lower in fat than dark meat. Remove the skin from chicken before cooking it. Turkey can be cooked with the skin to prevent it from drying out, but remove the skin before eating it.

DAY 3: CONFESS YOUR SINS

Today's the day to take a look at all the foods you've eaten over the past two days and play "Find the Fat." So pull out the pad on which you've scribbled down everything you ate and let's review your sins.

You knew the ½ cup of ice cream you ate last night after the 10 o'clock news was high in fat. But now, checking the fat table you bought on Day 1, you find that it had almost 12 grams of fat—one-fifth the maximum amount of fat a 5-foot 1-inch, 109-pound woman should eat in an entire day!

You also knew that your dinner, consisting of two hot dogs (13 grams of fat each), rolls (3 grams each), potatoes au gratin (9 grams for ½ cup), peas (good choice—less than 1 gram of fat) and low-fat milk (a glass of 2 percent milk has almost 5 grams of fat) might be a little heavy. And it was. The total fat you ate at that one meal—even though you resisted that second helping of potatoes—was 46 grams.

Forty-six grams of fat for dinner might not have been too bad—even with your 12-gram "snack"—if you'd had a light lunch. But no, you went shopping with your friends and stopped at the local deli. All you had was a cheese sandwich (14 grams of fat), a salad with blue cheese dressing (16 grams of fat) and an iced tea (0 grams), but that "light" lunch—which really didn't have very much food—actually contained 30 grams of fat.

FIND YOUR IDEAL CALORIE LEVEL

Use this table to determine the number of calories you should be eating daily, based upon your height, weight, bone structure and activity level.

Adult Females

			Calorie Level Based on Physical Activity			
Height without Shoes	Frame Size	Desirable Weight (Range)	Very Light	Light	Moderate	Heavy
5'0"	Small	106 (102–110)	1,400	1,600	1,800	2,100
	Medium	113 (107–119)	1,450	1,700	1,900	2,250
	Large	123 (115–131)	1,600	1,850	2,100	2,450
5'1"	Small	109 (105–113)	1,400	1,650	1,850	2,200
	Medium	116 (110–122)	1,500	1,750	1,950	2,300
	Large	126 (118–134)	1,650	1,900	2,150	2,500
5'2"	Small	112 (108–116)	1,450	1,700	1,900	2,250
	Medium	119 (113–126)	1,550	1,800	2,000	2,400
	Large	129 (121–138)	1,700	1,950	2,200	2,600
5'3"	Small	115 (111–119)	1,500	1,750	1,950	2,300
	Medium	123 (116–130)	1,600	1,850	2,100	2,450
	Large	133 (125–142)	1,750	2,000	2,250	2,650
5'4"	Small	118 (114–123)	1,550	1,750	2,000	2,350
	Medium	127 (120–135)	1,650	1,900	2,150	2,550
	Large	137 (129–146)	1,800	2,050	2,350	2,750
5'5"	Small	122 (118–127)	1,600	1,850	2,050	2,450
	Medium	131 (124–139)	1,700	1,950	2,250	2,600
	Large	141 (133–150)	1,850	2,100	2,400	2,800
5'6"	Small	126 (122–131)	1,650	1,900	2,150	2,500
	Medium	135 (128–143)	1,750	2,050	2,300	2,700
	Large	145 (137–154)	1,900	2,200	2,450	2,900
5'7"	Small	130 (126–135)	1,700	1,950	2,200	2,600
	Medium	139 (132–147)	1,800	2,100	2,350	2,800
	Large	149 (141–158)	1,950	2,250	2,550	3,000
5'8"	Small	135 (130–140)	1,750	2,050	2,300	2,700

Height without Shoes	Frame Size	Desirable Weight (Range)	Calorie Level Based on Physical Activity			
			Very Light	Light	Moderate	Heavy
	Medium	143 (136–151)	1,850	2,150	2,450	2,850
	Large	154 (145–163)	2,000	2,300	2,600	3,100
5'9"	Small	139 (134–144)	1,800	2,100	2,350	2,800
	Medium	147 (140–155)	1,900	2,200	2,500	2,950
	Large	158 (149–168)	2,050	2,350	2,700	3,150
5'10"	Small	143 (138–148)	1,850	2,150	2,450	2,850
	Medium	151 (144–159)	1,950	2,250	2,550	3,000
	Large	163 (153–173)	2,100	2,450	2,750	3,250

Adult Males

Height without Shoes	Frame Size	Desirable Weight (Range)	Very Light	Light	Moderate	Heavy
5'5"	Small	129 (124–133)	1,700	1,950	2,200	2,600
	Medium	137 (130–143)	1,800	2,050	2,350	2,750
	Large	147 (138–156)	1,900	2,200	2,500	2,950
5'6"	Small	133 (128–137)	1,750	2,000	2,250	2,650
	Medium	141 (134–147)	1,850	2,100	2,400	2,800
	Large	152 (142–161)	2,000	2,300	2,600	3,050
5'7"	Small	137 (132–141)	1,800	2,050	2,350	2,750
	Medium	145 (138–152)	1,900	2,200	2,450	2,900
	Large	157 (147–166)	2,050	2,350	2,650	3,150
5'8"	Small	141 (136–145)	1,850	2,100	2,400	2,850
	Medium	149 (142–156)	1,950	2,250	2,550	3,000
	Large	161 (151–170)	2,100	2,400	2,750	3,200
5'9"	Small	145 (140–150)	1,900	2,200	2,450	2,900
	Medium	153 (146–160)	2,000	2,300	2,600	3,050
	Large	165 (155–174)	2,150	2,500	2,800	3,300
5'10"	Small	149 (144–154)	1,950	2,250	2,550	3,000
	Medium	158 (150–165)	2,050	2,350	2,700	3,150
	Large	169 (159–179)	2,200	2,550	2,850	3,400
5'11"	Small	153 (148–158)	2,000	2,300	2,600	3,050
	Medium	162 (154–170)	2,100	2,450	2,750	3,250
	Large	174 (164–184)	2,250	2,600	2,950	3,500

Adult Males

Calorie Level Based on Physical Activity

Height without Shoes	Frame Size	Desirable Weight (Range)	Very Light	Light	Moderate	Heavy
6'0"	Small	157 (152–162)	2,050	2,350	2,650	3,150
	Medium	167 (158–175)	2,150	2,500	2,850	3,350
	Large	179 (168–189)	2,350	2,700	3,050	3,600
6'1"	Small	162 (156–167)	2,100	2,450	2,750	3,250
	Medium	171 (162–180)	2,200	2,550	2,900	3,400
	Large	184 (173–194)	2,400	2,750	3,150	3,700
6'2"	Small	166 (160–171)	2,150	2,500	2,800	3,300
	Medium	176 (167–185)	2,300	2,650	3,000	3,500
	Large	189 (178–199)	2,450	2,850	3,200	3,800
6'3"	Small	170 (164–175)	2,200	2,550	2,900	3,400
	Medium	181 (172–190)	2,350	2,700	3,300	3,850
	Large	193 (182–204)	2,500	2,900	3,300	3,850

NOTE: From 1959 Metropolitan Life Insurance Company, New York City. These tables are based on 1959 rather than 1983 Metropolitan Life Insurance Company height-weight tables because the earlier tables specify lower weights, more appropriate to health-related concerns.

So yesterday's evening snack, dinner and light lunch totaled 88 grams of fat. And what about breakfast? Again, you didn't eat a lot of food, but what you ate was dense: a danish and coffee racked up 24 grams of fat—and the coffee was merely an innocent bystander.

The fat bill for yesterday's menu: 112 grams of fat—an okay amount if you're a 6-foot 2-inch man who digs ditches or plays basketball for a living.

DAY 4: LIMIT MEAT TO LESS THAN SIX OUNCES

Okay, now you know the worst. You know the maximum amount of fat you can eat in a day if you want to stay healthy, and wise. And you know from your food log the amount of fat you actually eat.

So today you're going to begin eating lean meat and limiting the amount of meat you eat to less than six ounces (after cooking) a day.

How? Try mixing the select meat you bought the other day at the supermarket with pasta and vegetables so that you can have a belly-filling serving of food but a small serving of meat, suggests Scott. That way, the meat you bought will stretch over several meals.

Use meat as a flavor enhancer. "Instead of plunking a half-dozen meatballs on top of spaghetti," says Scott, "use an ounce or two of very lean ground meat to flavor the sauce." If you're the type who needs to see a big, beefy steak on your plate, she adds, make sure you have a meatless lunch and breakfast, then hold your dinnertime meat portion at six ounces.

DAY 5: SWEAR OFF PROCESSED MEATS

"For the most part, luncheon meats are among the fattiest meats available," says Scott. "Several low-fat varieties are available. But both the high- and low-fat varieties are usually high in salt."

You can sometimes find a freshly cooked turkey breast that hasn't been salted at a neighborhood deli or market where it's made right on the premises, adds Scott.

Or, once a week, you can turn your own kitchen into the neighborhood deli: Cook a turkey, chicken or lean roast, remove the skin or trim the fat and slice the meat into thin layers. Then slip it into self-locking storage bags and toss it in the freezer. Whenever you're planning on sandwiches, pull out a bag and defrost.

DAY 6: EAT MORE FISH

Remember that six-ounce limit of cooked meat per day? Well, now that you've eaten that amount for a couple of days, it's time to think fish. In fact, you might want to consider having fish not just today but two to three times a week, since it's naturally low in both total fat and saturated fat.

"Most finfish has only a gram or two of fat per serving," says Scott. You can sauté fish quickly and easily in a pan prepared with no-stick cooking spray or brushed with olive oil. Try leaving the skin on while you cook it, then remove it just before serving. Or you steam it over boiling water into which you've dropped a handful of lemon peel and herbs. In either case the fish is ready as soon as the translucent flesh becomes opaque.

DAY 7: PIZZA DAY

It's been a pretty full week. You've figured the maximum amount of fat you should eat and how much fat you actually eat. You've learned how to select low-fat cuts of meat and to limit your meat consumption. You've also curtailed processed meats and started eating more fish.

So, besides already starting to feel good, here's an additional reward: Sometime today you're going to make your very first totally healthy, totally great-tasting pizza.

The recipe? Unless you've been to pizza school and have a professional oven, buy a crust at your local supermarket, says Scott. Then buy a spaghetti sauce that lists zero grams of fat per serving on the label, some grated part-skim mozzerella cheese and a little meat—little meaning a handful of very lean ground beef. You'll have to live without pepperoni; its content of total fat and saturated fat is just too high for dietitians to recommend.

Cook and drain the meat well, directs Scott. Smear tomato sauce over the crust, sprinkle with mozzerella and top with meat. Add as many mushrooms, green peppers and onions as you like. Bake at 350° until the crust is brown and the cheese melts, about 20 minutes.

Week 2: Attack Fat, Phase Two

DAY 8: PLAY AROUND IN THE KITCHEN

Start the second week of your healthier life by taking a few hours to experiment with preparing lower-fat meats in new ways.

Since lower-fat meats are occasionally less tender, for example, try marinating them in an acid-based marinade—citrus or tomato juice, vinegar and soy sauce, for example—to break down those hard-to-chew fibers before cooking. Then thinly slice the meat and stir-fry with vegetables in a wok.

Or instead of roasting a lower-fat cut of meat in the oven, try braising it. Brown the meat, then simmer it in liquid for at least an hour.

And think about making some stock. Whether it's chicken or beef, cover the bones (you can get them from your butcher) with cold water, toss in any vegetable parings and onion skins you may have svaed, season as you please. Bring to a boil, then reduce heat and simmer for at least three to five hours for beef and two to three hours for chicken. Strain the stock and refrigerate immediately. (For rapid cooling or larger quantities, divide the stock into one-quart portions.) The fat will rise to the top, where you can easily skim it off and discard it. Freeze whatever you won't use within a couple of days. Use the defatted stock when cooking rice or vegetables to add robust flavor.

DAY 9: PUT YOUR MILK ON A DIET

Now that you've reduced the amount of fat you get from meat, turn your attention to milk.

"Most people are already savvy anough to be drinking milk that has 2 percent fat rather than whole," says Scott. "But a really healthy diet means cutting back even further." So today pick up a container of 1 percent fat milk and start using it both for drinking and in cooking. If ½ percent fat milk is available in your area, adds Scott, try switchimg to that instead. Skim milk—which has almost no fat at all—is the preferred choice. However, if you don't enjoy drinking it, milk with 1 percent or less is fine.

And don't be confused by labeling. As with meat, the "percent" in ½ or 1 or 2 percent milk refers to the amount of fat by weight rather than calories.

To compare products, check the ingredient label for the actual number of grams of fat. Two percent milk has 4.7 grams of fat per cup, 1 percent milk has 2.6 grams, ½ percent milk has 1 gram, skim milk has 0.6 gram.

DAY 10: TURN YOUR ATTENTION TO CHEESE

Cheese may be an excellent source of calcium and protein, but too much high-fat cheese can clog your arteries over time.

"Cut back on fat by eating only cheeses that have five grams of fat or less per ounce," suggests Scott. The part-skim mozzarella you ate on Day 7's pizza is a perfect choice to use in place of high-fat cheese.

Check the fat table you bought on Day 1 to find other low-fat cheeses that satisfy your five-gram limit. And check labels at your supermarket. There are at least 50 or 60 different kinds, says Scott, who has listed them all in *The Living Heart Brand Name Shopper's Guide,* a continually updated book of which she was coauthor.

Be aware, however, that most popular cheeses—Cheddar,

Swiss and American, for example—tilt the fat scales at a hefty eight or nine grams of fat per ounce. And, once again, make sure you check the claims on the label. "Reduced fat" does not necessarily mean "low fat."

DAY 11: ENJOY SOUR CREAM'S RICHNESS WITHOUT THE FAT

Most cooks agree that sour cream is one of the most versatile foods in the kitchen. It's used as the basis for dips, toppings, sauces—you name the category and some Sour Cream Sarah has created a recipe to fit it.

But sour cream has six grams of fat in two tablespoons, and most of its calories from fat.

The alternative? Today you're going to make your own healthier version. Puree low-fat cottage cheese with an equal amount of nonfat yogurt, then add a squeeze of lemon. The resulting swirl is so creamy and rich that you'll never again be tempted by regular sour cream.

DAY 12: USE A WHIPPED TOPPING

That's right. Today you are *ordered* to use a whipped topping. And, yes, there is a catch: You have to make it yourself and, no, it's not made from cream.

Pour $\frac{1}{3}$ cup skim milk into a small stainless steel bowl. Stick it in the freezer until ice crystals just begin to form—15 to 20 minutes. Then pull it out and quickly thicken by beating in $\frac{1}{3}$ cup instant nonfat dry milk with an electric mixer. Whip on high until soft peaks begin to form—about two minutes. Flavor with a bit of sugar and vanilla and beat until stiff peaks form again, about 2 minutes. Use within 20 minutes. It's perfect over berries or other fruits, and you simple won't believe the taste.

DAY 13: BEGIN THE COUNTDOWN

Today you're going to start using all that arithmetic you learned in grade school. You're going to start counting every single gram of fat and saturated fat you put into your mouth, then subtract it from those grams-of-fat totals. You *do* remember your fat maximum, don't you—that you memorized on Day 1?

Let's say your height, weight and bone structure have dictated that you should eat 1,650 calories a day. As you learned on Day 1 when you memorized your fat numbers from the table on page 723, that means you can eat a maximum of 53 grams of fat a day—of which 18 can be saturated fat.

So stick your fat-content-of-foods table in your handbag or pocket, along with a pencil, and prepare to count every gram of fat and saturated fat throughout the day. Add them to your fat numbers as you go. When you get near the maximum in either column, you've reached your limit.

If you stop at a Mexican restaurant for an iced tea and enchilada at lunch, for example, you need to count the enchilada's hefty 17.6 grams of total fat and 9.1 grams of saturated fat toward your daily allotment.

By the way, after you've completed this six-week program, you might decide you're ready to cut back on fat even more. The table on page 160 shows daily limits to aim for that can bring your total fat intake down another notch—from 30 to 25 percent of total calories.

DAY 14: USE JUST A SWIRL OF CREAM

Is there anyone who doesn't like the rich taste of cream? Probably not on this planet. So today's step toward a healthier diet—and your reward for the past two weeks of healthy eating—is to learn how to use it in a healthy way.

"The trick," says Dieter Doppelfeld, chef instructor at the Culinary Institute of America, "is to give people the satisfaction of cream without the substance." Like an impressionist artist who paints a soul-satisfying "impression" of a country landscape rather than every rock, tree and leaf he sees, Doppelfeld relies on a brief "impression" of cream, rather than a full measure, to caress and satisfy your palate.

When preparing cream soups, for example, he substitutes evaporated skim milk for cream in the basic recipe, then garnishes each bowl with a single swirl of heavy cream right across the top.

The result? Your tongue senses cream with every spoonful, explains Doppelfeld, so you have the feel and taste of cream—with only three grams of fat per serving (see recipe below).

High-Nutrition Recipe

SWEET POTATO SOUP

Here's how Chef Dieter Doppelfeld uses his just-a-hint-of-cream technique when making sweet potato soup. The soup is delicious either hot or cold.

½ cup diced onions
⅓ cup diced celery
1 leek (white part only), diced and rinsed well
1 clove garlic, minced
2½ cups defatted chicken stock
2 large sweet potatoes (about 1 pound), peeled and chopped
¼ teaspoon grated nutmeg
⅛ teaspoon ground cinnamon
⅓ cup evaporated skim milk
1 tablespoon maple syrup
¼ teaspoon salt (optional)
2 tablespoons heavy cream, whipped
1 tablespoon currants
1 tablespoon toasted slivered almonds

In a 3-quart saucepan over medium heat, slowly cook the onions, celery, leeks and garlic in about ¼ cup of the stock for 5 minutes, or until the vegetables are translucent.

Add the sweet potatoes, nutmeg, cinnamon and the remaining 2¼ cups stock. Bring to a boil, then cover and simmer for 20 minutes, or until the sweet potatoes arc tender. Let cool for 5 minutes.

Puree the sweet potato mixture in batches, since it probably won't all fit in the blender at one time. Transfer each batch to a bowl as it's pureed, then stir the milk, syrup and salt, if desired, into the whole batch in the bowl. If desired, refrigerate until cold.

To serve, ladle into individual bowls and garnish each serving with a swirl of whipped cream and a sprinkle of currants and almonds.

Serves 6
Per serving: *155 calories, 3.3 g. fat (19% of calories), 2.9 g. dietary fiber, 7 mg. cholesterol, 69 mg. sodium*

Week 3: Crack Down on Cholesterol

DAY 15: LET THE DOG HAVE YOUR YOLKS

Now that you have fat under control, it's time to tackle cholesterol, says Scott.

Your goal is to consume less than 300 milligrams of cholesterol a day. Since egg yolk is the most concentrated source of cholesterol, it means limiting egg yolks to no more than three a week.

Just three eggs a week sounds like an impossible limit when you consider the fact that the recipe for nearly everything you bake—casseroles, pancakes, bread, meat loaf—seems to call for an egg or two to hold things together. But you can make up a batch of cholesterol-free egg substitute, keep it handy in the refrigerator or freezer and use it whenever a recipe calls for eggs.

Preparing the egg substitute is simple: Separate six eggs. Whip the whites and ¼ cup powdered milk with 1 tablespoon oil until smooth, then refrigerate for up to a week or freeze until needed. One-quarter cup equals one egg.

Cook and refrigerate the yolks, then use them to augment your pet's—or your neighbor's pet's—canned or bagged food. For healthy animals, the fur will likely develop a healthy sheen, and *you'll* probably have a little more zip in your step. And you don't have to worry about your dog's cholesterol level. Dogs' arteries aren't affected by cholesterol the way humans are.

DAY 16: MEET YOUR FISHMONGER

You've already substituted fish for meat at least one day a week. Now you might want to think about doing it even more often, because not only can certain species of fish help limit your intake of fat, they can also curb your cholesterol.

Meat and poultry both have about 25 milligrams of cholesterol per ounce, says Scott, so if you are eating six ounces of either one a day, you are getting nearly half your daily allotment of cholesterol. By comparison, many fish have as little as 12 to 15 milligrams of cholesterol per ounce.

So today you're going to take a trip to your local fish market, get to know your fishmonger and learn how to select fish.

Your best bets? Fillets of bass, croaker, grouper, halibut, king mackerel, monkfish, ocean perch, orange roughy, pike, salmon (except fresh sockeye) shark, snapper, swordfish, tuna and whitefish are all terrific choices.

DAY 17: HAVE A VEGETARIAN LUNCH

An easy way to drop your cholesterol consumption is to regularly schedule some meals with no meat, poultry or even fish in them at all.

"You may not want to become a vegetarian," says Scott, "but having several vegetarian meals each week will help keep your cholesterol, fat and saturated fat intake low. Dried beans, peas and legumes, along with a glass of 1 percent or skim milk and whole-wheat bread, makes an excellent meal with plenty of protein.

DAY 18: TAKE IT OFF—TAKE IT ALL OFF!

If you're not already doing so, start taking the skin off any chicken or turkey you eat and tossing it in the garbage. It's so full of fat it's simply not fit for man or beast.

DAY 19: RESUPPLY YOUR PANTRY WITH LOW-CHOLESTEROL BASICS

One of the simplest tricks to keeping cholesterol levels low in both your food and your body is to get rid of the high-cholesterol basics many of us have tucked away on our kitchen shelves. Then lay in a supply of lower-cholesterol or cholesterol-free alternatives.

You can get rid of baking chocolate, for example, and keep cocoa on hand instead. (Three tablespoons of cocoa plus 1 teaspoon of oil equals 1 square of chocolate.) Canned evaporated skim milk can replace cream in almost every way. Canola oil can replace shortening, and artificial bacon bits can replace salt pork for seasoning vegetables.

Day 20: Season Vegetables with Nut Butters

One of the harder cholesterol-laden habits to give up is drizzling butter over vegetables. But once you've dotted a pile of cooked carrots with a teaspoon of unsalted cashew butter, or—in the Indonesian manner-dotted a pile of green beans with peanut butter, you'll wonder why you thought the stuff from cows was so great. Nut butters still contain fat, however, so don't go—uh—nuts. Each teaspoon contains approximately two grams of fat.

Check your supermarket shelves to see what other nut butters you can find. Then take them home and experiment. Who knows? Almond butter could make spinach a tempting treat; and nut butters have no cholesterol.

Day 21: Salmon Day

Congratulations! You've completed three weeks on the Eating Light, Eating Right Program. You've dumped a load of fat and cholesterol out of your diet and probably several pounds off your body. Here's your reward!

High-Nutrition Recipe

Salmon Wrapped in Phyllo

This recipe is an adaptation of one Philadelphia chef and food consultant Robin Rifkin prepares. It's simple, elegant and healthy. Although phyllo recipes are generally loaded with fat (thanks to all the butter), this dish requires only a minimum amount of light margarine. Most of the fat in this recipe comes from the salmon, which is a good source of healthy omega-3 fatty acids. Phyllo is available in supermarket freezer sections. Thaw it in the refrigerator before using.

8 sheets phyllo dough	4 teaspoons coarse-grain mustard
1½ tablespoons light margarine, melted	1 box (10 ounces) frozen chopped spinach, thawed and squeezed dry
4 salmon fillets (4 ounces each), skin removed	

Place 1 sheet of phyllo dough horizontally on a dry countertop in front of you. Top it with a second sheet. Wrap the remaining sheets tightly in plastic to prevent them from drying out; set them aside.

Using a pastry brush, lightly brush the right-hand side of the top phyllo sheet with a little margarine. Fold the right portion over the left half, making a rectangle about 12" × 18". Lightly brush the top of the dough with a little more margarine.

Lay a salmon fillet in the center of the phyllo. Spread 1 teaspoon of the mustard over the salmon. Top with ¼ of the spinach in a thin layer. Fold the top and bottom sections of the phyllo over the salmon; fold in the two sides to make a neat packet that encases the salmon.

Lightly brush the packet with margarine. Coat a baking sheet with no-stick spray; place the packet on the sheet.

Repeat the procedure three times, using the remaining phyllo, salmon, mustard and spinach.

Bake at 425° for 8 to 10 minutes, or until the phyllo begins to brown.

Serves 4
Per serving: *308 calories, 12 g. fat (33% of calories), 1.8 g. dietary fiber, 59 mg. cholesterol, 204 mg. sodium*

Week 4: Fortify with Grains

DAY 22: MAKE THE CHOICE

Now that you've zapped the fat and cholesterol from your diet, you're probably losing a few pounds and getting a bit hungry. In fact, you've probably started to add some food here and there to fill the gaps left by the fat.

The goal for any healthy diet, according to both Alphin and Scott, is 6 to 11 servings a day of breads, cereals and pasta. So if you're trying to lose weight, that means keeping your starches at around 6 servings a day—whole-wheat toast or a bowl of cereal at breakfast, a couple of slices of whole wheat bread at lunch, a potato or cup of pasta at dinner. "But if you don't want to lose any more weight," says Alphin, "start by adding 1 or 2 starch servings a day until your hunger stops or until you *either* reach 11 servings or start to put on pounds."

Eleven servings a day sounds like a lot. But when you look at a whole day's meals, it isn't really as much food as it seems, says Scott. "If you eat cereal and toast at breakfast, that's two to four. If you have a sandwich at lunch, there's another two. Then if you have some soup that has potatoes, or a salad with crackers, that's another one or two.

"Then at night, it's easy to eat a potato or a half-cup of pasta. A cup of pasta is equal to two slices of bread. And most of us can easily eat a cup and a half—that's 3 servings of starch." Add a hot roll and an ear of corn, says Scott, and you've eaten 9 to 11 servings over the course of a day.

DAY 23: BEGIN WITH WHOLE WHEAT

If you need to add starches to bring your diet up to the 6 to 11 recommended servings a day, begin with whole-wheat breads and bagels first, says Alphin. "Bread is usually among the first things to go when people are dieting," she explains. "So when they hear that they can include it, they feel like they're getting a treat." It really perks them up.

Besides, whole-wheat breads are high in fiber, she adds. And increasing fiber as you withdraw fat is a good strategy. The fiber fills you up in the places where less fat has made you feel empty.

DAY 24: ADD CEREALS AS YOU NEED THEM

Whole-grain cereals are not just for breakfast. They can be crushed as a topping over casseroles, used as an extender in meat loaf, sprinkled over salads to add crunch or eaten right out of the box as a healthy snack.

"Use cereals as needed to boost your fiber intake," suggests Alphin. "Just make sure you read and compare the labels. Buy those cereals that have the least amount of salt and sugar and the most amount of fiber."

DAY 25: INVESTIGATE THE PASTABILITIES

Once you've added more breads and cereals to your diet, think about using pasta to round out your starches, says Scott.

Spaghetti, fettuccine, ziti or just plain noodles are all great. But you might want to try some whole-grain pastas, too, for extra fiber. And you may find the pastas combined with vegetables—beets, spinach or artichokes, for example—add a cheerful splash of color to your plate.

DAY 26: REPLACE FAT WITH FIBER

You've been eating cheese with less than five grams of fat per ounce for a couple of weeks. So you're comfortable with the taste. You're so comfortable, in fact, that if someone crumbled some high-fat Cheddar into a salad when you weren't expecting it, you probably wouldn't enjoy it. It would taste too strong and feel too heavy.

So now you're ready to switch to an even lower-fat cheese: three grams of fat per ounce. And before you start squealing, remember how you felt on Day 10 when you switched from those high-fat Cheddars and blues to the five-gram cheeses. Thought you'd never get used to the difference, did you?

Yet it not only happened, but you now *prefer* the lower-fat cheese. Trust us. The same thing will happen as you move to cheeses with three grams of fat per ounce. So head for your supermarket and take some time to check out the cheeses that claim to be low-fat. Check the labels until you find a few that have three grams of fat or less per serving and toss them in your cart. And to make sure you don't feel deprived, also pick up a loaf of unsliced whole-wheat bread.

Why unsliced? Because you're going to replace that missing fat with fiber. When you get home, cut two *thick* slices of whole-wheat bread and top each with a slice of low-fat cheese. Then either melt the cheese in the microwave or broil it in the oven. Either way, the warm, sweet softness of this extra-thick bread will help you make the switch to lower-fat cheese with delight. For a special taste treat, try topping it with some Mexican salsa.

DAY 27: DRINK PLENTY OF WATER

As you add whole-grain products to your diet, make sure you're drinking eight 8-ounce glasses of water a day to help bulk up all that fiber and keep it moving through your digestive tract.

DAY 28: VISIT ANOTHER COUNTRY

Today you're going to have lunch at a restaurant that serves Middle Eastern food. Ask questions, sample dishes, then come home and put your own innovative juices to work. Your challenge? To combine several different types of starches into one stimulating dish. You might decide to make an eggplant stuffed with tomato, rice, nuts and bulgur wheat, for instance.

Week 5: Drain the Oil

DAY 29: GIVE ANY NONDAIRY CREAMER IN THE HOUSE TO A CAT

Give it to your cat, the neighbor's cat, any cat. Because only an animal with nine lives can possibly survive the repeated daily imbibing of a product that derives most of its substance from hydrogenated oils. Not only are these creamers full of fat, they're full of *bad* fat—the kind that congeals on an unwashed plate and turns your arteries into stiff, narrow straws that are easily clogged.

If you simply must have something white in your coffee or tea, try some more low-fat milk like you bought on Day 9.

DAY 30: MAKE HEALTHY CHOICES AT A FAST-FOOD RESTAURANT

If this suggestion to eat at a fast-food restaurant appalls you, you're probably thinking of what you ordered there in the past: fried chicken, greasy french fries, gloppy coleslaw. In short, a healthy person's nightmare.

But today, eating at a fast-food restaurant should be a pleasure because you're going to make healthy choices, like a giant bowl of greens topped with lean chunks of chicken, carrots, broccoli and cauliflower. And for a dressing, you're going to ignore every plastic package they try to hand you unless it's labeled "low fat." Not "reduced-fat" or "lite," but "low fat." Top off the meal with a roll, some pasta or another starch.

DAY 31: SWITCH FROM OIL TO VINEGAR

You need to start thinking about oil the way you think about salt: You only eat it when you can't avoid it. And you certainly don't add it to anything it hasn't managed to work its way into naturally.

Starting today, try sprinkling red-wine vinegar and a pinch of oregano over a salad at lunch instead of the usual squirt of oil. Or experiment with some of the flavored vinegars—tarragon, basil, rosemary—that are beginning to appear on supermarket shelves. You'll be surprised how quickly your taste buds will actually prefer the sharp brisk taste of foods that are no longer slathered in oil.

DAY 32: SAY GOOD-BYE TO FRIED FOODS FOREVER

If you've been filling your menus with fried foods on a regular basis, you might want to treat yourself to a cooking course that emphasizes steaming, baking and broiling. Check with your local Y or hospital about taking a course in the basics. Then ask the chef at your favorite restaurant if he'd be willing to give you—and maybe some of your friends—an after-hours graduate course in La Nouvelle American Cuisine.

DAY 33: USE BROTH INSTEAD OF OIL

Most of us have sprayed or slathered oil or butter over the surface of any pan we use since we first learned to cook—mostly to keep what we were cooking from sticking. Today, however, dietitians suggest that you skip the fat and increase flavor by substituting defatted chicken broth.

You can use homemade stock (see Day 8) or canned low-fat stock from the supermarket. If you're making your own stock, freeze some in an ice-cube tray. Then whenever you need a couple of tablespoons to coat a pan, just warm the pan on the stove and toss in a cube.

DAY 34: RETHINK YOUR SNACK FOODS

Potato chips, tortilla chips, corn chips and just about every other chip in your supermarket are loaded with oil. If you really need a crunch food to snack on, make your own chips by cutting up a tortilla and baking the pieces in an oven until the chips dry out. Or pick up some low-sodium pretzels or rice cakes as an alternative.

The rice cakes in particular may be something of a surprise. Once a glued-together version of puffed rice cereal, today's rice cakes are flavored with everything from sour cream and onion to teriyaki sauce—but without the fat.

DAY 35: FRISK YOUR MUFFINS

"I love it," says Alphin. "People are saying, 'I eat a bran muffin every morning.' But their muffin is so moist it has enough oil to last for the next four days!"

Bran is good, muffins are good, but the oil most muffin recipes call for is not good. So today you're going to frisk your muffins for oil. Check the grams-of-fat listing on any commercially made muffins you buy and check the amount of oil called for in any muffins you make.

Fortunately you can substitute an equal amount of nonfat yogurt—fruit-flavored or vanilla—for the oil and eggs in your muffin recipes. (Figure one egg is equivalent to ¼ cup.)

Or, if you want to add a chunk of fiber while you're draining the oil, you can smoosh some prunes in the blender and substitute an equal amount of prune puree for the oil. Your muffins will not be quite as light, but you'll have exactly the same richness and—believe it or not—even more flavor.

High-Nutrition Recipe

MAGIC MOLASSES MUFFINS

To celebrate your completion of five weeks on the Eating Light, Eating Right Program, here's a magic muffin created by JoAnn Brader of the Rodale Food Center. It will please every taste bud in your family—and it has just three grams of fat. For best results, use a nugget-type bran cereal such as Bran Buds.

1½ cups nugget-type bran cereal
½ cup apple juice
⅓ cup raisins
1 cup unbleached flour
1½ teaspoons baking soda

1 cup nonfat or low-fat lemon yogurt
¼ cup fat-free egg substitute
¼ cup molasses
2 tablespoons canola oil

In a large bowl, combine the cereal, juice and raisins. Let stand for 10 minutes.

In a small bowl, combine the flour and baking soda.

In another small bowl, mix the yogurt, egg, molasses and oil.

Lightly stir the flour mixture into the bran bowl, mixing it only slightly. Stir in the yogurt mixture. Mix with a large rubber spatula until all the flour is moistened; do not overmix.

Coat 12 muffin cups with no-stick spray. Spoon the batter into the cups, filling them about ¾ full. Bake at 400° for 20 minutes. Cool on a wire rack for 5 minutes before removing the muffins from the pan. Serve warm or cold.

Makes 12 muffins
Per serving: *129 calories, 2.7 g. fat (17% of calories), 3.4 g. dietary fiber, <1 mg. cholesterol, 191 mg. sodium*

Week 6: Crack Down on Calories

DAY 36: INCLUDE MORE VEGETABLES

Now that you've cut back on the fat, cholesterol and oil in your diet while boosting grains, it's time to start thinking about vegetables.

Vegetables are naturally low in calories. So the total number of calories in your diet will gradually fall as vegetables begin to play a larger part in what you eat.

Your goal, says Scott, is to eat five servings of vegetables a day (raw vegetables, whenever possible). You should lean heavily toward the cancer-fighting cruciferous vegetables—broccoli, cauliflower, cabbage, brussels sprouts—and others that are good sources of beta-carotene—carrots, sweet potatoes, pumpkin, squash and spinach.

So today why don't you begin including more veggies by putting a new twist on an old before-dinner favorite?

Empty an eight-ounce carton of plain, nonfat yogurt into a bowl and mix in a packet of dried salad dressing seasoning, like ranch, to make a rich-tasting dip, Scott suggests. Surround the bowl with raw vegetables and encourage the children to join in on the munching. They'll disappear within minutes.

DAY 37: INCREASE YOUR FRUIT INTAKE

Starting today, you're going to eat four servings of fruit a day, says Scott. Slice it on top of cereal, add it to salads or work it into desserts.

But remember that calories add up quickly in dried fruit, she adds. With the water removed, dried fruits seem like smaller portions than they really are, and people tend to overindulge. Unfortunately, dried fruit has only lost its water, not its calories.

DAY 38: MAKE YOUR FRUITS AND VEGETABLES WORK TWICE

Despite the recommendation that you eat at least nine servings a day of fruits and vegetables, some of us simply can't afford even those extra calories.

That's why you really have to eat smart, says Alphin. If you can't eat as many servings of fruits and vegetables as you should, then make sure the servings you do eat satisfy several nutrient requirements at once.

Many experts suggest, for example, that you eat a lot of carotenoids. Others suggest that you fill up with foods that are rich in vitamin C. But why not eat foods that have both? Fruits and vegetables that contain a double-barreled shot of both beta-carotene and vitamin C include oranges, cantaloupe, raspberries, apricots, carrots, winter squash, yams, spinach, sweet potatoes, broccoli and chard.

Day 39: Talk to the Produce Person at Your Market

This person does more than just keep the potato bin stocked. He or she is also a goldmine of information about the produce for sale there.

You can find out what makes an apple crisp and whether the one you're about to buy is the right choice. You may also learn that the sweetest carrots are the ones with their foliage intact and that large onions are sweeter than small ones. There's no better way to encourage yourself—and your family—to eat more vegetables and fruits than to put the freshest, most flavorful ones on the table.

Day 40: Develop Your Own Culinary Signature

Sad to say, some of us never learn how to cook vegetables in a way that delivers every ounce of flavor and nutrition. So today your assignment is to visit the local library, check out a bunch of cookbooks that espouse healthy eating and study the vegetable sections.

Note the different ways expert cooks work with vegetables. They usually end up steaming or stir-frying (in broth, not fat), but preparation and seasoning techniques vary so much from one cook to another that each person literally creates his or her own culinary signature. That's typically done by adding an aromatic such as garlic, fresh gingerroot, caraway seeds or fresh herbs such as rosemary, thyme or sage.

What's your culinary signature going to be? Study the cookbooks, then go experiment in the kitchen. It's the only way you'll ever find out.

Day 41: Make the Final Adjustments

Today you're going to run a happiness check. Close your eyes, put your hands on your tummy, and ask yourself: "How do I feel?"

"If you find you're feeling hungry all the time or low in energy, then add more starches, fruits and vegetables," says Al-phin. If not, then turn on the cruise control and continue en-joying your new way of eating.

DAY 42: GLAZE YOUR BROCCOLI WITH LEMON

Congratulations! You've spent six weeks eliminating fat, slashing cholesterol, sifting out salt, fortifying with grains, cutting down on calories and increasing fruits and vegetables. To send you off on your own with a reminder of precisely how delicious healthy eating can be, we've include this final recipe for broccoli with lemon glaze (see below).

You're probably feeling a whole lot better—maybe a few pounds lighter—than when you started the program. But these past six weeks have been just a beginning. And the rest is up to you.

High-Nutrition Recipe

BROCCOLI WITH LEMON GLAZE

Here's a recipe from the Culinary Institute of America as demonstrated by Chef Dieter Doppelfeld. Please note that the lemon glaze is also delicious served with other vegetables, such as asparagus.

1½ cups defatted chicken stock

2 tablespoons lemon juice

1½ teaspoons grated fresh ginger

1½ teaspoons arrowroot or cornstarch

2 tablespoons water

1 head broccoli (about 1 pound)

1½ teaspoons grated lemon   2   teaspoons toasted
   rind   sesame seeds
¼ teaspoon ground black
   pepper

In a 2-quart saucepan over medium-high heat, boil the stock, lemon juice, ginger, lemon rind and pepper until the mixture is reduced to about ½ cup, about 10 to 15 minutes.

In a cup, dissolve the arrowroot or cornstarch in the water. Whisk into the stock mixture and cook over medium heat, stirring constantly, until thickened, about 2 minutes. Strain into a small bowl.

Meanwhile, trim the broccoli and cut into thin stalks. Steam until tender, about 5 minutes. Serve drizzled with the glaze and sprinkled with the sesame seeds.

Serves 4
Per serving: *59 calories, 1.5 g. fat (19% of calories), 3.5 g. dietary fiber, 0 mg. cholesterol, 62 mg. sodium*

Index

NOTE: Page references in *italic* indicate tables.